Basic Conce...
HEAD AND NECK SURGERY
AND ONCOLOGY

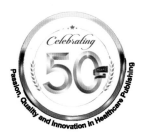

Basic Concepts in
HEAD AND NECK SURGERY AND ONCOLOGY

SECOND EDITION

Editors

Krishnakumar Thankappan MS DNB MCh
Professor
Department of Head and Neck Surgery and Oncology
Amrita Institute of Medical Sciences
Kochi, Kerala, India

Subramania Iyer MS MCh FRCS
Professor and Head
Department of Head and Neck Surgery and Oncology
Amrita Institute of Medical Sciences
Kochi, Kerala, India

Forewords

Alok Thakar
Moni Abraham Kuriakose

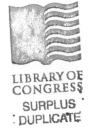

JAYPEE BROTHERS MEDICAL PUBLISHERS
The Health Sciences Publisher
New Delhi | London | Panama

Jaypee Brothers Medical Publishers (P) Ltd.

Headquarters
Jaypee Brothers Medical Publishers (P) Ltd.
4838/24, Ansari Road, Daryaganj
New Delhi 110 002, India
Phone: +91-11-43574357
Fax: +91-11-43574314
Email: jaypee@jaypeebrothers.com

Overseas Offices

JP Medical Ltd.
83, Victoria Street, London
SW1H 0HW (UK)
Phone: +44 20 3170 8910
Fax: +44 (0)20 3008 6180
E-mail: info@jpmedpub.com

Jaypee-Highlights Medical Publishers Inc.
City of Knowledge, Bld. 235, 2nd Floor, Clayton
Panama City, Panama
Phone: +1 507-301-0496
Fax: +1 507-301-0499
E-mail: cservice@jphmedical.com

Jaypee Brothers Medical Publishers (P) Ltd.
Bhotahity, Kathmandu, Nepal
Phone: +977-9741283608
E-mail: kathmandu@jaypeebrothers.com

Website: www.jaypeebrothers.com
Website: www.jaypeedigital.com

Basic Concepts in Head and Neck Surgery and Oncology

First Edition: 2015

Second Edition: **2019**

ISBN: 978-93-5270-896-3

Printed at: Samrat Offset Pvt. Ltd.

Dedicated to all our patients

Krishnakumar Thankappan, Subramania Iyer

CONTRIBUTORS

Abhijeet N Wakure DNB
Consultant
Department of Plastic Surgery
Lakeshore Hospital and Research Center
Kochi, Kerala, India

Adharsh Anand MS MCh
Assistant Professor
Department of Surgical Oncology
Malabar Cancer Center
Kannur, Kerala, India

Akshay Kudpaje MS MCh
Consultant Head and Neck Surgeon
Department of Surgical Oncology
MVR Cancer Center
Kozhikode, Kerala, India

Anoop R MD
Assistant Professor
Department of Radiation Oncology
Amrita Institute of Medical Sciences
Kochi, Kerala, India

Chaya Prasad MD
Assistant Professor
Department of Pathology
Amrita Institute of Medical Sciences
Kochi, Kerala, India

Chinmay Kulkarni DNB
Associate Professor
Department of Radiodiagnosis
Amrita Institute of Medical Sciences
Kochi, Kerala, India

Deepak Balasubramanian MS DNB MCh
Associate Professor
Department of Head and Neck Surgery and Oncology
Amrita Institute of Medical Sciences
Kochi, Kerala, India

Divya GM DLO DNB
Assistant Professor
Department of ENT
Government Medical College
Kozhikode, Kerala, India

K Pavithran MD DM
Professor
Department of Medical Oncology/Hematology
Amrita Institute of Medical Sciences
Kochi, Kerala, India

Krishnakumar Thankappan MS DNB MCh
Professor
Department of Head and Neck Surgery and Oncology
Amrita Institute of Medical Sciences
Kochi, Kerala, India

Mahamaya Prasad Singh MS MCh
Consultant Head and Neck Surgeon
North East Cancer Hospital and Research Institute
Guwahati, Assam, India

Mayuri Mohan Rajapurkar MS MCh
Consultant Head and Neck Oncologic and
Reconstructive Surgeon
Aster Medcity Hospital
Kochi, Kerala, India

Mohit Sharma MS MCh
Professor
Department of Plastic Surgery
Amrita Institute of Medical Sciences
Kochi, Kerala, India

Prameela CG MD
Associate Professor
Department of Radiation Oncology
Amrita Institute of Medical Sciences
Kochi, Kerala, India

P Shanmuga Sundaram DRM DNB MNAMS
Head and Clinical Professor
Department of Nuclear Medicine and PET-CT
Amrita Institute of Medical Sciences
Kochi, Kerala, India

Pushpaja KU DMRT DNB
Assistant Professor
Department of Radiation Oncology
Amrita Institute of Medical Sciences
Kochi, Kerala, India

Rajsekar CS DNB MNAMS
Assistant Professor
Department of Radiodiagnosis
Amrita Institute of Medical Sciences
Kochi, Kerala, India

Salima Rema Windsor MS DLO DNB
Assistant Professor
Department of ENT
Government Medical College
Kollam, Kerala, India

Sandya CJ MD
Associate Professor
Department of Radiodiagnosis
Amrita Institute of Medical Sciences
Kochi, Kerala, India

Shashikant Vishnubhai Limbachiya MS MCh
Consultant Head and Neck Surgical Oncologist
Narayana Health
Ahmedabad, Gujarat, India

Shibu George MS DNB
Professor and Head
Department of ENT
Government Medical College
Kottayam, Kerala, India

Shreya Bhattacharya MS MCh
Fellow-Head and Neck
Department of ENT
Sir Charles Gairdner Hospital
Nedlands, Western Australia

Sivakumar Vidhyadharan MS DNB
Assistant Professor
Department of Head and Neck Surgery and Oncology
Amrita Institute of Medical Sciences
Kochi, Kerala, India

Smitha NV DCP DNB
Associate Professor
Department of Pathology
Amrita Institute of Medical Sciences
Kochi, Kerala, India

Subramania Iyer MS MCh FRCS
Professor and Head
Division of Reconstructive Surgery
Department of Head and Neck Surgery and Oncology
Amrita Institute of Medical Sciences
Kochi, Kerala, India

Vasantha Nair MD
Professor
Department of Endocrinology
Amrita Institute of Medical Sciences
Kochi, Kerala, India

FOREWORD TO THE SECOND EDITION

It has been only a few years since the first edition of *Basic Concepts in Head and Neck Surgery and Oncology* by Thankappan and Iyer was first brought out in 2015. The book has had significant success, and in keeping with the expectations of its readers, the authors' have now brought out a second edition, which incorporates the recent developments in the subject

The second edition retains the strengths and the style of the first edition. It is simply written, comprehensive, and yet concise in its inclusion of the must-know and essential facts in the subject. Basic and fundamental concepts in the subject are very well covered, and the principles of evaluation and management well elucidated. The book is essentially a compilation of the current state of knowledge in the subject, which is distilled with the very considerable experience of the Head-Neck Team at the Amrita Institute of Medical Sciences at Kochi.

Specific inclusions and updates in the current edition include the current AJCC 8th Edition staging system, new chapters on parathyroid tumors, temporal bone tumors, and cutaneous cancers, and the current hot topics in the subject including Robotic surgery, and the promise of monoclonal antibodies and Immunotherapy. The reader shall find the book to be a sufficient resource to the fundamental knowledge necessary to practice evidenced based management of head and neck cancers.

My congratulations to the authors for their enthusiasm and commitment in bringing out this excellent textbook, which will certainly prove very useful and educative for all aspiring students in the subject.

Alok Thakar MS FRCSEd
Professor
Department of Otolaryngology
All India Institute of Medical Sciences
New Delhi, India

FOREWORD TO THE FIRST EDITION

It is indeed a great honor for me to write the foreword for the textbook *Basic Concepts in Head and Neck Surgery and Oncology*, edited by Dr Krishnakumar Thankappan and Professor Subramania Iyer. This book has its origin as a manual for the ever-popular Annual Head and Neck Oncology Education Program of Amrita Institute of Medical Science (AHEAD). This was started over 10 years ago primarily meant for trainees and junior faculty. The increasing number of delegates attending the program every year attests the popularity and need for such an educational event. The manual of this program is meant as a companion to this educational program. It is now expanded and made into an independent textbook. The contents and primary focus of the book are to simplify the concepts into day-to-day clinically applicable information. In this way, this book is quite distinct from all the other currently available textbooks in head and neck surgery and oncology. It is not meant as detailed textbook. In this book, the information is distilled into what is essential to practice the art and science of head and neck oncology. Another unique feature of this book is that each chapter is written by a leading expert in the field along with a trainee. Thereby, at every level from choosing the topics, to contents of these chapters, the end-users point-of-view is kept in mind. The book is divided into seven sections; thyroid, salivary gland, parapharyngeal space, neck, paranasal sinuses, oral cavity, oropharynx, larynx, hypopharynx, nasopharynx, and general topics. Each section is divided into pathology, imaging and practical management guidelines. The 34 concise chapters of this book provide fundamental knowledge necessary to practice evidence-based management of head and neck cancer. Both the editors of this book, Dr Krishnakumar Thankappan and Professor Subramania Iyer, have proven track record of establishing one of the finest head and neck training programs of the country. This book not only attests their experience but also exemplifies their commitment in excelling in head and neck oncology training. I am confident that many trainees and junior faculties in the head and neck surgery, surgical oncology, otolaryngology and maxillofacial surgery will find this manual very useful.

Moni Abraham Kuriakose MD FRCS
Professor and Director
Department of Surgical Oncology
Mazumdar-Shaw Cancer Center
Narayana Health City
Bengaluru, Karnataka, India

PREFACE TO THE SECOND EDITION

Management of head and neck cancer has changed over the last few decades. This change has occurred due to the better understanding of the pathology and better delineation of the tumor by advances in imaging and diagnostic techniques. The management of these cancers has improved greatly with increased knowledge on the tumor behavior and its response to the therapeutic regimens. This is a result of the integration of the three modalities namely surgery, radiation and chemotherapy as applied to the management of these cancers. Function and organ preservation by surgery or chemoradiation and better rehabilitation by appropriate reconstructive surgery have made the quality of the treatment acceptable. The factor that has brought in the difference is the emergence of multidisciplinary approach in the research, diagnosis and management of these cancers. This short book is aimed at giving the reader an overview of the subject to reflect all these changes based on the contemporary knowledge in various subspecialties involved in the management of these cancers. The book does not claim to be an exhaustive reference book but as an easy revision manual for the practicing physicians and the trainees. Each of the subsites has been dealt with separately emphasizing on the diagnosis and management. Separate chapters have been added to discuss areas like radiation, chemotherapy, reconstruction and molecular biology. The contents of this book have been, in a much smaller way given as handout to the annual instructional course in head and neck surgery conducted by the Amrita Institute of Medical Sciences, Kochi, Kerala, India for the past several years.

The second edition reflects the advances that have occurred in the recent past, especially the changes in the staging system as reflected in the American Joint Cancer Committee (AJCC) 8th edition. The impact on the management of oral cavity, thyroid and occult primary cancers, due to these changes, has been highlighted. Newer modalities of treatment like robotic surgery and immunotherapy, which have taken their place in the treatment armamentarium, are also updated. Other additions in this edition include management of Human Papillomavirus (HPV) positive tumors, facial nerve issues, melanoma and skin cancers, tumors of infratemporal fossa and practical issues related to tracheostomy. The book still maintains its simplicity in dealing the subject, but at the same time, tries to reflect the contemporary knowledge.

Krishnakumar Thankappan
Subramania Iyer

PREFACE TO THE FIRST EDITION

Management of head and neck cancer has changed over the last few decades. This change has occurred due to the better understanding of the pathology and better delineation of the tumor by advances in imaging and diagnostic techniques. The management of these cancers has improved greatly with increased knowledge on the tumor behavior and its response to the therapeutic regimens. This is a result of the integration of the three modalities namely surgery, radiation and chemotherapy as applied to the management of these cancers. Function and organ preservation by surgery or chemoradiation and better rehabilitation by appropriate reconstructive surgery have made the quality of the treatment acceptable. The factor that has brought in the difference is the emergence of multidisciplinary approach in the research, diagnosis and management of these cancers.

This short book is aimed at giving the reader an overview of the subject to reflect all these changes based on the contemporary knowledge in various subspecialties involved in the management of these cancers. The book does not claim to be an exhaustive reference book but as an easy revision manual for the practicing physicians and the trainees. Each of the subsites has been dealt with separately emphasizing on the diagnosis and management. Separate chapters have been added to discuss areas like radiation, chemotherapy, reconstruction and molecular biology. The contents of this book has been, in a much smaller way given as handout to the annual instructional course in head and neck surgery conducted by the Amrita Institute of Medical Sciences, Kochi, Kerala, India for the past several years. The book still maintains its simplicity in dealing the subject, but at the same time, tries to reflect the contemporary knowledge.

Krishnakumar Thankappan
Subramania Iyer

ACKNOWLEDGMENTS

We would like to express our sincere gratitude to the Medical Director, Principal and the management of Amrita Institute of Medical Sciences, Kochi, Kerala, India, for their immense support to make this book a reality. The fellows, trainees and staff of the Department of Head and Neck Surgery and Plastic Surgery have also helped immensely. Special word of appreciation also goes to Bri Abhirami, Mr Dinesh and other staff, Department of Graphics of the Institute, for their help in the preparation of illustrations.

We are thankful to Shri Jitendar P Vij (Group Chairman), Mr Ankit Vij (Managing Director), Ms Chetna Malhotra Vohra (Associate Director—Content Strategy), and Ms Nikita Chauhan (Senior Development Editor) of M/s Jaypee Brothers Medical Publishers (P) Ltd, New Delhi, India, for giving a go-ahead at the very beginning and helping us in every way possible to bring out this book.

CONTENTS

SECTION 3: NECK

SECTION 4: PARANASAL SINUSES

SECTION 5: ORAL CAVITY AND OROPHARYNX

SECTION 6: LARYNX, HYPOPHARYNX AND NASOPHARYNX

SECTION 7: GENERAL TOPICS

Section 1

Thyroid

Chapters

Thyroid

CHAPTER 1

Pathology of Thyroid Tumors

Smitha NV

• INTRODUCTION

Thyroid tumors account to 1% of all malignancies in developed countries and 0.2% of cancer deaths. They are the most common malignancies of the endocrine system and pose a significant challenge to pathologists, surgeons, and oncologists. Most of the carcinomas affect young and middle-aged adults and are indolent malignancies with a 10-year survival that exceeds 90%. There has been an increase in the incidence rate of these tumors worldwide which can be largely attributed to more sophisticated diagnostic methods and a change in diagnostic practices with an increasing number of smaller tumors being detected of late. Thyroid tumor pathology is an area replete with diagnostic challenges. Though there are typical morphological patterns described, overlaps with non-neoplastic entities pose diagnostic difficulties. Updates in this field include ancillary and research aiming at techniques that can further narrow down our diagnosis from the different "indeterminate/gray zone" lesions detected on screening.

• CLASSIFICATION

The conventional classification based on morphology and clinical features is largely supported by molecular data currently available. Genetic profiles of four main categories appear distinctly different from each other with a few areas of overlap.

The classification of thyroid tumors modified from WHO classification (2004) is as follows:

Tumors of Follicular Epithelium

- Follicular adenoma (including Hurthle cell adenoma)
- Hyalinizing trabecular adenoma
- Follicular carcinoma (including Hurthle cell carcinoma)
  - Minimally invasive
  - Widely invasive
- Papillary carcinomas
- Poorly differentiated carcinoma
- Anaplastic carcinoma
- Squamous cell carcinoma
- Mucoepidermoid carcinoma
- Sclerosing mucoepidermoid carcinoma with eosinophilia
- Mucinous carcinoma.

Tumors with C Cell Differentiation

Medullary carcinoma.

Tumors with Mixed Differentiation

- Collision tumor—follicular/papillary or follicular/medullary
- Mixed differentiated carcinoma inter-mediate type.

Tumors Showing Thymic or Related Branchial Pouch Differentiation

- Ectopic thymoma
- Spindle epithelial tumor with thymus-like element (SETTLE)
- Carcinoma showing thymus-like element (CASTLE).

Tumors of Lymphoid Cells

- Malignant lymphoma
- Plasmacytoma.

Mesenchymal Tumors

- Smooth muscle tumors
- Peripheral nerve sheath tumors
- Paragangliomas
- Solitary fibrous tumors
- Follicular dendritic cell tumors
- LCH
- Angiosarcoma.

Teratomas

Secondaries

● FINE NEEDLE ASPIRATION CYTOLOGY (FNAC)

Thyroid FNAC is a minimally invasive low-risk procedure commonly performed in a euthyroid patient with a clinically relevant thyroid nodule. Ultrasound guidance is generally recommended for thyroid nodule FNA. For FNA, 22 to 26-gauge needles can be used; most commonly used is a 24-gauge needle. As the name indicates, the biopsy technique uses aspiration to obtain cells or fluid from a mass. Another technique, fine needle nonaspiration (FNNA) biopsy, avoids aspiration but still permits cytologic review of thyroid masses.

The slides for wet fixation should be placed immediately in 95% alcohol for staining with the Papanicolaou stain. For Giemsa staining, air-dried smears are necessary, and prepared slides are left unfixed and transported to the laboratory. Usually, 3–6 aspirations are made. For cystic lesions, the fluid should be completely aspirated and FNA attempted on residual tissue. Sonological localization helps to see solid areas. Aspirated fluid should be placed in a plastic cup and saved for cytologic evaluation. Cell block preparation is occasionally done.

Bethesda system is used to categorize the results of cytology. Six categories as given in **Table 1** are possible with increasing chance of malignancy. 2017 update of the system gives two columns of the risk of malignancy considering noninvasive follicular thyroid neoplasm with papillary like nuclear features (NIFTP) as malignancy and not.

The diagnostic accuracy of thyroid FNA for technically satisfactory specimens is greater than 95%, with positive predictive values of 89–98% and negative predictive values of 94–99%. Sensitivities for thyroid FNA range from 43% to 98%, and specificities range from 72% to 100%. For the evaluation of cystic thyroid lesions, FNA is reported to have a low sensitivity (40%).

Limitations

False-negative rates generally vary from 1.5% to 11.5% (average, <5%). The false-negative rate is defined as the percentage of patients with benign cytology in whom malignant lesions are later confirmed on thyroidectomy. False-positive rates vary from 0% to 8% (average, 3%). A false-positive diagnosis indicates that a patient with a malignant FNA result was found on histologic examination to have benign lesions. Interpretive or sampling errors account for false diagnoses. Hashimoto thyroiditis is probably the most common cause of false-positive cytology. Inadequate specimens are labeled nondiagnostic or unsatisfactory and account for 2–20% of specimens (average, 10%). Several factors influence nondiagnostic rates for FNA results, including the skill of the operator, vascularity of the nodule, criteria used to judge

Table 1: Bethesda classification, risk of maliganacy and management.

Diagnostic category	Diagnostic category	Risk of malignancy if NIFTP is not carcinoma (%)	Risk of malignancy if NIFTP is carcinoma (%)	Usual management
I	Nondiagnostic or Unsatisfactory	5–10	5–10	Repeat FNA with ultrasound guidance
II	Benign	0–3	0–3	Clinical and sonographic follow-up
III	Atypia of undetermined significance or follicular lesion of undetermined significance	6–18	Approx 10–30	Repeat FNA, molecular testing, or lobectomy
IV	Follicular neoplasm or suspicious for a follicular neoplasme	10–40	25–40	Molecular testing, lobectomy
V	Suspicious for malignancy	45–60	50–75	Total thyroidectomy or lobectomy
VI	Malignant	94–96	97–99	Total thyroidectomy or lobectomy

(NIFTP: Noninvasive follicular thyroid neoplasm with papillary like nuclear features; FNA: Fine needle aspiration)

adequacy of the specimen, and the cystic component of the nodule. It is not possible to diagnose follicular carcinoma by FNAC as the full specimen needs to be studied to see the capsular and vascular invasion.

● PAPILLARY CARCINOMA

This is the most common malignant tumor of the thyroid gland and comprises 80–85% of all malignancies. It is common in countries having iodine sufficient or iodine excess diets. They tend to be biologically indolent and have an excellent prognosis. Papillary carcinoma can occur at any age, but most of them are diagnosed in third and fifth decades of life. Women are more frequently affected (2–4: 1). Multifocality is common. Most important etiological role is that of radiation. It was frequently diagnosed in patients who are treated with low dose radiation to head and neck for benign diseases. It was also recognized in survivors of atomic bomb explosion in Japan. Survivors of other cancers who were treated with radiation were also found to develop papillary carcinomas as second primaries. Dietary iodine concentration appears to influence incidence

and in some cases, the morphology of papillary carcinomas **(Figs. 1 and 2)**.

Pathology

Papillary carcinoma shows varied gross features. Majority of the cases present as a solid irregular and firm gray white growth with granular cut surface. Scarring may be very prominent in some of the cases. Calcification is a common finding. It can also present as a small scar in the subcapsular location. Some lesions may be completely cystic with a solid mural nodule attached.

Papillary thyroid carcinoma (PTC) is characterized by unique nuclear features which are diagnostic of this entity. Typical cytological findings include cells in papillae with anatomical borders and monolayered sheets showing swirling. They have ovoid, overlapping nuclei with grooves, and intranuclear inclusions. Studies have shown that presence of a combination of papillae, intranuclear inclusions, and metaplastic squamoid cytoplasm is 98% predictive of papillary carcinoma in cytology material. Nuclear grooves are also

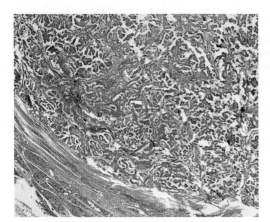

Fig. 1: Papillary thyroid carcinoma showing cells in complex and branching papillae (H & E, 2X).

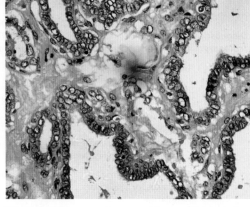

Fig. 2: Papillary carcinoma with overlapping clear "Orphan Annie nuclei" with nuclear grooves and inclusions (H & E, 40X).

seen in thyroiditis, HTA, and adenomatous hyperplasias while intranuclear inclusions are encountered in medullary carcinomas, HTAs, and paragangliomas. Histological sections show overlapping and clearing of nuclei typically described as Orphan Annie nuclei.

Depending on different patterns, cell types, and clinical features, different variants have been described. Except for oncocytic and hobnail variants, all others should have more than 50% of the tumors showing their unique patterns along with nuclear features for their diagnosis. An oncocytic variant shows oncocytic morphology in ≥75%; hobnail variant shows hobnailed nuclei in ≥30%.

Among the variants, specific prognostic significance is connoted to the following types:

- Tall cell variant
  - Cells should be 3 times taller than their width
  - Accounts for 10% of PTC cases
  - More seen in elderly
  - Usually large and show extrathyroid extension and recurrences more frequently
  - 10-year survival rate is 70%
  - Less sensitive to radioactive iodine (RAI) therapy
  - High prevalence of BRAF mutation
- Diffuse sclerosing variant
  - More seen in children and young adults
  - Clinically aggressive
  - All cases are associated with lymph node metastasis at the time of presentation
  - Diffusely infiltrating tumor with sclerotic stroma showing squamous morules, psammoma bodies, and associated thyroiditis
  - Lung metastasis is also more common at presentation (25%)
- Columnar cell variant
  - Very rare
  - High columnar cells with pseudo-stratification, supra and subnuclear vacuolations reminiscent of early secretory endometrium
  - Clinically aggressive
- Solid variant
  - Mimics solid type of poorly differentiated carcinoma, but do not have its guarded prognosis

- Cribriform morular variant
  - Seen typically in patients of familial adenomatous polyposis (FAP) and Gardner's syndrome (APC mutations)
  - Shows cribriform features, solid and spindle areas with squamoid morphology
  - Usually multifocal
- Clear cell variant
  - Recognition of this variant at metastatic sites can be problematic without immunostains
- Hobnail variant
  - Recently described entity
  - Clinically aggressive
- Oncocytic variant
  - Resistant to RAI therapy
  - Clinically aggressive.
- Follicular variant
  - Unique variant with different genetic profile
  - Often diagnosed as follicular neoplasms in FNA due to microfollicular arrangement and equivocal nuclear features
  - Percentage of tumor to be involved by this pattern is still debated
  - Subcategorized into unencapsulated, encapsulated/well-demarcated and diffuse/multinodular variants
  - Encapsulated—akin to follicular neoplasms, better prognosis
  - Diffuse type more aggressive.

Noninvasive Follicular Thyroid Neoplasm with Papillary-like Nuclear Features

Noninvasive encapsulated follicular variant of PTC has been established in the literature as a clinically indolent tumor. Despite this, it was traditionally treated like all other PTCs. In an attempt to reduce overtreatment of this entity, a panel of experts reclassified this entity as NIFTP. It is a low-grade tumor with an indolent clinical course. The removal of NIFTP from the carcinoma category has significantly lowered the rates of malignancy in thyroid fine-needle aspiration diagnostic categories and rates of adverse oncologic events in PTC. NIFTP is characterized as a low-to-intermediate suspicion nodule on ultrasound, often shows an indeterminate preoperative cytology diagnosis and demonstrates molecular alterations characteristic of low-grade thyroid follicular tumors. The set of criteria to diagnose this entity is follicular growth with less than 1% papillae, nuclear score of 2–3, absence of psammoma bodies and necrosis, less than 3 mitoses per 10 high per fields and less than 30% solid growth. Management recommendations for NIFTP are very similar to low-risk PTC measuring less than 4 cm. Most studies agree that nodules with nuclear features suggestive of NIFTP or small PTC should get lobectomy without radioactive iodine.

Papillary Microcarcinoma

It is not a specific variant but includes all papillary carcinomas that measure 1 cm or less in dimension (stage IA).

Clinical Markers for Potential Aggressiveness

- Nonincidental presentation
- Positive preoperative FNA
- Lymph node metastasis
- Positive family history
- Nodules in contralateral lobes
- Male gender.

Histological Markers for Aggressiveness

- Multifocal/bilateral
- Size ≥6 mm
- Extrathyroidal extension

- Desmoplastic fibrosis
- Presence of poorly differentiated components
- Lymphovascular emboli.

Prognosis

Prognosis of papillary carcinoma is excellent. Ten year survival rate is over 90% and for young patients, over 98%. Tall cell and columnar cell variants have a less favorable prognosis than conventional papillary carcinomas.

● FOLLICULAR CARCINOMA

It is a malignant epithelial tumor showing follicular cell differentiation and lacking diagnostic nuclear features of papillary carcinoma. It accounts for 10–15% of thyroid malignancies. It is more common in women in the fifth decade. Incidence is higher in iodine deficient areas. Follicular carcinomas most commonly present as large asymptomatic thyroid nodules which are typically cold on scintigraphy. Distant metastasis is seen in up to 20% during presentation. Oncocytic variants typically occur 10 years later than the conventional types and show greater propensity for recurrence and local invasion. Follicular carcinomas are usually encapsulated with gray tan to brown bulging cut surface. Widely invasive carcinomas may show extensive permeation of the capsule. Rarely thyroid veins and superior vena cava may be involved. Multifocality is uncommon. Distal metastasis to the lung and bones are common **(Figs. 3 and 4)**.

Cytology

Aspirates will be hypercellular and show repetitive microfollicles and scant colloid. Atypical nuclear features do not denote malignancy. Demonstration of capsular or vascular invasion is needed for the diagnosis of follicular carcinoma.

Histology

Follicular carcinomas show variable morphology with cells arranged in follicles, solid or trabecular patterns. They are divided into two major categories—minimally invasive and widely invasive. While conceptually simple, there is no consensus as to the definition of capsular invasion. Some authorities require complete transgression of the capsule, while other authorities do not require complete transgression of the capsule. Minimally invasive carcinomas have limited capsular and/or vascular invasion. Widely invasive carcinomas

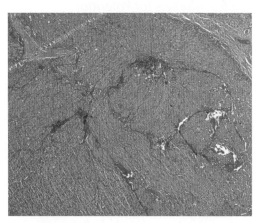

Fig. 3: Follicular carcinoma (H & E, 10X).

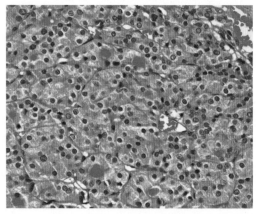

Fig. 4: Follicular carcinoma with cells in closely packed microfollicular pattern (H & E, 40X).

have widespread invasion of thyroid tissue and/ or blood vessels. The probability of aggressive behavior increases with the extent of vascular invasion. The term "grossly encapsulated angioinvasive follicular carcinoma" has been suggested for those tumors that demonstrate vascular invasion only.

Variants

- Oncocytic
- Clear cell
- Mucinous.

Prognosis

Minimally invasive follicular carcinomas have very low long-term mortality (3–5%). Widely invasive carcinomas have 50% mortality. Oncocytic carcinoma behaves more aggressively than conventional types with higher frequencies of extrathyroidal extension, local recurrence, and nodal metastasis. Adverse prognostic factors include age more than 45 years, oncocytic tumor type, extrathyroidal extension, tumor size greater than 4 cm, and presence of distant metastasis.

● POORLY DIFFERENTIATED CARCINOMA

They are defined as follicular cell neoplasms that show limited evidence of follicular cell differentiation and occupy both morphologically and behaviorally an intermediate position between differentiated and undifferentiated carcinomas. Turin proposal (2006) remains so far the most accepted criteria for diagnosing this entity. According to this proposal poorly differentiated carcinomas (PDTCs) are defined by: (1) presence of trabecular/insular/solid (TIS) architecture, with (2) at least one of the following features—convoluted nuclei, mitotic figures of >3/hpf, or coagulative necrosis; (3) absence of conventional nuclear features of papillary carcinoma. PTDCs can be seen as

component of well-differentiated carcinomas and as little as 10% is sufficient to confer an aggressive biological behavior. Most tumors present as cold nodules with or without enlarged lymphadenopathy. Lung and bone metastases are also relatively frequent at the time of diagnosis. Extrathyroidal extension is less commonly seen than in anaplastic carcinomas.

Focal TP53 positivity, increased ki67 index (10–30%), and absence of E-cadherin membrane expression are important immuno-histochemical features. They show reactivity for both thyroglobulin and TTF1, although thyroglobulin positivity may be focal.

These patients respond poorly to radioiodine therapy. The prognosis depends primarily on TNM staging, completeness of surgery, and response to radioactive iodine therapy.

● ANAPLASTIC (UNDIFFERENTIATED) CARCINOMA

Anaplastic carcinomas are highly malignant tumors that histologically appear wholly or partially composed of undifferentiated cells that exhibit immunohistochemical or ultra-structural features indicative of epithelial differentiation. It affects mainly the elderly age group with higher incidence reported in endemic goiter regions. It has a high mortality rate (90%) with a median survival rate of up to 6 months after diagnosis. Patients typically present with rapidly expanding neck mass with pressure symptoms like hoarseness and dysphagia. Tumors are hard and fixed, and frequently invade the surrounding structures. Lymph node involvement as well as distant metastasis is seen in up to 40% of cases. All anaplastic carcinomas are staged as T4 (T4a—intrathyroidal, T4b—extrathyroidal extension) **(Fig. 5)**.

Cytologically, smears are cellular with highly pleomorphic cells seen singly and in clusters. Three types of cells are observed—spindle,

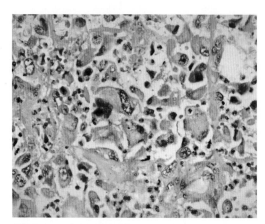

Fig. 5: Anaplastic thyroid carcinoma showing bizarre cells (H & E, 40X).

giant cell, and squamoid. There is increased mitosis and necrosis with the background characteristically showing polymorphonuclear leukocytes. There may be an associated differentiated component in some of the cases. Variants described are: (1) osteoclastic, (2) carcinosarcoma, (3) paucicellular, and (4) lymphoepithelioma and the likes.

These tumors are negative for thyroglobulin and TTF1, and show variable positivity with epithelial markers. Immunohistochemistry is used to differentiate them from other mesenchymal tumors, melanomas, and lymphomas.

Prognostic factors are related primarily to the extent of disease at presentation. Prognosis depends on the size of the undifferentiated component and the efficacy of eradicative surgery. Five-year survival rate ranges from 0% to 14%.

● MEDULLARY CARCINOMA

Medullary thyroid carcinoma is a malignant tumor showing C cell differentiation. It constitutes 5–10% of all thyroid malignancies. Up to 25% cases are heritable, caused by germ-line mutations in RET proto-oncogene. Mean age at presentation is 50 years for sporadic cases. MEN II B patients present in infancy or early childhood while MEN IIA associated tumors occur in late adolescence or early adulthood. Patients with FMTC present at an age of 50 years. Tumors typically are located in the middle third of the lobes. They present as cold nodules with more patients presenting with nodal metastasis (50%) and up to 15% with distant metastasis. Virtually all MTCs produce calcitonin, and serum levels are typically increased. Paraneoplastic syndromes may occur due to production of other peptides and amines. Cytologically smears show loosely cohesive cells with polygonal, bipolar, or spindle shapes. Plasmacytoid cells are common and multinucleated giant cell morphology is occasionally encountered. MGG stains show characteristic red cytoplasmic granules. Amyloid may be found in 50–70% of the cases **(Figs. 6 to 8)**.

Histologically, cells with salt and pepper chromatin are arranged in sheets, nests or trabeculae in an organoid fashion. Necrosis is infrequent. Variants include spindle cell, small cell, giant cell, oncocytic, clear cell, etc. (12 variants are described). Occasional cases may show more pleomorphic features.

Cells are positive for calcitonin, CEA, chromogranin, synaptophysin, TTF1, and low molecular weight keratin. C cell hyperplasia can be seen in surrounding thyroid tissue adjacent to the invasive tumor and also in prophylactic thyroidectomies in hereditary cases. "Neoplastic C cell hyperplasia" is a precursor lesion for heritable medullary carcinomas and is composed of groups of intrafollicular atypical C cells while "reactive C cell hyperplasias" seen in variety of other pathophysiological conditions is characterized by an increased number of normal appearing C cells.

Five and ten-year survival rates are 83.2% and 73.7%, respectively. Older age, male gender, and extent of local tumor invasion are associated with reduced survival. Presence of distant metastasis is also an independent

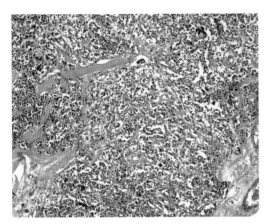

Fig. 6: Medullary carcinoma with cells in nesting pattern (H & E, 10X).

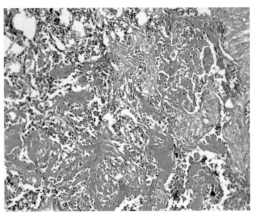

Fig. 7: Salt and pepper chromatin in medullary carcinoma (H & E, 10X).

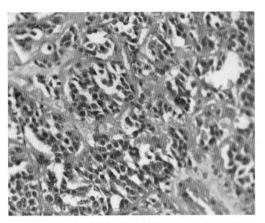

Fig. 8: Amyloid deposits in medullary carcinoma (H & E, 40X).

predictor of poor prognosis. Children with MEN IIB present at an earlier age and have a higher risk for aggressive forms when compared with MEN IIA cases. Presence of necrosis, squamous metaplasia, <50% of calcitonin reactive cells or CEA reactive cells in the absence of calcitonin has also been considered as a poor prognostic feature.

● MOLECULAR GENETICS

Alterations of follicular cells that lead to carcinogenesis are caused by unopposed activation of either the mitogen-activated protein (MAP) kinase pathway or the phosphatidylinositol-3-kinase (PI3K)/AKT pathway. Specifically, the MAP kinase pathway (encompassed by the MEK and ERK kinase cascade) is regulated by the RET, RAS, and BRAF genes. Point mutations in the BRAF and RAS genes or RET/PTC translocation can lead to unopposed cellular proliferation and to a carcinogenic environment via the MAP kinase pathway.

BRAF gene alterations are present in about 30–45% of patients with PTCs and, on average, in 15% (range, 12–47%) of patients with PDTCs. The BRAF gene is a marker of adverse prognostic factors, including disease aggressiveness, decreased radioiodine trapping, tumor recurrence, lymph node or distant metastatic disease, and extrathyroidal extension. RET/PTC rearrangements seen in 30% of PTC ultimately result in the unopposed activation of the MAP kinase pathway.

PAX8: PPARγ rearrangements are almost always associated only with follicular carcinomas. Such rearrangements are almost never expressed in patients with PDTCs.

RAS gene alterations are present in about 40–50% of patients with FTCs and, on average, in

35% (range, 20–50%) of patients with PDTCs and ATCs. It is a marker of tumor dedifferentiation and adverse prognostic outcome. TP53 gene alterations are rarely associated with WDTCs; however, they are highly prevalent in patients with PDTCs (about 28%; range, 17–38%) and in patients with ATCs (64%; range, 20–88%). Unlike the RAS and BRAF gene alterations, p53 mutations possess an exclusive function in triggering tumor dedifferentiation and evolution to PDTC and ATC.

The molecular genetics of medullary carcinoma is well-established, showing mutations in the *RET* proto-oncogene. Germline *RET* mutations are associated with hereditary medullary carcinomas, including familial medullary carcinoma (familial MTC) and the multiple endocrine neoplasia syndromes (MEN2a and 2b). However, it must also be noted that sporadic tumors may also harbor *RET* mutations (30–66%). Sporadic tumors may also harbor *HRAS* or *KRAS* mutations as well (up to 25%).

In familial setting, prophylactic total thyroidectomy is performed for family members based on positive mutational analysis.

Table 2 summarizes the prevalence of genetic alteration in patients with various thyroid carcinomas.

Molecular testing in indeterminate thyroid nodule: Molecular testing for thyroid nodules helps improve the diagnostic accuracy of thyroid cytology for indeterminate cases and potentially to guide the extent of surgery as initial therapy for suspected thyroid malignancies. Diagnostic test accuracy must also be considered, with evaluation of test sensitivity, specificity, and the underlying disease prevalence in the population. Diagnostic tests with high sensitivity and high negative predictive value (NPV) are good tests to "rule out" the presence of disease, depending on the disease prevalence within the population, suggesting that a negative test result has high accuracy (approximately 95%) to reassure patients that cancer is not present in the thyroid nodule evaluated. Diagnostic tests with a high specificity and high positive predictive value (PPV) are good to "rule in" disease, suggesting that a positive test result has high accuracy to confirm that a nodule is indeed cancerous,

The "rule in" tests assess for the presence of single gene point mutations (BRAF or RAS) or gene rearrangements (RRET/PPTC, PAX8// PPPARγ) which have been shown to increase the ability to predict cancer, while the "rule out" test (Afirma Gene Expression Classifier) utilizes a proprietary gene expression classifier (RRNA expression) specifically designed to maximize the ability to define a process as benign. None of the presently available tests is associated with a 100% negative or positive predictive value (NNPV or PPV). Thus, no currently available molecular test identifies the absence or presence of malignancy in all indeterminate nodules.

Table 2: Summary of the prevalence of genetic alterations in patients with various thyroid carcinomas.

Altered gene	PDTC (%)	PTC (%)	FTC (%)	ATC (%)
RET/PTC	0	20	0	0
TP53	20–30	0	0	65–70
BRAF	15	45	0	20–25
RAS	30–35	10–15	45	50–55
β-catenin	20–25	0	0	65
PAX8: PPARγ	0	0	35	0

(PDTC: Poorly differentiated thyroid carcinoma; PTC: Papillary thyroid carcinoma; FTC: Follicular thyroid carcinoma; ATC: Anaplastic thyroid carcinoma)

● ANCILLARY TESTING

Ancillary testing can be used for diagnostic, prognostic, and, to some extent, therapeutic purposes in thyroid cancer. While several markers are now commonly used in patient management, they are not yet a "universal standard of care."

A number of immunohistochemical markers has been proposed to confirm the diagnosis of papillary carcinoma, allowing for distinction from other lesions/tumors in the differential diagnosis. These markers include HBME-1, galectin 3, CITED-1, HMWCK, CD56, and cytokeratin 19. The literature has demonstrated a high sensitivity and specificity with various combinations of these markers for the diagnosis of papillary carcinoma and is particularly useful in resolving the diagnosis for follicular patterned lesions. However, these panels are not infallible as there are false-positives and false-negatives. With regard to the rare but important cribriform morular variant of papillary carcinoma, nuclear beta catenin accumulation is essentially a defining feature that is diagnostically invaluable.

● FURTHER READING

1. College of American Pathologists (CAP). (2014). CAP guidelines for thyroid cancer reporting. [online] Available from: http://webapps.cap.org/apps/docs/committees/cancer/cancer_protocols/2014/Thyroid_14Protocol_3100.pdf. [Accessed Jan., 2019].
2. Crippa S, Mazzucchelli L, Cibas ES, et al. The Bethesda system for reporting thyroid fine-needle aspiration specimens. Am J Clin Pathol. 2010;134(2):343-4.
3. Demellawy DE, Nasr A, Alowami S. Application of CD56, P63 and CK19 immunohistochemistry in the diagnosis of papillary carcinoma of the thyroid. Diagn Pathol. 2008;3:5.
4. Fischer S, Asa SL. Application of Immunohisto-chemistry to thyroid neoplasms. Arch Pathol Lab Med. 2008;132(3):359-72.
5. Hannallah J, Rose J, Guerrero MA. Comprehensive literature review: Recent advances in diagnosing and managing patients with poorly differentiated thyroid carcinoma. Int J Endocrinol. 2013;2013:317487.
6. Legakis I, Syrigos K. Recent advances in molecular diagnosis of thyroid cancer. J Thyroid Res. 2011; 2011:384213.
7. LiVolsi A. Papillary thyroid carcinoma: An update. Mod Pathol. 2011;24(Suppl 2):S1-9.
8. RC Path guidelines for thyroid cancer reporting; 2014.
9. WHO Bluebooks. Endocrine organs, 3rd edition. WHO Bluebooks; 2004.
10. Xing M, Haugen BR, Schlumberger M. Progress in molecular-based management of differentiated thyroid cancer. Lancet. 2013;381(9871):1058-69.

CHAPTER 2

Guidelines in the Management of Differentiated Thyroid Cancer

Shreya Bhattacharya, Krishnakumar Thankappan

● INTRODUCTION

Differentiated thyroid cancer (DTC) comprises around 90% of all thyroid malignancies. By far, the most common presentation of DTC is as a solitary thyroid nodule.

● DIAGNOSTIC EVALUATION

Thyroid function testing of TSH with or without free T4 is done. These are generally normal in malignant cases. The utility lies in detection of a toxic nodule which has a very low likelihood of malignancy, reducing the index of suspicion for the clinician. **Flowchart 1** shows the sequence of diagnostic evaluation.

Fine Needle Aspiration Cytology

Fine needle aspiration cytology (FNAC) is the single most useful study in assessment of a solitary thyroid nodule or the dominant nodule of multinodular goiter. Ultrasound guidance

Flowchart 1: Sequence of diagnostic evaluation.

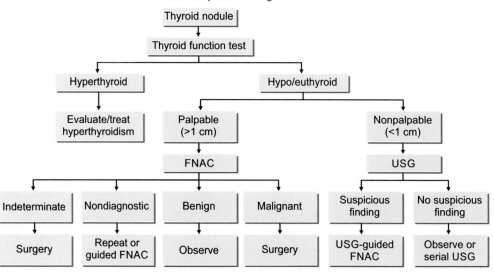

(FNAC: Fine needle aspiration cytology; USG: Ultrasonography)

is preferred for small, posteriorly located or cystic nodules. FNAC is categorized as benign, malignant, suspicious, or insufficient. Suspicious diagnosis may represent follicular lesions or follicular variant of papillary carcinoma. Insufficient aspirates may require re-aspiration with or without ultrasound guidance.

The Bethesda system for reporting thyroid cytopathology includes:

- *Nondiagnostic*—may require repeat FNAC with ultrasound guidance
- *Benign*—clinical follow-up
- *Atypia of undetermined significance (AUS)*—repeat FNAC, molecular testing or lobectomy
- *Suspicious for a follicular neoplasm/follicular neoplasm*—may require lobectomy or molecular testing
- *Suspicious for malignancy*—requires surgical intervention (Total thyroidectomy or lobectomy/hemithyroidectomy)
- *Malignant*—surgical intervention (Total thyroidectomy or lobectomy/hemi-thyroidectomy)

Imaging

Ultrasound is the most commonly used single imaging study for thyroid nodules. The overall risk of malignancy in detected nodules is around 15%. Suspicious ultrasound features are irregular shape, jagged borders, microcalcifications, presence of internal echoes, and absence of peripheral echoes. The status of cervical lymph nodes is also assessed. **Table 1** shows the ultrasound characteristics of a benign and malignant thyroid nodule. Thyroid cancers may require additional imaging like chest X-ray, CT, MRI, and PET scans. Chest X-ray may reveal tracheal compression or deviation and substernal extension. CT/MRI is done when invasion of visceral structures is suspected. The use of iodinated contrast in CT imaging should be carefully considered

Table 1: Ultrasound characteristics of benign and malignant thyroid nodule.

Benign	Malignant
• Hyperechoic	• Hypoechoic
• Peripheral vascularity	• Central vascularity
• Spongiform appearance	• Entirely solid
• Comet-tail shadowing	• Microcalcifications
• Purely cystic	• Size 2 cm or greater
	• Irregular margins
	• Incomplete halo
	• Nodule taller than wide

as it may reduce the radioiodine uptake later. MRI with gadolinium contrast is an effective alternative. PET scan mainly has a role in follow up in localizing disease when radioiodine scans are negative. Another probable use of PET is in lesions of indeterminate cytology. Studies differ in opinion whether PET can distinguish benign from malignant lesions in such cases. Thyroid incidentalomas are defined as nonpalpable thyroid nodules discovered on sonography in asymptomatic adults. These nodules are often detected when sonography is performed for parathyroid disease, carotid stenosis, or other nonthyroid-related neck problems. These are usually followed up by an ultrasound imaging. Further, FNAC is done in lesions more than 1 cm in size. Smaller lesions are put on serial ultrasound follow-up.

TNM Staging

The eighth edition of AJCC has introduced few new changes in the staging system and they are summarized in **Table 2**. **Table 3** shows the revised TNM staging and **Table 4** shows the overall staging.

● TREATMENT

Surgery is the first-line therapy for DTC. **Flowchart 2** shows the treatment algorithm.

Table 2: Major changes in TNM staging in AJCC, 8th edition, for differentiated thyroid cancers.

- The age cutoff for staging was increased from 45 to 55 years at diagnosis.
- Minor extrathyroidal extension detected only on histologic examination was removed from the definition of T3 disease and has no impact on either T category or overall stage.
- N1 disease no longer upstages a patient to stage III; if the patient's age <55 years at diagnosis, N1 disease is stage I; if age is 55 years, N1 disease is stage II.
- T3a is a new category for tumors >4 cm confined to the thyroid gland.
- T3b is a new category for tumors of any size demonstrating gross extrathyroidal extension into strap muscles (sternohyoid, sternothyroid, thyrohyoid, and omohyoid muscles)
- Level VII lymph nodes, previously classified as lateral neck lymph nodes (N1b), were reclassified as central neck lymph nodes (N1a) to be more anatomically consistent and because level VII presented significant coding difficulties for tumor registrars, clinicians, and researchers.
- In differentiated thyroid cancer, the presence of distant metastases in older patients is classified as stage IVB disease rather than stage IVC disease; distant metastasis in anaplastic thyroid cancer continues to be classified as stage IVC disease.

(TNM: Tumor, node, and metastases; AJCC: American Joint Committee on Cancer)

Table 3: TNM staging (AJCC, 8th edition) for papillary, follicular, poorly differentiated, Hurthle cell, and anaplastic thyroid carcinomas.

T category	T criteria
TX	Primary tumor cannot be assessed
T0	No evidence of primary tumor
T1	Tumor less than or equal to 2 cm in greatest dimension limited to the thyroid
T1a	Tumor less than or equal to 1 cm in greatest dimension limited to the thyroid
T1b	Tumor >1 cm but less than or equal to 2 cm in greatest dimension limited to the thyroid
T2	Tumor >2 cm but less than or equal to 4 cm in greatest dimension limited to the thyroid
T3	Tumor >4 cm limited to the thyroid or gross extrathyroidal extension invading only strap muscles
T3a	Tumor >4 cm limited to the thyroid
T3b	Gross extrathyroidal extension invading only strap muscles (sternohyoid, sternothyroid, thyrohyoid, or omohyoid muscles) from a tumor of any size
T4	Includes gross extrathyroidal extension into major neck structures
T4a	Gross extrathyroidal extension invading subcutaneous soft tissues, larynx, trachea, esophagus, or recurrent laryngeal nerve from a tumor of any size
T4b	Gross extrathyroidal extension invading prevertebral fascia or encasing carotid artery or mediastinal vessels from a tumor of any size
N category	**N criteria**
NX	Regional lymph nodes cannot be assessed
N0	No evidence of regional lymph nodes metastasis
N0a	One or more cytologic or histologically confirmed benign lymph node
N0b	No radiologic or clinical evidence of locoregional lymph node metastasis
N1	Metastasis to regional nodes
N1a	Metastasis to level VI or VII (pretracheal, paratracheal, or prelaryngeal/Delphian, or upper mediastinal) lymph nodes; this can be unilateral or bilateral disease
N1b	Metastasis to unilateral, bilateral, or contralateral lateral neck lymph nodes (levels I, II, III, IV, or V) or retropharyngeal lymph nodes
M category	**M criteria**
M0	No distant metastasis
M1	Distant metastasis

(TNM: Tumor, node, and metastases; AJCC: American Joint Committee on Cancer)

Table 4: Stage guide (differentiated thyroid cancer).

When age at diagnosis is ...	And T is ...	And N is ...	And M is ...	Then the stage group is ...
<55 years	Any T	Any N	M0	I
	Any T	Any N	M1	II
More than or equal to 55 years	T1	N0/NX	M0	I
	T1	N1	M0	II
	T2	N0/NX	M0	I
	T2	N1	M0	II
	T3a/T3b	Any N	M0	II
	T4a	Any N	M0	III
	T4b	Any N	M0	IVA
	Any T	Any N	M1	IVB

Flowchart 2: Treatment algorithm.

FNAC

↓

- USG thyroid and neck
- Vocal cord evaluation
- CT/MRI for fixed, bulky/substernal lesions

↓

Thyroidectomy

- Size >4 cm
- Gross extrathyroidal extension (cT4)
- Clinical nodes (cN+)

- Size >1 cm <4 cm
- No extrathyroidal extension
- No clinical evidence of lymph nodes (cN0)

- Size >1 cm
- No extrathyroidal extension
- cN0
- Unifocal
- No h/o prior head and neck RT
- No family h/o thyroid cancer

Total thyroidectomy

Total Thyroidectomy
- Older age (>45 years, >55 years according to recent data)
- Contralateral nodules
- History of radiation to head and neck
- Family history of DTC

Thyroid lobectomy/ hemithyroidectomy
- Low, risk papillary/follicular
- Carcinomas

Thyroid lobectomy or Hemithyroidectomy

(FNAC: Fine needle aspiration cytology; USG: Ultrasonography; RT: Radiotherapy)

Extent of Thyroidectomy

Surgery for thyroid cancer is an important component of the treatment approach. Previous guidelines have endorsed total thyroidectomy as the primary initial surgical treatment option for nearly all differentiated thyroid cancers >1 cm with or without evidence of locoregional or distant metastases. This was based on retrospective data suggesting that a total thyroidectomy would improve survival, decrease recurrence rates, allow for routine use of radioiodine remnant ablation, and facilitate detection of recurrent/persistent disease during follow-up. However, recent data have demonstrated that in properly selected patients, clinical outcomes are very similar following unilateral (thyroid lobectomy/hemithyroidectomy) or bilateral thyroid surgery (total thyroidectomy).

The American Thyroid Association (ATA, 2015) recommendations are as below:

- For patients with thyroid cancer >4 cm, or with gross extrathyroidal extension (clinical T4), or clinically apparent metastatic disease to nodes (clinical N1) or distant sites (clinical M1), the initial surgical procedure should include a near-total or total thyroidectomy and gross removal of all primary tumors unless there are contraindications to this procedure.
- For patients with thyroid cancer >1 cm tand <4 cm without extrathyroidal extension, and without clinical evidence of any lymph node metastases (cN0), the initial surgical procedure can be either a bilateral procedure (near-total or total thyroidectomy) or a unilateral procedure (lobectomy). Thyroid lobectomy alone may be sufficient initial treatment for low-risk papillary and follicular carcinomas; however, the treatment team may choose total thyroidectomy to enable radioactive iodine (RAI) therapy or to enhance follow up based upon disease features and/or patient preferences.
- If surgery is chosen for patients with thyroid cancer <1 cm without extrathyroidal extension and cN0, the initial surgical procedure should be a thyroid lobectomy unless there are clear indications to remove the contralateral lobe. Thyroid lobectomy alone is sufficient treatment for small, unifocal, and intrathyroidal carcinomas in the absence of prior head and neck radiation, familial thyroid carcinoma, or clinically detectable cervical nodal metastases.

Completion Thyroidectomy

Completion thyroidectomy should be offered to those patients for whom a total thyroidectomy would have been recommended, had the diagnosis been available before the initial surgery. This may be necessary when the diagnosis of malignancy is made following lobectomy for an indeterminate or nondiagnostic biopsy. Some patients with malignancy may require completion thyroidectomy to provide complete resection of multicentric disease and to allow radioiodine therapy. The surgical risks of two-stage thyroidectomy (lobectomy followed by completion thyroidectomy) are similar to those of a total thyroidectomy.

Management of Neck Disease

The primary echelon nodes in central compartment (level VI) drain into the middle and lower deep jugular nodes (levels III and IV) and to the nodes in the lower posterior triangle (level Vb). **Flowchart 3** shows the algorithm for management of neck.

Management of Node-positive Neck

Node-positive neck, either clinically, radiologically, or if found intraoperatively, will need a neck dissection. Extent of neck dissection is determined by the extent of neck disease. Central compartment nodes require

Flowchart 3: Management of neck in differentiated thyroid cancer.

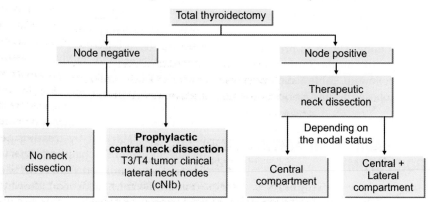

central compartment clearance. Extensive central compartment clearance requires en bloc dissection of nodes between the hyoid bone and innominate vein and from one carotid to the other. This is associated with risk to the nerve and parathyroid. Thus, many authors prefer limited dissection in the central compartment as per the disease. For low-risk cases, the dissection may be confined medial to the nerve. Nodes along jugular chain merit a central and lateral neck dissection with or without posterior triangle clearance. Levels II–IV are most commonly involved. Level I is rarely involved and can be omitted. The need for inclusion of level IIb is controversial and recommended if nodal disease at IIa is identified.

Management of Node-negative Neck

The role of prophylactic central compartment neck dissection is controversial. Evidence suggests that central compartment node dissection increases the proportion of patients who appear disease free with unmeasurable thyroglobulin (Tg) levels postoperatively. Other studies have demonstrated higher morbidity, primarily recurrent laryngeal nerve injury, and transient hypoparathyroidism. For patients with small, noninvasive, apparently node-negative tumors, the balance of risk and benefit may favor total thyroidectomy with close intraoperative inspection of the central compartment with compartmental dissection only in the presence of obviously involved lymph nodes.

American Thyroid Association (ATA, 2015) Recommendations

- Therapeutic central compartment (level VI) neck dissection for patients with clinically involved central nodes should accompany total thyroidectomy to provide clearance of disease from the central neck.
- Prophylactic central compartment neck dissection (ipsilateral or bilateral) should be considered in patients with papillary thyroid carcinoma with clinically uninvolved central neck lymph nodes (cN0) who have advanced primary tumors (T3 or T4) or clinically involved lateral neck nodes (cN1b), or if the information will be used to plan further steps in therapy.
- Thyroidectomy without prophylactic central neck dissection is appropriate for small (T1 or T2), noninvasive, clinically node-negative PTC (cN0), and for most follicular cancers.
- Therapeutic lateral neck compartmental lymph node dissection should be performed for patients with biopsy-proven metastatic lateral cervical lymphadenopathy.

● RISK STRATIFICATION

After the surgery is done, based on the clinical and the surgical pathology details, an initial risk stratification is done. This is to prognosticate as well as to decide on the further adjuvant treatment and follow up. **Table 5** shows the risk stratification proposed by the American Thyroid Association.

● ROLE OF RADIOIODINE AFTER THYROIDECTOMY

Depending on the postoperative risk stratification of the individual patient, the primary goal of postoperative administration of RAI after total thyroidectomy may include:

(1) RAI remnant ablation (to facilitate detection of recurrent disease and initial staging by tests such as Tg measurements or whole-body RAI scans), (2) RAI adjuvant therapy (intended to improve disease-free survival by theoretically destroying suspected, but unproven residual disease, especially in patients at increased risk of disease recurrence), or (3) RAI therapy (intended to improve disease-specific and disease-free survival by treating persistent disease in higher risk patients). This is carried out in TSH-stimulated state (TSH more than 30 micro IU/mL), achieved either by thyroid hormone withdrawal or administration of recombinant human TSH. The radioiodine dose required is typically 30–100 mCi for ablation of

Table 5: ATA initial risk stratification (ATA, 2009, with proposed modifications in ATA, 2015).

ATA low risk	• Papillary thyroid cancer (with all of the following):
	  – No local or distant metastases
	  – All macroscopic tumor has been resected
	  – No tumor invasion of locoregional tissues or structures
	  – The tumor does not have aggressive histology (e.g. tall cell, hobnail variant,
	  – Columnar cell carcinoma)
	  – If ^{131}I is given, there are no RAI-avid metastatic foci outside the thyroid bed on the first post-treatment whole-body RAI scan
	  – No vascular invasion
	  – **Clinical N0 or less than or equal to 5 pathologic N1 micrometastases (<0.2 cm in largest dimension)**
	  – **Intrathyroidal, encapsulated follicular variant of papillary thyroid cancer**
	  – **Intrathyroidal, well-differentiated follicular thyroid cancer with capsular invasion and no or minimal (<4 foci) vascular invasion**
	  – **Intrathyroidal, papillary microcarcinoma, unifocal or multifocal, including BRAFV600E mutated (if known)**

ATA intermediate risk	• Microscopic invasion of tumor into the perithyroidal soft tissues • RAI-avid metastatic foci in the neck on the first post-treatment whole-body RAI scan • Aggressive histology (e.g. tall cell, hobnail variant, columnar cell carcinoma) • Papillary thyroid cancer with vascular invasion • **Clinical N1 or >5 pathologic N1 with all involved lymph nodes <3 cm in largest dimension** • **Multifocal papillary microcarcinoma with ETE and BRAFV600E mutated (if known)**
ATA high risk	• Macroscopic invasion of tumor into the perithyroidal soft tissues (gross ETE) • Incomplete tumor resection • Distant metastases • Postoperative serum thyroglobulin suggestive of distant metastases • **Pathologic N1 with any metastatic lymph node more than or equal to 3 cm in largest dimension** • **Follicular thyroid cancer with extensive vascular invasion (>4 foci of vascular invasion)**

Note: 2015 modifications in **bold**.
(ATA: American Thyroid Association; RAI: Radioactive iodine)

thyroid remnant only and 100–200 mCi in cases with residual disease, aggressive histology, or extrathyroidal spread. The role of radioiodine in the management of differentiated thyroid cancers is discussed in detail in one of the following chapters.

ATA 2015 Recommendations

- RAI remnant ablation is not routinely recommended after thyroidectomy for ATA low-risk DTC patients.
- RAI remnant ablation is not routinely recommended after lobectomy or total thyroidectomy for patients with unifocal papillary microcarcinoma, in the absence of other adverse features.
- RAI remnant ablation is not routinely recommended after thyroidectomy for patients with multifocal papillary microcarcinoma in absence of other adverse features.
- RAI adjuvant therapy should be considered after total thyroidectomy in ATA intermediate-risk level DTC patients.
- RAI adjuvant therapy is routinely recommended after total thyroidectomy for ATA high-risk DTC patients.

● DISTANT METASTASIS

At presentation warrants thyroid surgery for locoregional control and radioiodine treatment for distant disease with dose range of 150–200 mCi. Micronodular pulmonary metastasis responds well to radioiodine. The exceptions to this are solitary brain and bone metastasis compressing the spinal cord, which should be considered for resection and local radiation.

● EXTERNAL BEAM RADIOTHERAPY (EBRT)

The role of radiation therapy in DTC is limited. ATA recommends no role for routine adjuvant

EBRT to the neck in patients with DTC after initial complete surgical removal of the tumor. However, it may have some role in certain individual patients undergoing multiple and frequent serial neck re-operations for palliation of locoregionally recurrent disease. EBRT using modern techniques such as intensity modulated radiotherapy and stereotactic radiation, is considered for locoregional recurrence that is not surgically resectable or with extranodal extension or involvement of soft tissues, particularly in patients with no evidence of distant disease.

TSH suppression is discussed in a separate chapter.

● FOLLOW-UP

It is recommended that serial stimulated thyroglobulin (Tg) measurement should be the principal test in the follow-up of DTC. Imaging studies in patients with elevated Tg levels should aim at localizing the recurrence. Neck ultrasound and diagnostic radioiodine scanning are the routinely employed modalities. Combination of stimulated Tg measurements and ultrasound scan have been shown to have the highest sensitivity for monitoring of treated DTC patients. Outcome patients with DTC do well with overall survival in excess of 90% in multiple series.

● RECURRENT DTC

The discovery of increase in stimulated thyroglobulin level warrants further and/or diagnostic radioiodine scan. Approximately, two-thirds of recurrences occur in the neck. Recurrence of significant size requires surgery, commonly a neck dissection. The surgical risks to the recurrent laryngeal nerve and the parathyroid glands should be understood in such re-surgery cases. Thyroid bed recurrences with invasion of aerodigestive tract structures require more aggressive resections. Small volume disease (less than 1 cm), visualized on radioiodine scans, can be treated with radioiodine therapy. In cases of distant recurrences, the site of disease impacts the management. Osseous metastases should be considered for intravenous zoledronic acid therapy. Empiric radioiodine therapy has been advocated by many authors in the management of thyroglobulin-positive, radioiodine scan-negative patients. Literature reports mortality of 50% at 10 years in recurrent DTC.

● **FURTHER READING**

1. Haugen BR, Alexander EK, Bible KC, et al. 2015 American Thyroid Association Management guidelines for adult patients with thyroid nodules and differentiated thyroid cancer: The American Thyroid Association Guidelines Task Force on thyroid nodules and differentiated thyroid cancer. Thyroid. 2016;26(1):1-133.

2. Tuttle RM, Haugen B, Perrier ND. Updated American Joint Committee on cancer/tumor-node-metastasis staging system for differentiated and anaplastic thyroid cancer (Eighth edition): What changed and why? Thyroid. 2017;27(6):751-6.

CHAPTER 3

Guidelines in the Management of Medullary and Anaplastic Thyroid Cancers

Shreya Bhattacharya, Krishnakumar Thankappan

MEDULLARY THYROID CANCERS

● INTRODUCTION

Medullary thyroid cancer (MTC) arises from the parafollicular or C cells of thyroid. Seventy-five percent cases are sporadic and 25% occur in familial form, associated with multiple endocrine neoplasia type 2 (MEN2) syndrome.

- *Familial (10-30%):* The patients with familial variety have MTC as an autosomal dominant trait in one of the three distinct clinical syndromes that are associated with specific mutation of RET oncogene located on chromosome 10 most commonly. RET mutations have been described within exons 11, 13, 14, 15 also.
  - *Familial MTC*—presents only with MTC without extrathyroidal manifestations.
  - *Associated with MEN2A*—presents with MTC, pheochromocytoma or hyperparathyroidism. Hirschsprung's disease and cutaneous lichen amyloidosis are less common.
  - *Associated with MEN2B*—presents with MTC and pheochromocytoma. This may be associated with ganglioneuroma of the oral and gastrointestinal mucosa and a marfanoid body habitus.
- Sporadic (70-90%).

● DIAGNOSTIC EVALUATION

Laboratory Tests

Serum calcitonin is a useful marker and routinely done when MTC is suspected. False positive elevation has been reported in Hashimoto's thyroiditis, hyperthyroidism, and goiter. Pentagastrin or calcium stimulation test can be done to rule out the above. Some authors advocate routine calcitonin testing in patients with thyroid nodules. ATA guidelines neither recommend nor are against this. However, this has not been widely used. Basal serum calcitonin concentrations usually correlate with tumor mass, but also reflect tumor differentiation, and they are almost always high in patients with a palpable tumor. Most MTCs also secrete carcinoembryonic antigen (CEA), which, like calcitonin, can be used as a tumor marker. Even in the absence of family history, MEN2 syndrome should be ruled out in all patients, as they may represent the index case of previously undiagnosed kindred. Twenty-four-hour urine, vanillylmandelic acid and metanephrines should be done before any surgical intervention to rule out pheochromocytoma. Serum calcium and parathormone levels should also be determined to exclude hyperparathyroidism, seen in MEN2A, so that surgery can address both the thyroid and parathyroid diseases as appropriate.

Fine needle aspiration cytology (FNAC):
Immunohistochemistry for calcitonin can aid
in the FNA diagnosis of MTC.

Imaging

Ultrasonography (USG) is the single most
useful imaging modality in evaluating a thyroid
nodule. CT/MRI head, neck, and chest may be
required when invasion of visceral structures,
cervical and mediastinal nodal disease is
suspected. Cross-sectional imaging of lungs and
liver can be done to exclude distant metastases.
Sometimes, adrenal imaging may be done for
pheochromocytoma.

RET Germline Testing

All patients with MTC merit testing for RET
oncogene mutation. The prevalence of RET
mutations in apparently sporadic cases is
reported to be 7.3%. DNA-based testing will
identify mutations in about 95% of MEN2
cases and 85% of familial cases. When a patient
is identified carrying a mutation, genetic
screening of first-degree relatives should be
done. Gene-positive cases should then be
offered prophylactic surgery.

● TNM STAGING

See **Tables 1 and 2**.

● TREATMENT

See **Flowchart 1**.

Sporadic or Inherited Cases Presenting with Clinical Disease

Meticulous surgery is the first-line treatment
option. The aim is to achieve both clinical and
biochemical cures. It is important to rule out
pheochromocytoma before surgery. If present,
it should be operated upon first before the
thyroid surgery. Total thyroidectomy with at
least a central compartment neck dissection

is recommended. In cases of hyperparathyroidism, excision of parathyroid adenoma or subtotal parathyroidectomy or
autotransplantation is done.

Management of Neck

Ipsilateral lateral neck dissection is
recommended for clinical or radiological
evidence of nodal disease. Prophylactic lateral
neck dissection should be considered if there is
significant central neck disease.

RET Germline Mutation and Prophylactic Thyroidectomy

Mutations of codons 883, 918 and 922 are
associated with MEN2B. Surgical intervention
is merited in the first year of life.

Mutations of codons 611, 618, 620 and 634
are associated with MEN2A. Surgery is merited
before the age of 5 years.

Mutations of codons 768, 790, 791, 804 and
891 are associated with familial MTC. Surgery is
merited before the age of 10 years.

Radiotherapy

Role of external beam radiotherapy is unclear.
NCCN guidelines recommend radiation to be
considered for T4 tumors.

Follow-up

Patients are put on thyroid hormone
replacement. Lifelong follow-up is mandatory
with serum basal calcitonin measurements.
Cases of MEN2 require multidisciplinary
approach.

Recurrent MTC

Recurrent MTC is detected by elevation in
serum calcitonin levels. Further evaluation
requires imaging like USG neck, MRI, CT head,
neck, chest, abdomen and pelvis, FDG-PET
scan, MDP bone scan and GA DOTATATE scans.

Table 1: TNM staging, AJCC, 8th edition, medullary thyroid cancer.

T category	T criteria
TX	Primary tumor cannot be assessed
T0	No evidence of primary tumor
T1	Tumor less than or equal to 2 cm in greatest dimension limited to the thyroid
T1a	Tumor less than or equal to 1 cm in greatest dimension limited to the thyroid
T1b	Tumor >1 cm but less than or equal to 2 cm in greatest dimension limited to the thyroid
T2	Tumor >2 cm but less than or equal to 4 cm in greatest dimension limited to the thyroid
T3	Tumor >4 cm limited to the thyroid or gross extrathyroidal extension invading only strap muscles
T3a	Tumor >4 cm limited to the thyroid
T3b	Gross extrathyroidal extension invading only strap muscles (sternohyoid, sternothyroid, thyrohyoid, or omohyoid muscles) from a tumor of any size
T4	Includes gross extrathyroidal extension into major neck structures
T4a	Gross extrathyroidal extension invading subcutaneous soft tissues, larynx, trachea, esophagus, or recurrent laryngeal nerve from a tumor of any size
T4b	Gross extrathyroidal extension invading prevertebral fascia or encasing carotid artery or mediastinal vessels from a tumor of any size
N category	**N criteria**
NX	Regional lymph nodes cannot be assessed
N0	No evidence of regional lymph nodes metastasis
N0a	One or more cytologic or histologically confirmed benign lymph node
N0b	No radiologic or clinical evidence of locoregional lymph node metastasis
N1	Metastasis to regional nodes
N1a	Metastasis to level VI or VII (pretracheal, paratracheal, or prelaryngeal/Delphian, or upper mediastinal) lymph nodes; this can be unilateral or bilateral disease
N1b	Metastasis to unilateral, bilateral, or contralateral lateral neck lymph nodes (levels I, II, III, IV, or V) or retropharyngeal lymph nodes
M category	**M criteria**
M0	No distant metastasis
M1	Distant metastasis

(TNM: Tumor, node, and metastasis; AJCC: American Joint Committee on Cancer)

Table 2: Overall staging.

When T is ...	And N is ...	And M is ...	Then the stage group is ...
T1	N0	M0	I
T2	N0	M0	II
T3	N0	M0	II
T1-3	N1a	M0	III
T4a	Any N	M0	IVA
T1-3	N1b	M0	IVA
T4b	Any N	M0	IVB
Any T	Any N	M1	IVC

Flowchart 1: Algorithm for the management of medullary thyroid carcinoma.

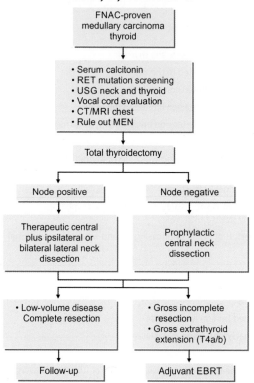

(FNAC: Fine needle aspiration cytology; MEN: Multiple endocrine neoplasia; EBRT: External beam radiotherapy)

Liver metastasis is an area of concern in this scenario, seen in approximately 25% cases. This may require laparoscopy and hepatic angiography. Re-operation should be considered whenever feasible. Radiation can be given for unresectable cases. Recently, vandetanib has been approved for aggressive MTC by FDA.

● PROGNOSIS

MTC accounts for 10–15% of deaths due to thyroid cancer. Literature reports 5- and 10-year survival rates of 69–97% and 56–96%, respectively. Biochemical cure after surgery

has been associated with excellent survival rates. Published data indicates the presence of somatic RET mutation, advanced disease stage, tumor size, extent of nodal metastases, distant metastases, less extensive surgery, and extrathyroidal spread confer adverse outcomes.

ANAPLASTIC CARCINOMA

● INTRODUCTION

Anaplastic carcinoma is the most aggressive of all thyroid malignancies with a natural history of progressive aerodigestive tract compromise. It commonly presents with extrathyroidal spread and distant metastasis. It appears to be associated with preexisting long-standing goiter or may arise from dedifferentiation of differentiated thyroid cancer. The presentation is of an elderly patient with rapidly growing neck mass, compressing the trachea and esophagus. This must be differentiated from lymphoma which may present in the same manner.

● STAGING

Unlike previous editions, where all anaplastic thyroid cancers were classified as T4 disease, anaplastic cancers will now use the same T definitions as differentiated thyroid cancer. Intrathyroidal disease is stage IVA, gross extrathyroidal extension or cervical lymph node metastasis is stage IVB, and distant metastasis is stage IVC. Overall staging is given in **Table 3**.

● MANAGEMENT

Typically, surgery is not feasible due to extensive extrathyroidal infiltration. Sometimes, airway compromise may require resection of thyroid isthmus and adjacent tumor. Rarely, cases presenting early can be treated with surgery for locoregional control. When the diagnosis is known only on final pathology, there is no role for completion thyroidectomy. A differentiated

Table 3: Overall staging, anaplastic carcinoma.

When T is ...	And N is ...	And M is ...	Then the stage group is ...
T1-T3a	N0/NX	M0	IVA
T1-T3a	N1	M0	IVB
T3b	Any N	M0	IVB
T4	Any N	M0	IVB
Any T	Any N	M1	IVC

thyroid cancer with areas of anaplastic transformation also merits a more aggressive treatment.

External beam radiotherapy (EBRT) to the thyroid bed and neck is commonly used for locoregional control. Chemotherapy in combination with RT has been used. Doxorubicin is the single most effective agent.

Despite all measures, prognosis is very poor with reported locoregional control of 45% and overall survival of 28% at 1 year.

• FURTHER READING

1. Cooper DS, Doherty GM, Haugen BR, et al. American Thyroid Association (ATA) Guidelines Taskforce on Thyroid Nodules and Differentiated Thyroid Cancer. Revised American Thyroid Association management guidelines for patients with thyroid nodules and differentiated thyroid cancer. Thyroid. 2009;19(11):1167-214.
2. Edge S, Byrd DR, Compton CC, Fritz AG, Greene F, Trotti A (Eds). AJCC Cancer Staging Manual, 7th edition. New York, NY: Springer-Verlag; 2010. pp. XIX, 718.
3. NCCN. (2012). Thyroid Carcinoma V.2.2012: NCCN Clinical Practice Guidelines in Oncology. [online] Available from: www.nccn.org. [Accessed Jan., 2019].
4. Sherman EJ, Lim SH, Ho AL, et al. Concurrent doxorubicin and radiotherapy for anaplastic thyroid cancer: A critical re-evaluation including uniform pathologic review. Radiother Oncol. 2011;101(3):425-30.
5. Smallridge RC, Copland JA. Anaplastic thyroid carcinoma: Pathogenesis and emerging therapies. Clin Oncol (R Coll Radiol). 2010;22(6):486-97.

CHAPTER 4

Principles of Thyroid Surgery

Shreya Bhattacharya, Krishnakumar Thankappan

● INTRODUCTION

There are only two surgical procedures to be considered in patients presenting with a potential thyroid malignancy, hemithyroidectomy, and total thyroidectomy. Several other surgical procedures have been carried out on the thyroid gland historically.

Hemithyroidectomy or lobectomy: Complete removal of one lobe of thyroid and the isthmus. A subsequent completion thyroidectomy is safe because the contralateral lobe is not dissected. This may be suggested in "low-risk" cases as per the ATA guidelines.

Subtotal thyroidectomy: Bilateral removal of more than one half of the thyroid gland on each side plus the isthmus.

Near total thyroidectomy: Total lobectomy and isthmusectomy with removal of more than 90% of the contralateral lobe. Variable amounts of tissues over or under the recurrent laryngeal nerve are left as long as there is no concern of disease in that area. Apart from this, this is surgically same as total thyroidectomy

Total thyroidectomy: Complete removal of both thyroid lobes and the isthmus. This is typically done for malignant disease.

Completion thyroidectomy: A subsequent procedure to convert a lesser operation into a total thyroidectomy.

● SURGICAL ANATOMY

The thyroid gland is made of up two lateral lobes, which extend from the sides of the thyroid cartilage down to the sixth tracheal ring. These are joined together in the midline by the isthmus, which overlies the second to fourth tracheal rings. On either side, there are two important nerves: the external branch of the superior laryngeal nerve and the recurrent laryngeal nerve; both lie in close proximity to the gland and its blood supply.

The external branch of the superior laryngeal nerve lies deep to the upper pole of the gland as it passes in the sternothyrolaryngeal (Joll's) triangle. This triangle is formed laterally by the superior thyroid vessels, superiorly by the attachment of the strap muscles and deep investing layer of fascia to the hyoid and medially by the midline. Its floor is the cricothyroid muscle with the external laryngeal nerve running on it. Cernei et al. described three anatomical variations of the nerve. Type I nerve passes 1 cm above the superior pole. Type IIa nerve passes within 1 cm of superior pole and type IIb nerve passes below the level of superior pole, thus putting it at maximum risk of injury. The impact on phonation in injury to external branch of superior laryngeal nerve (EBSL) is subtle but affects professional voice users. Dissection in the avascular space between the upper pole and the cricothyroid muscle helps in identifying the nerve.

The recurrent laryngeal nerves run in, or lateral to, the tracheoeosophageal groove and have a variable relationship with the branches of the inferior thyroid artery, crossing deep to it in most cases. Here, the Beahr's triangle is formed by the nerve, inferior thyroid artery, and the common carotid artery. On the left side, the nerve hugs the tracheoesophageal groove as it ascends from the chest. However, on the right side the nerve is more superficial, being 45° to the tracheoesophageal groove. The common sites of injury are: (1) near the lower pole in case of anterior displacement, (2) point of crossing the artery, and (3) at the point of entry. The tubercle of Zuckerkandl is represented in all thyroid glands where the ultimobranchial body fuses with the main thyroid process. The nerve is at risk when nodules develop in this area.

Parathyroid glands lie outside the thyroid capsule beneath the pretracheal fascia. The superior glands are more constant in their location and usually lie near the cricothyroid joint close to the recurrent laryngeal nerve, cephalic to the inferior thyroid artery. The inferior glands are often more variable in their location, being caudal, the recurrent laryngeal nerve and the inferior thyroid artery.

● SURGICAL TECHNIQUE

Historically, Theodore Kocher described the classical techniques of thyroid surgery.

The review of surgical technique by L Delbridge stresses on four main steps in the procedure:
1. Exposure
2. Dissection of upper pole and superior laryngeal nerve
3. Dissection of lateral aspect of the lobes preserving the recurrent laryngeal nerve and parathyroid glands
4. Closure.

Exposure

A low anterior neck skin crease incision is made. It should not be displaced too much cephalic or caudal. Flaps are raised in subplatysmal plane. Strap muscles are separated in the midline. Routine division of strap muscle is not necessary; a partial division of the sternothyroid muscle helps the exposure of the upper pole and cricothyroid space.

Dissection of Upper Pole

The dissection and preservation of the external laryngeal nerve is now a routine practice. The cricothyroid space (space between the muscle and the gland) is usually avascular. The lateral aspect of the superior pole is freed from the sternothyroid muscles, which exposes the polar vessels and the nerve. The vessels are ligated and divided individually.

Lateral Dissection

Paracarotid tunnel is entered and the middle thyroid vein is ligated. Next, the inferior pole is freed and anterior surface of trachea exposed. The gland is gently mobilized medially. Subcapsular dissection is then used on the gland. The recurrent laryngeal nerve and the parathyroid glands are pushed laterally and away from the gland. The nerve is in danger at the point of entry to the larynx where it may be closely related to the gland. Once the nerve is clear off the gland, sharp dissection on the trachea frees that lobe and the isthmus. Same procedure is repeated on the other side and the specimen removed in toto. During hemithyroidectomy, one lobe and isthmus is removed and the cut end of the gland transfixed. The parathyroid glands should be inspected at end of procedure to ensure the vascularity. Autotransplantation of parathyroid gland is done when viability is suspected.

Closure

Closure is done only after ensuring meticulous hemostasis. A suction drain is secured. Careful approximation of skin is recommended since the scar is almost always visible.

● COMPLICATIONS OF THYROIDECTOMY

Hemorrhage

Significant hemorrhage usually occurs within the first few hours after the surgery, caused by uncoupling of ligature or from a small vessel near the entry point of the recurrent laryngeal nerve. Symptoms include stridor, prolific drain output and anterior neck swelling. Immediate attention is required with removal of sutures and evacuation of hematoma. Then the patient is shifted back to the operating room for control of the bleeding source.

Seroma

Wound seromas are seen after resection of large tumors. This may predispose to infection. Most seromas can be treated by repeated aspiration.

Laryngeal Nerve Paralysis

Recurrent laryngeal palsy is of more concern because of the resulting voice change. Reported incidence of permanent injury is around 1% and temporary paresis is around 2.5–5%. Most palsy is temporary due to stretch or devascularization of the nerve which may improve over variable periods of time. Malignant disease, reoperation and central compartment nodal disease are high risk factors for palsy. Unilateral palsy presents with a weak breathy voice with vocal cord paralyzed in paramedian position. Such cases may be observed for variable length of time for possible return of nerve function in neurapraxia or for compensation by the opposite cord. Permanent cases can undergo medialization

thyroplasty procedures. Bilateral palsies lead to airway compromise requiring immediate airway control like tracheostomy. Once airway is secured, they may be monitored for the return of nerve function. Surgical procedures like laser cordotomy may be beneficial to some patients.

Superior laryngeal nerve palsy is under reported as it causes mild voice change in the form of loss of upper range vocalization and some voice fatigue. Speech therapy may be helpful in these cases.

Hypoparathyroidism

It is the major cause of postoperative hypocalcemia. This may be due to ischemic damage or/and resection of the parathyroids. Transient hypocalcemia is the most common complication with reported incidence of 12–24%. Risk factors are total thyroidectomy, central compartment disease, and bilateral ligation of inferior thyroid artery. Incidence of permanent hypocalcemia is less, 1–10%. Typically, patients undergoing thyroid surgery are followed by calcium levels and careful watch for symptoms of hypocalcemia. Asymptomatic patients may be observed carefully without any therapy. Treatment should be tailored individually depending on the severity of calcium deficiency. In the setting of severe tetany, spasm or ECG changes, calcium gluconate 10 mL of 10% solution should be infused intravenously over 10 minutes. Continued support with 10% calcium gluconate in 500 mL of 5% dextrose should be adjusted based on serum calcium levels. Long-term oral vitamin D and calcium supplementation may be necessary for prolonged hypocalcemia.

Completion Thyroidectomy

Reoperation is associated with increased risk of complications, especially if that area is previously dissected. Careful attention to parathyroid preservation should be paid.

Neck Dissection

Central compartment dissection is associated with greater risk of hypoparathyroidism. Lateral compartment dissection may cause shoulder dysfunction due to the stretch or injury to the spinal accessory nerve. Chylous fistulas have been encountered with extensive neck dissections.

Remote Access Thyroidectomy

Incision is placed in a site remote from the neck, permitting thyroidectomy without a scar in the anterior neck. The amount of surgical invasiveness is usually more in case of these approaches. Multiple approaches are described; can be robotic or endoscopic, transaxillary or retroauricular. Mainly done for cosmetic indications to avoid an anterior neck scar.

CHAPTER 5

Role of Nuclear Medicine in Adjuvant Therapy and Follow-up of Differentiated Thyroid Cancer

P Shanmuga Sundaram

● INTRODUCTION

Differentiated thyroid carcinoma (DTC), arising from thyroid follicular epithelial cells, accounts for the vast majority of thyroid cancers. Of the differentiated thyroid cancers, papillary thyroid cancer (PTC) comprises about 85% of cases compared to about 10% of follicular histology and 3% of Hürthle cell or oxyphil cell types.[1,2] The prognoses of PTC and follicular thyroid cancer (FTC) are almost similar while certain histologic subtypes of PTC (like tall cell, columnar cell, and diffuse sclerosing variants) have a worse prognosis.

Total thyroidectomy is the mainstay of management in thyroid malignancies. It is followed by radioiodine uptake scan and therapy in those patients with DTC. Postoperative ^{131}I ablation of functioning thyroid tissue has become established in the management of differentiated thyroid cancer as the long-term risk of recurrence and death is reduced post-^{131}I therapy. This beneficial effect results from the destruction of potentially malignant cells or occult multifocal disease that may occur in up to 30% of patients with papillary tumors. Furthermore, the specificity of thyroglobulin as a tumor marker is increased and the sensitivity of subsequent whole body ^{131}I scans is improved as normal residual thyroid tissue may compete with recurrent or metastatic thyroid cancer cells for radioiodine (^{131}I) uptake. Indeed, it has been

demonstrated by Verburg et al. that patients with successful ablation of remnant thyroid tissue have a better prognosis than those with unsuccessful ablation (disease-free survival of 87% versus 49% after 10 years, while thyroid cancer-related survival was 93% versus 78%).[3] This suggests that it is important to achieve complete ablation as soon as possible after diagnosis in order to ensure the best possible prognosis for a DTC patient.

High dose ^{131}I ablation: Why we need to ablate? Radioiodine ablation refers to the total destruction of residual macroscopically normal thyroid tissue after complete gross surgical resection of cancer. Although ablation of the remaining lobe with radioactive iodine has been used as an alternative to completion thyroidectomy, the American Thyroid Association (ATA) does not recommend routine radioactive ^{131}I ablation in lieu of completion thyroidectomy. Radioiodine ^{131}I ablation is a simple and easy therapeutic procedure. It is administered orally in the form of ^{131}I sodium iodide solution or capsule. This treatment is given 3–4 weeks postoperatively and is beneficial for three reasons. First, it destroys any remaining normal thyroid tissue, thereby increasing the sensitivity of subsequent ^{131}I whole body scanning and the specificity of serum thyroglobulin measurements for the detection of persistent or recurrent disease. Second, ^{131}I therapy can destroy occult microscopic carcinoma, subsequently decreasing the long-term risk of recurrent disease. Third, the use of a large amount of ^{131}I for therapy permits postablative ^{131}I whole body scanning, a sensitive test for detecting persistent carcinoma.

The algorithm commonly followed in the management of DTC involves thyroidectomy (total/near total) followed by low dose ^{131}I/^{123}I whole body imaging and high-dose ^{131}I ablation or metastasis therapy. Goals of postoperative staging of thyroid cancer as proposed in ATA guidelines 2009[4] are: to permit prognostication of DTC patients; to tailor decisions regarding postoperative adjunctive therapy, including ^{131}I therapy and TSH suppression, to assess the patient's risk for disease recurrence and mortality; to take decisions regarding the frequency and time interval of follow-up, follow-up of poorly differentiated thyroid cancers (PDTC) and Hürthle cell cancers; and prognostication and follow-up after external beam radiation, surgical resection, embolization or systemic therapy.

● SELECTION OF PATIENTS FOR RADIOIODINE ^{131}I ABLATION

- Patients with multifocal, multicentric, and microscopic differentiated thyroid malignancy
- All patients with papillary, follicular, mixed, insular carcinoma with tumors more than 1.5 cm in size with and without capsular invasion
- Patients with ^{131}I concentrating distant metastases (lymph node, pulmonary, skeletal)
- Patients with residual thyroid tissue for whom revision surgery is not possible or patient is not willing.

There is new evidence now to support that patients with only a lobectomy or lumpectomy, can also successfully undergo ^{131}I lobar

ablation.[5] Success of ^{131}I ablation depends on various factors like histology of tumor, age of patient, size of lesion, presence or absence of lymph nodal, distant metastases, and lastly the patient preparation prior to therapy. Point to be remembered is that aggressive and undifferentiated tumors show poor radioiodine uptake, hence this subset of patients need not undergo ^{131}I scan or therapy as it will remain unresponsive.

Based on guidelines set by the ATA, evidence for radioiodine effectiveness is only available for high-risk patients; i.e. patients with age >45 years old with tumor size >4 cm and patients of any age with gross extrathyroidal extension (T4 disease), or any patient with distant metastasis. On the other hand, current evidence indicates that ^{131}I ablation is not effective in T1a tumors (microcarcinomas, <1 cm). For all patients in between these extremes, evidence for ^{131}I high dose therapy effectiveness is largely inconclusive, conflicting, or lacking.[6]

Who Should Not be Ablated

Patients with low-risk factors need not be ablated with radioiodine. They include patients with papillary carcinoma of thyroid of tumor size less than 1–1.5 cm with no capsular invasion or distant metastasis. Patients with neither papillary nor follicular histology subtypes need no high dose ^{131}I therapy. Postoperative metastatic or recurrent medullary thyroid carcinomas also need not be treated with radioiodine based on the fact that these cancers arise from parafollicular c cells which cannot concentrate radioiodine. Hence they need to be treated with ^{131}I labeled metaiodobenzylguanidine (MIBG).

Controversies in Ablation

The recommendation to withhold ^{131}I ablation in adults with micropapillary cancer and low-risk DTC, however, has been challenged on the following grounds:[7]

- Small amounts of ^{131}I (30 mCi or 1.11 GBq) can be administered to ablate remnant tissue in 90% of the patients after thyroidectomy.
- It is possible to use recombinant human TSH (rhTSH) in preparation for therapy to reduce total-body irradiation.
- Patients can be more reliably assured to be disease free when there is no clinical or ultrasound evidence of tumor and serum thyroglobulin is undetectable during both TSH suppression and stimulation when thyroglobulin antibody are not present.
- TSH can be maintained in the non-suppressed ranges when the patient is disease free.

As such, remnant ablation is routinely performed by some groups in adults and not by others.

Properties of Radioiodine

Both ^{131}I and ^{123}I are radioisotopes of iodine which are routinely used in thyroid imaging. Radioiodine is the radioactive form of naturally occurring stable iodine ^{127}I.

^{123}I is preferred for imaging because of its better image quality and less radiation burden to patient due to its short half-life (13 hours). As it is produced in a cyclotron and has a short half-life, its availability is limited. ^{131}I is popularly termed as "magic bullet". It gets organified in thyroid cells like stable iodine thereby exerting its cytotoxic effect on thyroid cells. ^{131}I has a half-life of 8 days. It emits therapeutically useful beta particle (with a higher energy) and a gamma ray of 364 KeV which is used for imaging.

Patient Preparation

It is important that patients undergoing an ^{131}I diagnostic thyroid and whole body scan or therapeutic procedure like ^{131}I ablation/metastatic therapy is weaned off from iodine containing drugs (like cough expectorants), iodinated contrast-based imaging procedures, and food stuffs (like sea foods and iodized salt)

for 3–4 weeks. It is mandatory to stop tablet thyroxine prior to ^{131}I imaging or therapy so that serum thyroxine level is elevated to more than 30 micro IU/mL. By following these salient instructions, the uptake of ^{131}I by thyrocytes gets accentuated, thereby achieving a higher therapeutic benefit to the patient.

Pretherapy Imaging Procedure

Amount of residual thyroid calculation is ideally performed using a thyroid uptake probe at 4, 6, and 24 hours after 25–50 microcurie ^{131}I oral administration. In the event of nonavailability of a thyroid uptake probe, ^{131}I low-dose imaging is performed (prior to therapy) using a conventional gamma camera 24–48 hours after the oral administration of ^{131}I **(Figs. 1A and B)**. Anterior and posterior whole body images along with images of anterior neck are conventionally obtained. Region of interest are drawn over the residual thyroid tissue and amount of remnant thyroid tissue is calculated.

Algorithm of Management of Differentiated Thyroid Carcinoma Patient Post-thyroidectomy

Conventionally 3–4 weeks after a total thyroidectomy, a residual thyroid low dose ^{131}I scintigraphy is performed to assess the presence of residual thyroid tissue. In presence of residual thyroid tissue, patients undergo ^{131}I ablation therapy. Two important determinants of the success of thyroid ablation are the mass of remaining thyroid tissue in the neck, and the initial dose rate to this tissue. Normal dosage of ^{131}I used to ablate residual thyroid tissue is in the range of 30–70 mCi (between 30,000 and 100,000 Rads is needed to be delivered to the remaining thyroid tissue) **(Flowchart 1)**.

Following the ^{131}I ablation therapy **(Fig. 2)**, patient is put on suppressive doses of tablet thyroxine. After 6 months, an ^{131}I whole body and neck scintigraphy is performed to assess

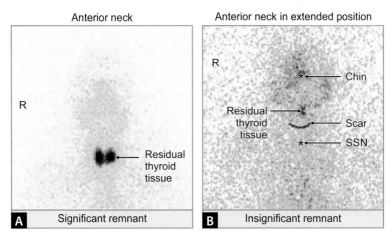

Anterior neck

Anterior neck in extended position

R

Residual thyroid tissue

R

Chin

Residual thyroid tissue

Scar

SSN

A   Significant remnant

B   Insignificant remnant

Figs. 1A and B: Diagnostic low-dose ^{131}I thyroid images in anterior projection: (A) Presence of significant residual thyroid tissue in both lobes; (B) Highlights a good surgery with negligible residual thyroid tissue.

Flowchart 1: Algorithm of management of differentiated thyroid carcinoma post-thyroidectomy.

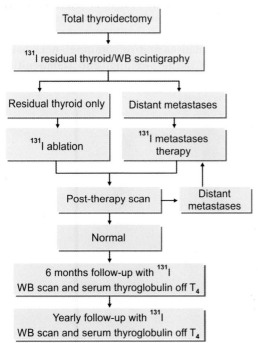

Total thyroidectomy

^{131}I residual thyroid/WB scintigraphy

Residual thyroid only

Distant metastases

^{131}I ablation

^{131}I metastases therapy

Post-therapy scan

Distant metastases

Normal

6 months follow-up with ^{131}I WB scan and serum thyroglobulin off T_4

Yearly follow-up with ^{131}I WB scan and serum thyroglobulin off T_4

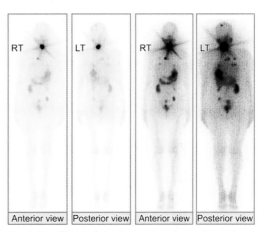

RT   LT   RT   LT

Anterior view | Posterior view | Anterior view | Posterior view

Fig. 2: Post ^{131}I whole body scintigraphy performed 5–8 days posttherapy—to look for successful ^{131}I uptake in residual thyroid tissue and also for any unsuspected metastases.

the success of ^{131}I ablation. A post-therapy ^{131}I whole body scintigraphy is routinely performed 5–7 days after ^{131}I thyroid residual ablation/ metastases therapy to identify unsuspected distant metastases.

Yearly follow-up of DTC is done with ^{131}I whole body scintigraphy, S. thyroglobulin and S. thyroglobulin antibody. It is mandatory that all these investigations be performed when the patient is off thyroxin at least for 3-4 weeks (Serum TSH should be over

30 micro-IU/mL). Nowadays, with the availability of recombinant human TSH injection (rhTSH marketed as Thyrogen), patients with extensive functioning metastases, poor compliance, psychiatric disorders can be treated with high dose ^{131}I therapy without thyroxine withdrawal. Patients treated with rhTSH typically receive 0.9 mg rhTSH intramuscular injections on 2 consecutive days, and after monitoring the rise of TSH above 30 micro-IU/mL, ^{131}I is given orally 24 hours later.

Patients presenting with distant metastases are recommended to undergo a high dose ^{131}I metastases therapy **(Fig. 3)**. Conventionally around 100–120 mCi of ^{131}I is administered orally in patients with lymph node metastases. Patients presenting with pulmonary metastases are treated in range of 150 mCi of ^{131}I and those with skeletal metastases are treated with 200 mCi. The limiting factor of ^{131}I dosage is that the radiation dose delivered to bone marrow and blood which should not be more than 2 Rads. Also the retained whole body activity of [131]I

should be no more than 120 mCi at 48 hours (or 80 mCi in patients with lung metastases to avoid potential complication of pulmonary fibrosis).

Patients undergoing a high-dose ^{131}I metastasis therapy or a residual thyroid ablation with a dosage of more than 30 mCi need isolation from general public to minimize the radiation exposure. Hence ^{131}I therapy isolation wards are mandatory for this type of specialized treatment. Once their exposure rate comes down to permissible levels, which is usually achieved within 2–3 days depending on the dose administered, they are allowed to move out of isolation.

● SIDE EFFECTS OF ^{131}I HIGH-DOSE THERAPY

Transient Side Effects

[131]I residual thyroid ablation or therapy can produce transient problems that include gastritis (nausea and/or vomiting), neck pain from soft tissue swelling, and sialadenitis.

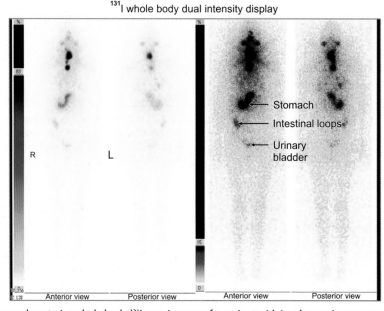

Fig. 3: Anterior and posterior whole body ^{131}I scan images of a patient with insular carcinoma presenting with ^{131}I concentrating residual thyroid tissue, lymph nodal and extensive skeletal metastases.

Sialadenitis is not uncommon in the first few days after therapy, with pain and enlargement of salivary glands but rarely progressing tochronic xerostomia. Prophylaxis usually takes the form of ingestion of large quantities of fluids and sialogogues, such as lemon juice or chewing gum. Some patients also complain of altered taste and discoloration of tongue due to destruction of tongue papillae. Temporary sterility in both sexes is also documented.

● LONG-TERM EFFECTS OF [131]I

Infertility, Gonadal Failure, and Genetic Effects

Administration of ^{131}I is strictly contraindicated in pregnant and lactating women.

Temporary sterility is noted in both sexes. In males, repeated radioiodine administration is associated with an impairment of spermatogenesis, increased levels of follicular-stimulating hormone, and decreased levels of inhibin B. In females, a transient ovarian failure, mainly in older premenopausal women has been reported. The notion that radiation is mutagenic and may affect germ cells (thereby resulting in genetic damage to offspring) has raised concern regarding the use of ^{131}I in the management of thyroid disorders in patients of childbearing ages.[8] Exposure to ^{131}I did not alter the likelihood of preterm birth, low birthweight, stillbirth, congenital malformations, death during the first year of life, thyroid disease, or nonthyroidal malignancies in offspring. On the basis of these data, there is no reason for patients exposed to radioiodine to avoid pregnancy.

Carcinogenic Effects

Incidence of leukemia and solid malignancies in post-^{131}I treated cases versus general public has been long debated. Follow-up studies of patients exposed to ^{131}I did not demonstrate any tumorigenic effect of ^{131}I on the thyroid gland in adults, but do exclude such an effect in children.

The dose delivered to other tissues is relatively low, and significant risk of cancer and leukemia has been found only in patients exposed to high cumulative activities of [131]I (>500–600 mCi). No genetic effect has been found in studies on the outcome of subsequent pregnancies in women treated with ^{131}I for thyroid carcinomas. When treated with ^{131}I, simple measures such as overall good hydration and use of laxatives help in reducing tissue radiation doses.

Absolute Contraindications to [131]I Therapy

- *Pregnancy:* It is recommended to delay conception for 1 year after high-dose ^{131}I therapy
- Lactating mother
- Patients with elevated urine iodine levels (over 200 µg/L) either from IV contrast or from dietary intake. Therapy should be postponed until levels return to normal.

● CONCLUSION

Postoperative DTC is followed up mainly with whole body ^{131}I scans and serum thyroglobulin. The use of radioactive ^{131}I ablation after thyroidectomy has shown reduced recurrence rates and prolonged survival in all patients with DTC who are high risk for recurrent disease and has been accepted as part of the standard of care for these patients. Radioiodine ^{131}I is the preferred modality of therapy for functioning thyroid metastases.

● REFERENCES

1. Koh KB, Chang KW. Carcinoma in multinodular goitre. Br J Surg. 1992;79(3):266-7.
2. Lam KY, Lo CY. Metastatic tumors of the thyroid gland: A study of 79 cases in Chinese patients. Arch Pathol Lab Med.1998;122(1):37-41.
3. Verburg FA, de Keizer B, Lips CJ, et al. Prognostic significance of successful ablation with radioiodine of differentiated thyroid cancer patients. Eur J Endocrinol. 2005;152(1):33-7.

4. Cooper DS, Doherty GM, Haugen BR, et al.; American Thyroid Association (ATA) Guidelines Taskforce on Thyroid Nodules and Differentiated Thyroid Cancer. Revised American Thyroid Association management guidelines for patients with thyroid nodules and differentiated thyroid cancer. Thyroid. 2009;19(11):1167-214.

5. Bal CS, Kumar A, Pant GS. Radioiodine lobar ablation as an alternative to completion thyroidectomy in patients with differentiated thyroid cancer. Nucl Med Commun. 2003;24(2):203-8.

6. Mäenpää HO, Heikkonen J, Vaalavirta L, et al. Low vs. high radioiodine activity to ablate the thyroid after thyroidectomy for cancer: A randomized study. PLoS One. 2008;3(4):e1885.

7. Mazzaferri EL. What is the optimal initial treatment of low-risk papillary thyroid cancer (and why is it controversial)? Oncology (Williston Park). 2009;23(7):579-88.

8. Robbins RJ, Schlumberger MJ. The evolving role of ^{131}I for the treatment of differentiated thyroid carcinoma. J Nucl Med. 2005;46(Suppl 1):28S-37S.

CHAPTER 6

Medical Management of Differentiated Thyroid Cancer

Vasantha Nair, Krishnakumar Thankappan

● INTRODUCTION

The role of a medical specialist or an endocrinologist is very important in the management of thyroid cancers. In the immediate postoperative state, medical expertise is essential for the management of hypocalcemia and thyroxine supplementation. Suppression of thyroid-stimulating hormone (TSH) as needed and periodic follow-up for evaluation of disease status are then needed and are the vital areas which need medical help. Initiation and management of patients on chemotherapeutic agents and the newer agents like tyrosine kinase inhibitors (TKIs) may also need a medical specialist involvement.

● GENERAL PRINCIPLES

Just as in the case of replacement therapy with T4 in hypothyroidism, certain general principles should be adhered to when prescribing the drug for differentiated thyroid cancer (DTC). T4 should be taken on an empty stomach. This is to aid absorption. If a patient just cannot tolerate it this way, adding a proton pump inhibitor before the evening meal may help. No medicine should be taken along with T4. Any food, be it coffee, tea or breakfast, should be taken after 1/2–1 hour only. T4 is prescribed as a single dose only, not in divided doses. Retesting to see the efficacy of the dose is done after 2 months only

as it takes that much time for the hypothalamic–pituitary–thyroid axis to come back to baseline. This applies to all situations whether drug is initiated after initial therapy or restarted after a nuclear scan. The dose is held on the day of testing and no fasting is needed.

● FOLLOW-UP AFTER INITIAL THERAPY

Once initial therapy is completed, the patients are started on thyroxine, at doses needed to maintain an appropriate level of TSH. These patients are staged using the American Joint Committee on Cancer (AJCC) System. Staging, however, predicts only death from the disease. In view of the need to judge risk for recurrence of disease, the American Thyroid Association (ATA) has introduced a risk categorization, which was updated in 2015. This helps to streamline patients better. First re-evaluation consists of a diagnostic whole-body iodine scan, a neck ultrasound scan, serum thyroglobulin, and thyroglobulin antibody under TSH stimulation. How often these tests are needed on follow-up is based on response to therapy as outlined in the ATA, 2015, guidelines. These can be used as early as 1–2 years after initial therapy and helps to avoid unnecessary, expensive tests in those where they are not required, at the same time, intensively following those who have a good chance for recurrence.

• T4 SUPPRESSION THERAPY

A clear-cut relationship exists between TSH levels and thyroid cancer. Moreover, considerable work in this field has shown survival benefit for patients on TSH suppression to less than 0.1 mIU/mL, when they fall in the high-risk category. Giving T4 to thyroid cancer patients is referred to as "suppression therapy" as against "replacement therapy" for hypothyroidism, as the aim here is to keep TSH below the normal range. T4 is begun after thyroidectomy, only after a radioiodine scan and ablation are completed. The starting dose is 2.5–3 g/kg body weight. Tailoring the initial dose to body weight avoids oversuppression. After a period of 2 months, TSH is checked to see if it has reached the goal. Further adjustments can be made at 2-month intervals, based on the TSH. Sensitivity to T4 varies considerably among patients and may be genetically determined. Therefore, one dose does not fit all.

Initial TSH Suppression

Initial T4 dose is based on the patient's risk for disease recurrence and death. Many guidelines exist, each differing from the other in a small way. After risk stratification of the patient into high, intermediate or low-risk as per an accepted guideline, the dose of T4 is adjusted with the TSH goal as in **Table 1**. In very low-risk patients (micropapillary thyroid carcinoma without high-risk features), TSH needs to be kept in the low normal range only as this entity is not, in the great majority of cases, associated with

Table 1: Risk levels and thyroid-stimulating hormone (TSH) goals.

Risk level	TSH goal
High risk	TSH <0.1 mIU/mL
Intermediate risk	0.1–0.5 mIU/mL
Low risk	Low normal
Very low-risk	Low normal

increase in recurrence or mortality. This degree of suppression is maintained till the patient is re-evaluated after 6 months with a nuclear scan, neck ultrasound, stimulated thyroglobulin, and antithyroglobulin antibody.

Ongoing TSH Suppression

As patients are followed up, the risk status may change. The disease may come under control and the patient may even become "disease-free" or it may progress locally or metastasize. These features of the disease would determine the degree of suppression needed for patients on follow-up. In patients who started out as high-risk, it is recommended that maintaining a TSH below 0.1 mIU/mL for 5–10 years is beneficial. As response to therapy is assessed, the T4 dose can be further adjusted in the low- and intermediate-risk groups, in patients with persistent or recurrent and progressive disease, TSH should be maintained at below 0.1 mIU/mL, if comorbidities exist, attempt should be made to optimally control them. Coronary artery disease, if present, should be addressed by a specialist and medications optimized. Elderly, postmenopausal women may be assessed for risk for fractures and given therapy for same in addition to supplementation with calcium and vitamin D. Thyrotoxic symptoms may be controlled with beta blockers. Tolerable dose of T4 should then be continued. Always, the risks should be balanced against the benefits.

Stopping T4

Thyroid carcinoma patients should be fully made aware of the fact that they need to continue on T4 for the rest of their lives. They should be conveyed that they would be instructed to stop the drug for 3–4 weeks in preparation for a nuclear scan and for radioactive iodine (RAI) therapy. They should be advised clearly as to when to restart T4. After a scan, T4 can be reinstated the next day, however; after the therapy, a few days interval is given as this would help for a full effect of the RAI given. This practice may vary from center to center. If serious side effects are experienced while on a dose, the concerned specialist should be contacted for advice.

● ROLE OF T3

This is another product of the thyroid gland and is the physiologically active hormone, formed by secretion from the gland and from deiodination of T4 at target tissues. Although not recommended for replacement therapy, T3 can be useful in preparing a thyroid cancer patient for scanning or RAI therapy. Withdrawal of T4 is needed for 3–4 weeks before performing a radioiodine scan or before RAI therapy during follow-up. Although most patients tolerate this iatrogenic hypothyroidism, some do not. The only alternative to stopping T4 is to use recombinant thyroid-stimulating hormone (rhTSH) for stimulation. rhTSH is prohibitively expensive and beyond the reach of many patients. To avoid the discomfort on withdrawing T4, T3 is an option. After stopping T4, T3 is given for 2 weeks and stopped. This reduces the period of hypothyroidism and its attendant symptoms to a shorter period of 2 weeks. Unfortunately, T3 is not freely available.

● POSTOPERATIVE HYPOCALCEMIA OR HYPOPARATHYROIDISM

It is the most common and often the most troubling consequence of thyroidectomy. It may be due to injury to the parathyroid glands or its blood supply, or an inadvertent removal of the parathyroid. Hypoparathyroidism following surgery can be temporary or permanent. The time cut-off to differentiate between the two is often taken as 12 months.

The clinical symptoms of hypoparathyroidism are:
- Subjective hyperesthesia of the distal extremities

- Peroral numbness or tingling
- Nocturnal leg cramps
- Chvostek or Trousseau signs.

The biochemical definitions are as below:
- Hypocalcemia is total calcium corrected to a serum albumin of 4.0 mg/mL, less than 8.5 mg/dL
- Ionized calcium, less than 1.15 mmol/L
- Hypoparathormonemia: Serum PTH (parathyroid hormone) values can vary from laboratory to laboratory. Usually, it is taken as hypoparathormonemia when less than 13 pg/mL.

The protocol followed in authors' department is given in **Flowcharts 1 to 3**.

● CHEMOTHERAPY

Cytotoxic chemotherapy has very little role in the management of DTC. New modalities of chemotherapeutic agents, however, are coming to the forefront. These drugs are known as TKIs. They target the molecular pathways in the thyroid follicular cell that propagates continued growth of the tumor. These are becoming available in India, are very expensive and not devoid of side effects. They may be tried for patient's refractory to RAI and having progressive and metastatic disease. TKI should only be prescribed under the close supervision of a medical oncologist. Even with these drugs, no dramatic effects are usually seen. TKIs available for the treatment of thyroid cancers are sorafenib, lenvatinib, vandetanib, and cabozantinib. Selumetinib is a redifferentiating agent used in radioiodine refractory patients.

● ADDRESSING COMORBIDITIES

Association with diabetes mellitus, hypertension, and dyslipidemia is fairly common, especially in the older patients. Along with thyroid cancer therapy, these issues should also be managed effectively. There is recent evidence for an increase in cardiovascular

Flowchart 1: Preoperative prophylaxis and postoperative hypocalcemia management based on serum calcium levels.

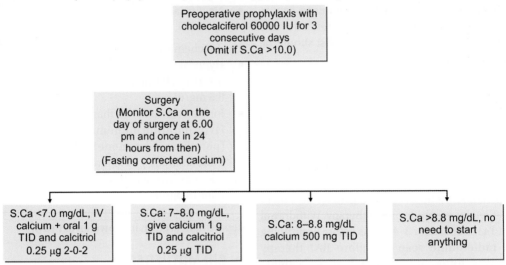

Preoperative prophylaxis with cholecalciferol 60000 IU for 3 consecutive days (Omit if S.Ca >10.0)

Surgery
(Monitor S.Ca on the day of surgery at 6.00 pm and once in 24 hours from then)
(Fasting corrected calcium)

| S.Ca <7.0 mg/dL, IV calcium + oral 1 g TID and calcitriol 0.25 µg 2-0-2 | S.Ca: 7–8.0 mg/dL, give calcium 1 g TID and calcitriol 0.25 µg TID | S.Ca: 8–8.8 mg/dL calcium 500 mg TID | S.Ca >8.8 mg/dL, no need to start anything |

Flowchart 2: Postoperative hypocalcemia management based on serum parathyroid hormone (PTH) levels.

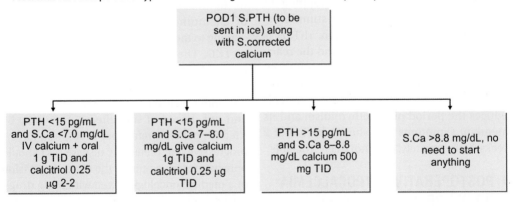

POD1 S.PTH (to be sent in ice) along with S.corrected calcium

| PTH <15 pg/mL and S.Ca <7.0 mg/dL IV calcium + oral 1 g TID and calcitriol 0.25 µg 2-2 | PTH <15 pg/mL and S.Ca 7–8.0 mg/dL give calcium 1g TID and calcitriol 0.25 µg TID | PTH >15 pg/mL and S.Ca 8–8.8 mg/dL calcium 500 mg TID | S.Ca >8.8 mg/dL, no need to start anything |

Flowchart 3: Postoperative hypocalcemia (persisting beyond 3 days and not responding to calcium and calcitriol) management based on serum magnesium levels.

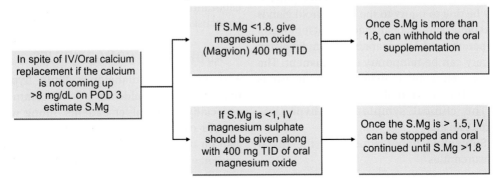

In spite of IV/Oral calcium replacement if the calcium is not coming up >8 mg/dL on POD 3 estimate S.Mg

If S.Mg <1.8, give magnesium oxide (Magvion) 400 mg TID

Once S.Mg is more than 1.8, can withhold the oral supplementation

If S.Mg is <1, IV magnesium sulphate should be given along with 400 mg TID of oral magnesium oxide

Once the S.Mg is > 1.5, IV can be stopped and oral continued until S.Mg >1.8

mortality in patients treated for DTC. This appears to be not related to the conventional cardiovascular risk factors but relates inversely with TSH. This makes it all the more important that unnecessary TSH suppression be avoided and an ongoing assessment of the T4 dose be made. Yearly evaluation for cardiovascular disease would help.

● FURTHER READING

1. Biondi B, Cooper DS. Benefits of thyrotropin suppression versus the risks of adverse effects in differentiated thyroid cancer. Thyroid. 2010;20(2).

2. Haugen BR, Alexander EK, Bible KC, et al. 2015 American Thyroid Association Management guidelines for Adult Patients with Thyroid Nodules and Differentiated Thyroid Cancer: The American Thyroid Association Guidelines Task Force on Thyroid Nodules and Differentiated Thyroid Cancer. Thyroid. 2016;26(1):1-133.

3. Klein Hesselink EN, Klein Hesselink MS, de Bock GH, et al. Long-term cardiovascular mortality in patients with differentiated thyroid carcinoma: An observational study. J Clin Oncol. 2013; 31(32):4046-53.

4. Stack BC Jr, Bimston DN, Bodenner DL, et al. American Association of Clinical Endocrinologists and American College of Endocrinology Disease State Clinical Review: Postoperative Hypoparathyroidism: Definitions and Management. Endocr Pract. 2015;21(6):674-85.

CHAPTER 7

Parathyroid Tumors: Evaluation and Management

Shibu George

• ANATOMY

Parathyroid glands are four small (20–40 mg) bean-shaped structures found near the posterior aspect of the thyroid gland; the number may vary with some patients having three, five, or more glands. They are smooth surfaced, encapsulated and light brown to tan in color. The glands are identified based on their location (superior or inferior) on either side.

The inferior glands are derived from the third pharyngeal pouch. They are usually located near the inferior pole of the thyroid on the posterior surface. The location of the inferior parathyroid glands exhibits more variability due to their migration with the thymus gland. They can lie anywhere along this path of descent like adjacent to or within the thymus in the mediastinum, within the carotid sheath or thyroid gland.

The superior glands derive their embryonal origin from the fourth pharyngeal pouch which also gives rise to the parafollicular, C cells of the thyroid gland. They are more consistent in location in contact with the posterior part of the middle third of the thyroid lobes; usually found 1 cm superior to the intersection of the inferior thyroid artery and the recurrent laryngeal nerve towards the cricothyroid joint. Because of their embryologic origin, the superior glands can be occasionally found within the substance of the thyroid gland or rarely in the retropharyngeal and retroesophageal space.

The inferior parathyroid gland is supplied by the inferior thyroid artery; if positioned low in the mediastinum, it may be supplied by a thymic branch of the internal thoracic artery or even a direct branch of the aortic arch. The superior parathyroid gland is also usually supplied by the inferior thyroid artery or by an anastomotic branch between the inferior thyroid and the superior thyroid artery.

The parathyroid glands are primarily responsible for maintaining extracellular calcium concentrations through their secretion of parathyroid hormone (PTH). The main effects of PTH are to increase the concentration of plasma calcium by increasing the release of calcium and phosphate from bone matrix, increasing calcium reabsorption by the kidney, and increasing renal production of vitamin D-3 (calcitriol), which increases intestinal absorption of calcium. The secretion of PTH is regulated directly by the plasma concentration of ionized calcium. Parathyroid hormone also causes phosphaturia, thereby decreasing serum phosphate levels.

• PRIMARY HYPERPARATHYROIDISM AND PARATHYROID ADENOMA

Primary hyperparathyroidism is a disease characterized by unregulated overproduction of PTH resulting in abnormal calcium homeostasis.

Epidemiology

The prevalence of the disease is low and annual incidence has been reported to be approximately 20 cases per 100,000. The mean age presentation and diagnosis is between 52 and 56 years with a female-to-male ratio of 3:1.

Etiology

In >85% cases, primary hyperparathyroidism is caused by a single parathyroid adenoma; multiple adenomas or hyperplasia with multiglandular involvement is seen in 10–15%. Rarely, primary hyperparathyroidism is caused by parathyroid carcinoma (<1%).

In most cases the etiology of adenomas or hyperplasia remains unknown. Familial cases can occur as either part of the multiple endocrine neoplasia syndromes (MEN 1 or MEN 2A), hyperparathyroid–jaw tumor (HPT-JT) syndrome, or familial isolated hyperparathyroidism (FIHPT).

Genetics

The molecular genetic basis of MEN 1 is an inactivating mutation of the *MEN1* gene, located on chromosome band *11q13*. MEN 2A is caused by a germline mutation of the *Ret* proto-oncogene on chromosome 10. Germline mutation of *HRPT2* gene localized on chromosome arm 1q is responsible for HPT-JT syndrome; FIHPT is genetically heterogeneous.

Pathophysiology and Clinical Manifestations

In parathyroid adenoma excess hormone production is due to the loss of feedback on PTH production by extracellular calcium; in parathyroid hyperplasia, increase in number of cells is the probable cause.

Parathyroid hormone excess causes symptoms due to osteopenia following excessive resorption of calcium from bone. This may result in osteitis fibrosa cystica, characterized by subperiosteal resorption of the distal phalanges, tapering of the distal clavicles, salt-and-pepper appearance of the skull, and brown tumors of the long bones. In addition, the chronically increased excretion of calcium in the urine can predispose to the formation of renal stones.

The other symptoms are nonspecific and due to the hypercalcemia; these include muscle weakness, fatigue, volume depletion, nausea and vomiting, coma, and even death in severe cases. Subtle neuropsychiatric manifestations like depression and confusion are common. Increased gastric acid secretion following hypercalcemia leads to peptic ulcer and pancreatitis. Cardiovascular manifestations like hypertension, bradycardia, and arrhythmias may also occur. (The clinical spectrum can hence be summarized by the age-old dictum "bones, stones, abdominal groans, and psychic moans.")

Local cervical examination is usually noncontributory. A palpable neck mass is not a feature of benign lesions; if present, it may indicate parathyroid cancer.

● ASYMPTOMATIC PRIMARY HYPERPARATHYROIDISM

A paradigm shift in the symptom profile of patients with hyperparathyroidism has been reported in literature. The introduction of calcium auto-analyzers deeply modified the clinical spectrum of the disease at diagnosis. Most new cases now present with biologically milder form of disease without overt hypercalcemia-related clinical features; but still significant risks of cardiovascular complications and increased risk of malignancy has been observed on long-term follow-up of these patients.

Investigations

Laboratory Evaluation

An elevated intact PTH level with an elevated ionized serum calcium level is diagnostic of primary hyperparathyroidism. Other laboratory findings in primary hyperparathyroidism include hypophosphatemia and mild to moderate increase in urinary calcium excretion rate.

Indications for Imaging

Imaging studies are unnecessary to make the diagnosis of primary hyperparathyroidism (usually based on laboratory evidence) or to decide on surgical therapy (usually based on clinical criteria). They are used to guide the surgeon after decision on surgery has been made. Imaging is not mandatory when complete parathyroid exploration with resection of all involved glands is done. But, if a limited parathyroid exploration is to be attempted, a localizing study is necessary. Imaging is also indicated in recurrent or persistent hyperparathyroidism after a previous surgical exploration, when planning for revision.

Ultrasonography of the Neck: It is widely used for rapid localization of abnormal parathyroid glands with accuracy rates of 75–80%.

Scintigraphy: Technetium-99m (99mTc) sestamibi scan is also another common technique. The radionuclide gets concentrated in thyroid and parathyroid tissue but quickly gets washed out of normal thyroid tissue; it persists in abnormal parathyroid tissue on delayed images as a persistent focus of activity. It has 60–90% sensitivity for detecting solitary adenomas with ability to detect ectopic parathyroid glands, particularly in the mediastinum; however, it is less sensitive in detecting multiglandular disease. Combination of sestamibi with SPECT allows better sensitivity and more precise anatomic localization than standard planar imaging.

CT Scan: Standard CT scans have inadequate sensitivity in detection of abnormal parathyroids; newer techniques with dynamic contrast images (4D-CT) have shown promise, with accuracy rates as high as 88%.

MRI Scan: MRI is useful in cases of recurrent or persistent disease and detection of ectopic locations such as the mediastinum.

Treatment

Medical

This is aimed at management of severe hypercalcemia prior to surgery; reduction of elevated serum calcium can be accomplished by intravascular volume expansion with sodium chloride and loop diuretics such as furosemide once the intravascular volume is restored.

Medical treatment may be considered for patients who do not fulfill criteria for surgery or those who are unsuitable for or decline surgery; but is not an alternative to parathyroidectomy. Medical treatment may improve bone mineral density and normalize serum calcium but does not improve long-term outcomes. Bisphosphonates (in particular alendronate) has been shown to improve the bone mineral density in patients with hyperparathyroidism; but it does not significantly lower serum calcium levels. Calcimimetic drug, Cinacalcet, effectively lowers and even normalizes serum calcium levels with substantial lowering of PTH levels; but no improvement in bone mineral density has been observed.

Surgery

The only permanent and curative treatment for primary hyperparathyroidism is surgical excision of the abnormal parathyroid glands. Indications for surgery are given in **Table 1**.

The standard operative approach is complete neck exploration with identification and removal of all abnormal parathyroid glands. However, this approach may result in unnecessary neck dissection since primary hyperparathyroidism is caused by a single adenoma in 85% cases. Therefore, directed parathyroidectomy has evolved which relies on preoperative imaging with either sestamibi scans or ultrasonography to localize the abnormal gland. However, since

Table 1: Indications for surgery in primary hyperparathyroidism.

A	**Symptomatic disease**	• All patients with symptoms
B	**Asymptomatic primary hyperparathyroidism** *(4th International Workshop on Asymptomatic Primary Hyperparathyroidism–2013).*	• Age younger than 50 years • Serum calcium >1 mg/dL above reference range • Creatinine clearance < 60 cc/min • 24 hrs urinary calcium excretion >400 mg/day and increased risk of calculus • Presence of nephrolithiasis or nephrocalcinosis on radiography, USG, or CT scan • Bone mineral density T-score at or below -2.5 (in peri/postmenopausal women and men 50 years or older) at lumbar spine, hip, femoral neck, or distal 1/3 radius • Vertebral fracture on radiography

(USG: Ultrasonography; CT: Computed tomography)

neither technique is reliable for detecting multiple abnormal glands intraoperative PTH assay also has been advocated to ensure that no other abnormal glands are present.

Follow-up

Structured follow up and monitoring is needed in asymptomatic patients who do not undergo surgery; this includes clinical assessment, annual serum calcium and creatinine testing, and bone mineral density evaluation every 1–2 years.

● PARATHYROID CARCINOMA

Parathyroid carcinoma is an extremely rare but aggressive neoplasm which can result in life-threatening form of primary hyperparathyroidism; however, it accounts for only less than 1% of cases of hyperparathyroidism, majority (>85%) of which is caused by parathyroid adenoma and hyperplasia.

Epidemiology

It is a rare disease; reported annual incidence according to the "Surveillance, Epidemiology and End Results" (SEER) cancer registry data is 5.73 per 10,000 million. This represents a prevalence of 0.005% of all cancers. There is no known racial predilection; it is seen equally in males and females, and present mostly in the 4th–5th decades of life.

Etiology

Exact etiology is unknown in majority of cases.

Head and neck irradiation has been associated with the development of parathyroid carcinoma.

Parathyroid cancer has also been reported in patients with hyperparathyroidism. An increased risk has also been reported in multiple endocrine neoplasia type 1 (MEN 1).

End-stage renal failure can promote clonal expansion of cells within the parathyroid glands that can progress to carcinoma.

Associations

Parathyroid cancer has reported associations with HPT–JT syndrome and FIHPT. HPT–JT is an autosomal dominant disease characterized by fibromas of the maxilla and mandible and tumors of the parathyroid. In this condition, 30% of the parathyroid tumors are parathyroid cancers.

Genetics

Several oncogenes and tumor suppressor genes have been linked to parathyroid carcinoma.
- *Cyclin D1* is an oncogene involved in cell cycle regulation and is located on

chromosome 11q13.10. It is overexpressed in 91% of parathyroid carcinoma and up to 61% of benign parathyroid tumors.

- *HRPT2* is a tumor suppressor gene on chromosome 1q25-q32, encoding the protein parafibromin which has anti-proliferative properties; parafibromin expression is decreased or absent in parathyroid cancers.

  Inactivating germline CDC73 mutation of the *HRPT2* gene is seen HPT–JT syndrome; the gene is defective in other sporadic parathyroid cancers as well.

  HRPT2 gene mutation also results in the upregulation of 4 proteins. These are histone H1 & H2, E-cadherin, and amyloid BA4 precursor protein; used as diagnostic markers for parathyroid carcinoma.

- These tumors are also associated allelic loss of the *Retinoblastoma protein* (on chromosome 13) and mutations of the *MEN1* gene.

● SECONDARY PARATHYROID MALIGNANCY

Two types are reported in literature: (1) contiguous extension from thyroid cancer/adjoining head and neck sites, and (2) metastatic disease from distant primaries like renal, breast, liver or lung. However, there are only limited data available; this is because search for parathyroid spread is often overlooked during thyroid surgery due to the desire to preserve parathyroid function. On the other hand, metastasis from distant sites likely indicates widespread metastatic disease.

Clinical Features

History

The history should focus on symptoms of hypercalcemia plus the other symptoms of hyperparathyroidism. The clinician should be aware of the differences in presentation between primary hyperparathyroidism due to

benign adenoma and parathyroid cancer to suit the management approaches.

- Patients with parathyroid cancer are typically younger than those with benign causes with equal sex incidence.
- The onset is usually more abrupt, and the symptoms more severe, in parathyroid cancer.
- Since majority (>90%) of parathyroid cancers are functioning tumors, symptoms are apparently similar to benign hyperparathyroidism. However, bone disease and renal involvement are much more common in parathyroid cancers (seen in 80–90%) and the presence of both has a strong positive predictive value for malignancy.
- Unusually severe hyperparathyroidism or a palpable neck mass should trigger suspicion for parathyroid carcinoma. Palpable neck mass is virtually never a presentation of benign adenomas or hyperplasia.

Clinical Evaluation

Majority of patients (>90%) show evidence of bone disease like bone pain, osteopenia, osteoporosis and pathologic fractures.

Symptoms of hypercalcemia include fatigue, weakness, confusion, depression constipation; less commonly patients may present with acute pancreatitis, peptic ulceration, and hypercalcemic crisis. Renal involvement (50–80% of patients) is characterized by ureteric calculi, nephrocalcinosis, or renal impairment.

Palpable neck mass may be the presentation in around 50–70% of patients; this may be the presentation of nonfunctioning tumors where symptoms of hypercalcemia are not that evident. Lymph node spread is uncommon and, when present, are localized in the central compartment.

Distant metastasis has been reported; up to 30% of patients already have metastases at initial presentation. The most common sites of metastatic spread are lungs, liver, and bone.

Laboratory Studies

Serum calcium and PTH are elevated in parathyroid carcinoma; calcium is much higher than in benign causes of hyperparathyroidism (>14 mg/dL). A PTH level 10 times the upper limit of normal carries a positive predictive value of 81% for parathyroid cancer.

Imaging

Neck Ultrasound: Highly sensitive, in comparison with benign disease, parathyroid carcinoma appears as larger (>15 mm), hypoechoic, hypervascular, heterogeneous, lobulated, and irregular lesions on USG. Associated local infiltration and calcification have added predictive value for identifying parathyroid malignancy. Tumor size, however, has no role in prognosis of the tumor.

Scintigraphy: 99mTC sestamibi scintigraphy is useful for localizing primary, recurrent, and metastatic parathyroid disease because of its affinity for parathyroid mitochondria; but, discrimination between benign and malignant disease is not possible.

CT Scan and MRI: Useful in determining extent of local infiltration of parathyroid cancer to plan surgery; PET-CT has been used in recurrent disease to know extent of locoregional spread or distant metastasis; MRI is useful for evaluation of mediastinal recurrence.

Plain Radiographs: Changes of hyperparathyroidism can be demonstrated; hand x-rays may show subperiosteal bone resorption of the distal phalanges. Skull radiographs demonstrate a characteristic "ground glass" or "salt and pepper" appearance. In severe cases bone cysts (brown tumors) may be demonstrable.

Genetic Testing

Genetic testing for germline *CDC73* mutation should be considered in patients with parathyroid carcinoma, to rule out HPT-JT syndrome.

Cytology

FNAC is not helpful in establishing a diagnosis of parathyroid cancer or differentiating from benign disease; on the contrary, it carries the risk of tumor dissemination. Ultrasound-guided FNAC may be useful in the evaluation of associated cervical lymphadenopathy, if present.

Histopathology

The tumor is usually encapsulated and often has fibrous septa extending into the gland. The parenchyma may show rosette-like cellular architecture with predominance of chief cells (which are larger than those seen in a benign adenoma). Vascular and extracapsular invasion with nuclear atypia and mitotic figures are usually evident. Proven lymphatic metastases, though uncommon, are a clear indication of malignancy.

Markers

Immunohistochemistry for molecular or genetic markers may prove useful in distinguishing parathyroid cancer from other lesions.

- Demonstration of the *HRPT2* mutation is relatively specific; *HRPT2* gene product, parafibromin, is often absent in parathyroid carcinoma and has >90% specificity in diagnosis. Loss of parafibromin expression is also associated with increased incidence of recurrence or metastasis.

- Increased expression *PGP9.5*, has also been shown to be highly specific for parathyroid carcinoma and complement parafibromin in the immunohistochemistry process.

Staging

Two staging systems have been developed for risk stratification in parathyroid carcinoma: Differentiated system **(Table 2)** and high/low risk system **(Table 3)**.

Table 2: The differentiated system: Divides patients into 4 "classes" of risk, based on typical TNM staging system.

T (Tumor)	N (Node)	M (Metastasis)
(Tx)—No information available	(Nx)—Lymph node not assessed	(Mx)—Distant metastases not
T1—Evidence of capsular invasion	N0—No regional lymph node	assessed
T2—Invasion of surrounding soft tissues	metastases	M0—No evidence of distant
(excluding the trachea, larynx, and esophagus)	N1—Regional lymph node	metastases
T3—Evidence of vascular invasion	metastases	M1—Evidence of distant
T4—Invasion of vital organs, such as the		metastases
hypopharynx, esophagus, larynx, trachea,		
recurrent laryngeal nerve, carotid artery		

Classes:
Class I—T1 or T2 N0 M0
Class II—T3 N0 M0
Class III—Any T, N1 M0
Class IV—Any T, Any N, M1

(TNM: Tumor node metastasis)

Table 3: High-/low-risk system.

Low risk	Capsular invasion combined with invasion of surrounding soft tissue
High risk	Vascular invasion and/or lymph node metastases and/or invasion of vital organs and/or distant metastases

Treatment

Medical Therapy

There is no effective medical therapy for parathyroid carcinoma; trials of chemotherapeutic agents have been generally disappointing and rarity of this tumor renders controlled trials impossible. Though several reports on use of dacarbazine, fluorouracil, cyclophosphamide, methotrexate, and doxorubicin have shown some success, there is no standard chemotherapy regime due to lack of adequate RCTs.

Medical care hence is limited to the control of hypercalcemia and renal dysfunction with correction of electrolyte imbalance (if needed); this is also useful to optimize the patient's condition prior to surgery. Treatment of hypercalcemia due to parathyroid cancer is similar to that due to other causes. For rapid treatment of severe hypercalcemia, volume expansion with normal saline and diuresis with a calcium-wasting loop diuretic like furosemide

is adequate. Bisphosphonates and calcitonin may also be used for short-term control of the hypercalcemia. However, hypercalcemia associated with parathyroid carcinoma may be often severe and refractory to medical treatment. Treatment with denosumab (120 mg/month) has been effective in controlling such resistant hypercalcemia. Severe hypercalcemia resistant to long-term medical management is usually the cause of death in patients with metastatic disease.

Surgery

Even in the presence of metastasis, mainstay of treatment in parathyroid carcinoma is surgical resection. However, the diagnosis of parathyroid carcinoma may not be known prior to surgery. Often, the first indication of parathyroid carcinoma is the discovery of suspicious mass during surgical exploration; usually appears as a large (often greater than 3 cm in maximal diameter) firm, gray-white mass adherent to adjacent tissue. Benign adenomas, in contrast, are smaller, softer and are reddish-brown in color.

The goal of the initial surgery is to remove the tumor en bloc with clear margins with any adherent tissue and ipsilateral thyroid lobectomy; care should be taken not to rupture the tumor capsule, as this increases the risk of seeding and recurrence. Management of enlarged lymph nodes should involve selective central compartment dissection; prophylactic lateral neck dissection is not indicated. Involvement of the overlying strap muscles, trachea, esophagus, or recurrent laryngeal nerve warrants their en bloc resection to provide the best chance of cure. Resection of recurrent laryngeal nerve is indicated only in cases where there is complete loss of function due to tumor infiltration or where it is involved circumferentially by malignancy; normally functioning nerve need not be sacrificed unless its preservation results in gross residual disease.

Postoperative Follow-up: All patients require both immediate monitoring and lifelong surveillance. Temporary hypocalcemia may occur in the early postoperative period due to secondary uptake of calcium into bones (hungry bone syndrome); this requires treatment with supplemental calcium and vitamin D. Estimation of serum PTH levels should also be done to ensure curative resection. Parathyroid hormone and serum calcium are monitored every 3 months. If these exhibit an increase in value, sites of recurrence should be evaluated with scintigraphy and anatomical imaging.

Management of patients with parathyroid carcinoma diagnosed only after initial surgery (by histology) is controversial; tumors showing minimal invasion and low malignant potential may be followed up at 3 monthly intervals while aggressive histopathological features like extensive capsular and vascular spread may require revision surgery for completion of resection.

Recurrence: Surgery is advisable for local and regional recurrence to provide palliation from hypercalcemia; this is true for even pulmonary or hepatic metastases. Locoregional recurrence most often occurs within 2–3 years of the initial surgery. Revision surgery in the neck is challenging due to scar tissue and distorted anatomical planes. Localization may be aided by injection of methylene blue (selectively taken up by parathyroid tissue) or technetium-99m injection with use of the gamma probe. Mediastinal exploration including thymectomy may also be indicated. Long-term cure after a recurrence is virtually unknown.

Radiotherapy

Parathyroid carcinoma has been considered radioresistant and there is lack of strong evidence for its routine use. But, sporadic reports do exist on the successful use of postoperative external beam radiation. Hence, it may be considered when surgical options have been exhausted especially in metastatic disease.

Prognosis and Survival

Parathyroid cancers are slow-growing tumors with overall survival rates of 85% at 5 years and 35–79% at 10 years. Most important factor affecting prognosis is adequacy of surgical resection. En bloc resection results in 90% long-term survival and 10–30% local recurrence rates; incomplete resection on the other hand results in a 50% recurrence rate and a mortality rate as high as 46%. Other adverse factors affecting prognosis include lymph node or distant metastases and nonfunctioning tumors.

Guidelines

The following are the recommendations for diagnosis and treatment of parathyroid carcinoma proposed by the American Association of Endocrine Surgeons (AAES) (proposed in guidelines for definitive management of primary hyperparathyroidism–2016).

- The diagnosis of parathyroid carcinoma to be considered in primary hyperparathyroidism with markedly elevated PTH levels and severe hypercalcemia.
- Primary hyperparathyroidism presenting with hypercalcemic crisis should be medically managed, followed by parathyroidectomy for suspected parathyroid carcinoma.
- Parathyroidectomy is indicated when clinical or biochemical evidence is consistent with parathyroid carcinoma because this is the only potentially curative treatment.
- Preoperative FNAC is not recommended for diagnosis of parathyroid carcinoma.
- Histologic diagnosis of parathyroid carcinoma relies on identification of unequivocal angioinvasion and can be assisted by biomarkers.
- Intraoperative suspicion of parathyroid carcinoma should be managed by complete resection avoiding capsular disruption; en bloc removal with resection of adherent tissues offers potential cure.
- There is insufficient evidence to recommend prophylactic central or lateral neck dissection.
- Adjuvant external beam radiotherapy after surgical resection is reserved for palliative care and is not indicated routinely.

● FURTHER READING

1. Asare EA, Sturgeon C, Winchester DJ, et al. Parathyroid carcinoma: An update on treatment outcomes and prognostic factors from the National Cancer Database (NCDB). Ann Surg Oncol. 2015;22(12):3990-5.
2. Bilezikian JP, Brandi ML, Eastell R, et al. Guidelines for the management of asymptomatic primary hyperparathyroidism: Summary statement from the Fourth International Workshop. J Clin Endocrinol Metab. 2014;99(10):3561-9.
3. Fang SH, Lal G. Parathyroid cancer. Endocr Pract. 2011;17(Suppl 1):36-43.
4. Siperstein A, Berber E, Barbosa GF, et al. Predicting the success of limited exploration for primary hyperparathyroidism using ultrasound, sestamibi, and intraoperative parathyroid hormone: Analysis of 1,158 cases. Ann Surg. 2008;248(3):420-8.
5. Talat N, Schulte KM. Clinical presentation, staging and long-term evolution of parathyroid cancer. Ann Surg Oncol. 2010;17(8):2156-74.
6. Wilhelm SM, Wang TS, Ruan DT, et al. The American Association of Endocrine Surgeons Guidelines for Definitive Management of Primary Hyperparathyroidism. JAMA Surg. 2016;151(10): 959-68.

Section 2

Salivary Glands and Parapharyngeal Tumors

Chapters

Salivary Glands and Parapharyngeal Tumors

Chapter

CHAPTER 8

Pathology of Salivary Gland Tumors

Chaya Prasad, Smitha NV

• INTRODUCTION

Salivary gland neoplasms occur frequently enough that even pathologists in small practices can expect to encounter them from time to time. A broad spectrum of tumors arises in this location; there is considerable morphologic overlap between some subtypes, and a substantial minority of tumors do not fit easily into existing diagnostic categories. The World Health Organization (WHO) classification stresses the distinction between benign and malignant tumors.

• WHO CLASSIFICATION

See **Table 1**.

• MALIGNANT TUMORS

Acinic Cell Carcinoma (ACC)

It is a malignant epithelial neoplasm of salivary glands in which at least some of the neoplastic cells demonstrate serous acinar cell differentiation, which is characterized by cytoplasmic zymogen secretory granules.

Epidemiology

This tumor is more common in women, and the peak incidence is in the fifth and sixth decades of life. Four percent of the patients are under 20 years of age.

Localization

ACC represents ~2% of salivary gland tumors, with approximately 90% arising in the parotid gland. The rest involve the submandibular, minor salivary glands, and rarely in ectopic salivary gland tissue involving periparotid lymph nodes.

Tumor Spread

ACC initially metastasizes to cervical lymph nodes and then to more distant sites, most commonly the lungs.

Macroscopy

Most tumors are 1–3 cm, usually circumscribed, solitary or multinodular in nature. The cut surface appears lobular and tan to red.

Microscopy

The pattern of growth may be predominantly solid, microcystic, papillary-cystic, or follicular. The most characteristic cell, known as acinic, has a cytoplasmic appearance (granular and basophilic) **(Fig. 1)**. Other cell types are intercalated duct, clear, vacuolated, and nonspecific glandular. When the clear cell component predominates, the tumor acquires a "hypernephroid" appearance reminiscent of renal cell carcinoma. Lymphoid follicles with germinal centers may be prominent at the periphery of the tumor which may be confused

Table 1: WHO classification of Salivary tumors

Malignant
- Acinic cell carcinoma
- Secretory carcinoma
- Mucoepidermoid carcinoma
- Adenoid cystic carcinoma
- Polymorphous adenocarcinoma
- Epithelial -myoepithelial carcinoma
- Clear cell carcinoma
- Basal cell adenocarcinoma
- Sebaceous adenocarcinoma
- Intraductal carcinoma
- Cystadenocarcinoma
- Adenocarcinoma NOS
- Salivary duct carcinoma
- Myoepithelial carcinoma
- Carcinoma expleomorphic adenoma
- Carcinosarcoma
- Poorly differentiated carcinoma
  - Neuroendocrine and non-neuroendocrine
  - Undifferentiated carcinoma
  - Large cell neuroendocrine carcinoma
  - Small cell neuroendocrine carcinoma
- Lymphoepithelial carcinoma
- Squamous cell carcinoma
- Oncocytic carcinoma

Borderline tumor
Sialoblastoma

Benign tumors
- Pleomorphic adenoma
- Myoepithelioma
- Basal cell adenoma
- Warthin tumor
- Oncocytoma
- Lymphadenoma
- Cystadenoma
- Sialadenoma papilliferum
- Ductal papilloma
- Sebaceous adenoma
- Canalicular adenoma and other ductal adenomas

Other epithelial lesions
- Sclerosing polycystic adenosis
- Nodular oncocytic hyperplasia
- Lymphoepithelial lesions
- Intercalated duct hyperplasia

Soft tissue lesions
- Hemangioma
- Lipoma/sialolipoma
- Nodular fasciitis

Hematolymphoid tumor
- Extranodal marginal zone lymphoma of MALT

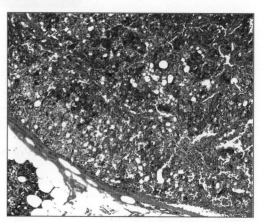

Fig. 1: Acinic cell carcinoma. The cells have an abundant cytoplasm filled with basophilic zymogen granules (H&E, 10X).

with lymph node metastasis. Also seen are psammoma bodies within the lumina. ACC is a well-differentiated tumor that lacks overt cytologic features of malignancy **(Fig. 2)**.

Immunoprofile

There is positivity for cytokeratin and also focal reactivity for amylase, α1-antichymotrypsin, transferrin, lactoferrin, IgA, secretory component, and proline-rich protein. A minor neuroendocrine component may also be present. DOG1 and SOX10 are the newly described immunomarkers.

Prognosis and Predictive Factors

Multiple recurrences, metastasis to cervical lymph nodes and distant metastasis indicate a poor prognosis. While tumors in the submandibular gland are more aggressive than those in the parotid gland, ACC in minor salivary glands are less aggressive than those in the major salivary glands. Features of prognostic importance are pain or fixation, gross invasion, deep lobe involvement, desmoplasia, cytologic atypia, increased mitotic activity, and adequacy of initial excision. Dedifferentiated acinic cell carcinoma may be seen, that requires adjuvant treatment. The cell proliferation marker Ki-67 predicts the biological behavior.

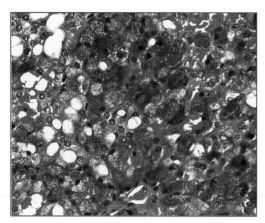
Fig. 2: Acinic cell carcinoma (H&E, 40X).

Mucoepidermoid Carcinoma (MEC)

It is a malignant glandular epithelial neoplasm characterized by mucus, intermediate and epidermoid cells, with columnar, clear cell, and oncocytoid features.

Synonyms

Mixed epidermoid and mucus-secreting carcinoma.

Epidemiology

Women are affected slightly more than men. The incidence tends to peak at approximately the fifth decade, but it is the most common salivary gland malignancy in childhood. Mean patient age is approximately 45 years. Sixty percent of palate lesions are in patients under 40 years of age.

Localization

These tumors represent ~5% of all salivary gland tumors, with ~67% arising in the parotid gland and 33% arising in the minor salivary glands. Occasionally, may arise within the mandibular, maxillary bones, intraparotid or periparotid lymph nodes, or they may be associated with a Warthin tumor.

Clinical Features

The low-grade tumors are well-circumscribed, often cystic masses. Slow painless growth is quite characteristic. High-grade variants are poorly delineated with lymph node metastasis, is fixed to the surrounding soft tissues. They are often painful as a result of facial nerve involvement.

Microscopy

The most common cell types are—squamous cells, mucus cells, cuboidal intermediate cells, and basaloid cells **(Figs. 3 and 4)**. The squamous cells form solid nests, and this component often predominates in high-grade tumors. The mucus cells are cuboidal, columnar or goblet-like and form solid masses or line cysts in one or more layers. Mucus cells often predominate in low-grade tumors. Mucus-filled cysts may rupture and elicit an inflammatory response. Intermediate cells are usually small with dark-staining nuclei but can be larger with a clear cytoplasm. Occasionally, MEC are composed of prominent clear cells or prominent oncocytic cells. A sclerosing variant has been described, containing numerous IgG4-positive plasma cells.

Grading

There is a marked difference in prognosis depending on the grade of the tumor, whether one uses the traditional two-tier system (low-grade and high-grade) or the three-grade scheme proposed by the Armed Forces Institute of Pathology (AFIP) authors, which is the one currently favored. This is based on a points system: Intracystic component greater than 20%, 2 points; neural invasion, 2 points; necrosis, 3 points; four or more mitoses per 10 high-power fields, 3 points; anaplasia, 4 points. A total score between 0 and 4 defines a low-grade tumor, a score of 5–6 applies to an intermediate-grade tumor, and a score of 7 or more indicates a high-grade tumor.

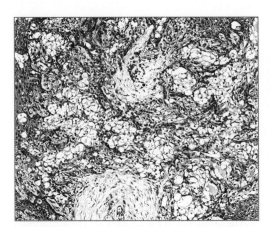

Fig. 3: Mucoepidermoid carcinoma. Mucus, squamous, and intermediate cells can be seen (H&E, 10X).

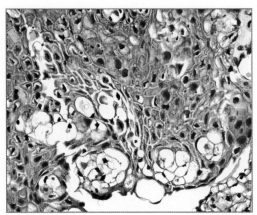

Fig. 4: Mucoepidermoid carcinoma. Mucus and intermediate cells can be seen (H&E, 40X).

Immunoprofile

Mucin stains and high molecular weight cytokeratins are useful. The mucins expressed are MUC1, MUC2, MUC4, MUC5AC, and MUC5B, but not MUC3. MUC1 predominates in the high-grade tumors, whereas MUC4 is more prevalent in low-grade tumors. The usual profile of MEC is CK7+/CK14+/CK20 –ve.

Cytogenetics

This tumor is associated with a balanced t(11;19) translocation that creates a fusion gene composed of portions of *MECT1* and *MAML2* genes.

Differential Diagnosis

Differential diagnosis includes various sebaceous neoplasms, clear-cell tumors, squamous cell carcinoma, chronic sialadenitis, and necrotizing sialometaplasia.

Prognosis and Predictive Factors

All MEC are malignant with metastatic potential, regardless of their microscopic appearance. Histological grading is agreed to be prognostically useful. Other techniques of prognostic value include the Ki-67 index, and the differential expression of membrane-bound mucins, MUC4 and MUC1.

Adenoid Cystic Carcinoma (AdCC)

It is a basaloid tumor consisting of epithelial and myoepithelial cells in variable morphologic configurations, including tubular, cribriform, and solid patterns **(Figs. 5 and 6)**.

Epidemiology

Patients' ages range from 20 to 84 years, with a median age of 52 years and there is no apparent sex predilection. It accounts for ~10% of all salivary gland tumors and 30% of epithelial minor salivary gland tumors.

Localization

This tumor is most common in the minor salivary glands. It has highest frequency in the palate, followed by the tongue, buccal mucosa, lip, maxillary sinus, and floor of mouth. Intramandibular AdCC are rare occurrences.

Clinical Features

It is a slow-growing but highly malignant neoplasm. Pain is present due to perineural invasion **(Table 2)**.

Macroscopy

It has infiltrative pattern of growth, few are well circumscribed.

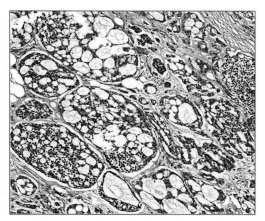

Fig. 5: Adenoid cystic carcinoma (H&E, 10X).

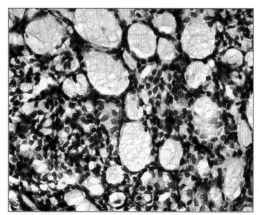

Fig. 6: Adenoid cystic carcinoma. Numerous "cylinders" containing a homogeneous acidophilic material can be seen (H&E, 10X).

Table 2: Differential diagnosis of adenoid cystic carcinoma.

Tumor type	Pattern	Cellular features	Perineural invasion
Basal cell adenoma	Syncytial noninvasive	Uniform, basaloid	No
Epithelial–myoepithelial carcinoma	Tubular/biphasic	Uniform, with clear outer cells	Rare
Basaloid squamous cell carcinoma	Syncytial	Marked pleomorphism focal keratinization	Rare
Basal cell adenocarcinoma	Syncytial/invasive	Mild pleomorphism/invasive	Yes
AdCC solid	Syncytial	Mild pleomorphism	Yes
AdCC tubular/cribriform	Ductal/cylindromatous	Uniform biphasic Mild pleomorphism	Yes Yes
PLGA	Tubular papillary pattern variable	Mild pleomorphism	Yes
Cellular PA	Syncytial	Uniform	No

(AdCC: Adenoid cystic carcinoma; PLGA: Polymorphous low-grade adenocarcinoma; PA: Pleomorphic adenoma)

Microscopy

Tumors consist of two main cell types—ductal and modified myoepithelial cells that have hyperchromatic, angular nuclei, and frequently clear cytoplasm. There are three patterns—tubular, cribriform and solid. Mitoses may be slightly increased in this variant, but marked nuclear pleomorphism and areas of necrosis are absent. Perineural and intraneural invasion is a common feature.

Immunoprofile

In differentiating between PLGA and AdCC, Ki-67 immunostaining may be helpful with much higher Ki-67 proliferation index in the former. DNA content, C-kit, and E-cadherin are associated with the biological behavior of these tumors. The p53 oncoprotein may also be an adverse prognostic marker in AdCC. ER, PR positivity has been reported in AdCC but the biological significance is currently unknown.

Genetics

These tumors have recurrent translocation t(6;9) (q22-23;p23-24) in at least 80–90% of cases of AdCC. There is overexpression of MYB-NFIB fusion proteins.

Prognosis and Predictive Factors

The prognosis of AdCC is influenced by its grading system. The solid or anaplastic type of AdCC is associated with a higher incidence of metastases and a rapid clinical course. Other factors that influence the prognosis are stage, presence of tumor at the margins, anatomic site, size of the primary lesion, degree of atypia, and lymph node metastases. Intraneural invasion is an independent predictor of poor prognosis. Reduced expression of E-cadherin expression correlates with an unfavorable prognosis. AdCC frequently metastasize to the lungs. Wide local and radical surgical excisions with and without postoperative radiation, is the treatment.

Salivary Duct Carcinoma

It is an aggressive adenocarcinoma which resembles high-grade breast ductal carcinoma.

Epidemiology

Salivary duct carcinoma (SDC) represents 9% of salivary malignancies. It is usually seen in elderly males (4:1 male to female ratio).

Localization

Most SDC (80%) occur in the parotid gland, and only 5% arise in intraoral minor salivary glands. Other rare sites are maxillary and larynx.

Macroscopy

SDC are firm, solid, tan, white with a cystic and invasive component.

Tumor Spread and Staging

For SDC, perineural spread (60%) and intravascular tumor emboli (31%) are common. Most patients present with stage III or IV disease, as lymph nodes are positive in 59% of patients.

Microscopy

It resembles in situ and invasive ductal carcinoma of the breast, whether comedo, solid, cribriform, apocrine, papillary, invasive micropapillary, mucinous (mucin-rich), the usual invasive form, or even sarcomatoid. Psammoma bodies, foci of squamous differentiation may be present. Mitotic figures are usually abundant. Perineural and lymphovascular invasions are frequently seen **(Figs. 7 and 8)**.

Immunoprofile

There is expression of keratin, HER2/neu, CEA, androgen receptors, estrogen receptor-beta, CD117 (cKIT) and GCDFP-15. A recent study proposed that SDC can be classified into three molecular subtypes analogous to that of breast cancer—luminal androgen receptor positive subtype (AR+, HER2 negative, CK5/6 negative); HER2 subtype (HER2 immunohistochemical expression 3+, HER2/neu gene amplified); basal phenotype (AR–, HER2–, CK5/6+) and the remainder were not classifiable.

Differential Diagnosis

Differential diagnosis includes metastatic breast and squamous carcinomas, oncocytic carcinoma and mucoepidermoid carcinoma.

Prognosis and Predictive Factors

The high-grade invasive form of this tumor is markedly aggressive, with frequent metastases to both regional nodes and distant organs, and a mortality rate of 70%. Conversely, the low-grade forms are accompanied by an excellent prognosis. The presence of a micropapillary component is said to be associated with an aggressive behavior. Tumor size, distant metastasis, and HER-2/neu overexpression

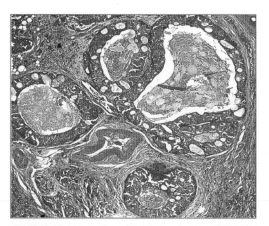

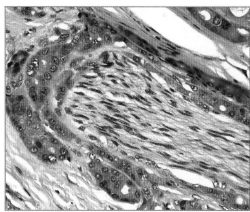

Fig. 7: High-grade ductal-type carcinoma of parotid gland. There is some degree of cytoplasmic apocrine-like change (H&E, 10X).

Fig. 8: High-grade salivary duct carcinoma showing perineural invasion (H&E, 40X).

are putative prognostic parameters for SDC. The pure intraductal tumors treated by simple excision recur frequently, either with the same intraductal pattern or as invasive tumor.

Polymorphous Adenocarcinoma (PAC)

It is a malignant epithelial tumor characterized by cytologic uniformity, morphologic diversity, an infiltrative growth pattern, and low metastatic potential.

Synonyms

Terminal duct carcinoma, lobular carcinoma, low-grade papillary adenocarcinoma and polymorphous low grade adenocarcinoma (PLGA).

Epidemiology

PAC is the second most common intraoral malignant salivary gland tumor, accounting for 26% of all carcinomas. This tumor is twice as common in women compared with men, and the average age at diagnosis is 57 years.

Localization

Approximately 60% of the cases have involved the palate. The buccal mucosa, lip, retromolar

triangle, cheek, tongue, lacrimal glands, nasopharynx, and nasal cavity may also be involved. Involvement of major salivary glands is extreme.

Clinical Features

A painless mass in the palate is the most common clinical sign.

Macroscopy

PAC usually appears as a firm, circumscribed, yellow-tan lobulated nodule, ranges in size from 1–5 cm, and usually has intact overlying mucosa.

Microscopy

The patterns include—tubular, lobular, trabecular, cribriform, papillary or papillary cystic, solid, and fascicular formations. The periphery of the tumor has invasive features, sometimes in an Indian-file pattern. Neurotropism and bone invasion may be seen. Mitotic activity is inconspicuous. The tumor cells are small to medium-sized with bland, minimally hyperchromatic, oval nuclei, and only occasional nucleoli. Foci of oncocytic, clear, squamous or mucous cells may be found. Stroma may show areas of mucinosis or hyalinization.

Immunoprofile

The tumor cells of PAC are immunoreactive with antibodies to cytokeratin (100%), vimentin (100%), S-100 (97%), CEA (54%), GFAP (15%), muscle-specific actin (13%), and EMA (12%). Staining for CD117 is stronger and more diffuse in adenoid cystic carcinoma than in PLGA, with S-100 protein showing the reverse.

Differential Diagnosis

Differential diagnosis include pleomorphic adenoma, basal cell adenoma, and adenoid cystic carcinoma.

Prognosis and Predictive Factors

The overall survival rate of patients with PAC is excellent. The behavior of this tumor is that of a low-grade malignancy. Tumors with a conspicuous papillary component are associated with a higher incidence of lymph node metastases. Treatment consists of complete surgical excision and neck dissection.

Myoepithelial Carcinoma

It is a neoplasm composed of tumor cells with myoepithelial differentiation, characterized by infiltrative growth and potential for metastasis. This tumor represents the malignant counterpart of benign myoepithelioma. The age range of patients is 14–86 years. Males and females are affected equally. It comprises <2% of all salivary gland carcinomas. Most cases (75%) arise in the parotid, but they also occur in the submandibular and minor glands. The tumors are painless and locally destructive. Perineural, bony, and vascular invasion may occur. Regional and distant metastases are uncommon at presentation, but may occur late in the course of the disease.

Macroscopy

Tumors are unencapsulated, may be well-defined with nodular surfaces. The cut surface is gray-white. Some tumors show areas of necrosis and cystic degeneration.

Microscopy

These tumors should have exclusive myoepithelial differentiation (morphologic and IHC) and clear-cut tumor infiltration into adjacent salivary gland or other tissues. The tumor cells are spindled, stellate, epithelioid, plasmacytoid (hyaline), or, occasionally, vacuolated with signet ring-like appearance. The tumor cells may form solid and sheet-like formations, trabecular or reticular patterns, but they can also be dissociated, often within plentiful myxoid or hyaline stroma. Pseudocystic or true cystic degeneration, foci of squamous differentiation may be noted. They also may have high mitotic activity with considerable variation and marked cellular pleomorphism. These tumors can be classified as high, intermediate, or low-grade based on the degree of nuclear atypia and the presence or absence of necrosis and mitosis. Reactivity for cytokeratin and at least one of the other myoepithelial markers, including P63, SMA, GFAP, CD10, calponin and SMA is required for diagnosis.

Differential Diagnosis

Differential diagnosis includes AdCC, PLGA, and tumors with clear-cell morphology, like hyalinizing clear-cell carcinoma, epimyoepithelial carcinoma, and metastatic renal cell carcinoma. Melanoma, high-grade lymphoma, or plasmacytoma must be ruled out when the tumor shows plasmacytoid differentiation. With spindle cell morphology, the most common differentials are sarcomatoid squamous carcinoma, spindle cell melanoma, and schwannoma.

Prognosis and Predictive Factors

Myoepithelial carcinoma of the salivary glands is a rare tumor. Approximately one-third of patients die of disease, another one-third have recurrences, mostly multiple, and the remaining one-third are disease-free. High-grade morphology and high proliferative activity correlate with a poor clinical outcome. The diagnosis is dependent on histology and immunohistochemistry. The tumor has a high rate of distant metastasis and high rate of lymph node metastasis in T3 to T4 cases. The treatment of myoepithelial carcinoma has been mainly surgical, including wide excision with free margins, with or without nodal dissection. The role of chemotherapy and radiotherapy has not yet been established.

Epithelial–Myoepithelial Carcinoma

A malignant tumor composed of two cell types, which typically form duct-like structures. The biphasic morphology is represented by an inner layer of duct lining, epithelial type cells and an outer layer of clear, myoepithelial-type cells.

Synonym

Adenomyoepithelioma.

Epidemiology

Epithelial–myoepithelial carcinoma (EMC) represents around 1% of the salivary gland tumors. It is more prevalent in women (F:M = 2:1). The patients range in age from 13 to 89 years, with the peak incidence in the 6th and 7th decades.

Localization

EMC occurs mostly in major salivary glands, mainly in the parotid (60%), but also in the minor glands of oral mucosa and the upper and lower respiratory tract.

Clinical Features

EMC forms a painless, slow-growing mass. Tumors arising in minor glands present as ulcerated, submucosal nodules, and have less well-defined margins. Rapid growth, facial nerve palsy and/or associated pain are suggestive of concomitant high-grade areas.

Macroscopy

EMC is a multinodular mass, with expansive borders and lacking a true capsule. Cystic spaces may be present.

Microscopy

The tumor has a well-defined capsule with a mixed tubular and solid architectural arrangement. Papillary and cystic areas are seen. Tumors show infiltration of surrounding tissues and there is ulceration of the overlying mucosa.

The hallmark of EMC histology is the presence of bilayered duct-like structures. The inner layer is formed by a single row of cuboidal cells, with dense, finely granular cytoplasm and central or basal, round nucleus. The outer layer may show single or multiple layers of polygonal cells, with well-defined borders **(Fig. 9)**. PAS-positive (Periodic-acid schiff-positive) basement membrane-like material surrounds the duct-like structures. Intratumoral hyalinization and cystification may be prominent features. The mitotic rate is low and necroses are found in about 20% cases. Unusual variants of EMC include Verocay-like bodies, sebaceous differentiation, oncocytic differentiation, dedifferentiation, myoepithelial "anaplasia," and tumors with a clear-cell ductal and myoepithelial ("double clear") appearance. Perineural, vascular, and bone invasion may occur.

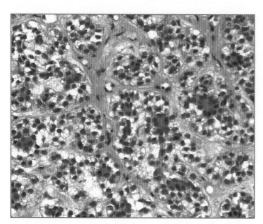

Fig. 9: Epithelial–myoepithelial carcinoma. The myoepithelial component is represented by the cells with clear cytoplasm (H&E × 10X).

Immunoprofile

The ductal epithelial cells react for cytokeratin, EMA, and occasionally S-100 protein. The clear myoepithelial cells react with cytokeratin, S-100, SMA, p63, CD10, and calponin. The surrounding stroma of basement membrane material stains with collagen type IV. The Ki-67 proliferative index is variable.

Differential Diagnosis

Differential diagnosis includes pleomorphic adenoma, myoepithelioma, oncocytoma, mucoepidermoid carcinoma, myoepithelial carcinoma, adenoid cystic carcinoma and clear cell carcinoma, not otherwise specified (NOS). Metastatic renal and thyroid carcinoma should be ruled out.

Cytogenetics

Few cases are positive for HRAS exon 3, codon 61 mutations.

Prognosis and Predictive Factors

EMC behaves as a low-grade malignancy with a high likelihood for local recurrence.

Regional lymph node and distant blood-borne metastases spread to lungs and kidneys. Poor prognostic features include positive margins, angiolymphatic invasion, necrosis, and myoepithelial anaplasia. EMC can occasionally transform to a high-grade myoepithelial neoplasm or adenocarcinoma.

New Entities

Mammary analogue secretory carcinoma and cribriform adenocarcinoma of the tongue and minor salivary glands.

Mammary Analogue Secretory Carcinoma: It is a new entity described. It was previously classified as a subset of acinic cell carcinoma. It is characterized by papillary-cystic pattern, abscence of DOG1 positivity and positivity for S-100 and Mammaglobin (versus acinic cell carcinoma). It is also called secretory carcinoma. The diagnostic translocation desribed is t(12;15).

Cribriform Adenocarcinoma of Salivary Glands (CASG): It is a new subset described in polymorphous adenocarcinoma, which shows an adenocarcinoma in cribriform pattern with nuclear features mimicking papillary thyroid carcinoma.

Intraductal Carcinoma: Also called cribrifrom cystadenocarcinoma low grade. Mostly seen in parotid gland. It has excellent prognosis. It shows a variety of growth patterns, both solid and cystic, ranging from cribriform to solid to micropaillary reminiscent of low-grade ductal carcinoma insitu or atypical ductal hyperplasia of the breast.

Carcinoma Ex-pleomorphic Adenoma

It is defined as a pleomorphic adenoma from which an epithelial malignancy is derived. Many of these result from the accumulation of genetic instabilities in long-standing pleomorphic adenomas. Malignant transformation occurs in approximately 2–7% of mixed tumors. The malignant component is a poorly differentiated adenocarcinoma or an undifferentiated carcinoma. Metastatic sites are lungs, bone, abdomen, and central nervous system. Tumor with capsular penetration of >1.5 mm is associated with a poor prognosis.

Other malignant tumors include small cell and large cell neuroendocrine carcinoma and lymphoepithelial carcinoma.

● BENIGN TUMORS

Pleomorphic Adenoma

It is a tumor of variable capsulation characterized microscopically by architectural rather than cellular pleomorphism. Epithelial and modified myoepithelial elements intermingle most commonly with tissue of mucoid, myxoid or chondroid appearance **(Fig. 10)**. It is most frequent in women in the fourth decade of life, but it can be seen in children and in elderly persons of either sex. In the parotid gland, most tumors arise within the superficial lobe, from either the tail (50%) or the anterior portion (25%). The remaining 25% arise from the deep lobe and often present as a pharyngeal mass without external evidence of tumor. These

are slow growing, mobile, discrete, painless masses. Although pleomorphic adenoma is a benign tumor, it can cause problems in clinical management due to its tendency to recur and the risk of malignant transformation **(Fig. 11)**.

Warthin Tumor

A tumor composed of glandular and often cystic structures, sometimes with a papillary cystic arrangement, lined by characteristic bilayered epithelium, comprising inner columnar eosinophilic or oncocytic cells surrounded by smaller basal cells. The stroma contains a variable amount of lymphoid tissue with germinal centers **(Fig. 12)**. This tumor commonly affects men in their sixth and seventh decades of life, probably because of smoking. Bilateral or multifocal tumor involvement is observed in approximately 10–15% of patients. Most patients present with a painless lobulated mass. On cross-section, it has a typical multicystic appearance, with fluid-filled spaces separated by grayish septa of varying thicknesses.

Other benign tumors include oncocytic tumors and myoepithelioma.

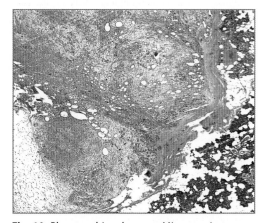

Fig. 10: Pleomorphic adenoma: Microscopic appearance of benign mixed tumor. Epithelial and myoepithelial cells can be easily distinguished (H&E, 4X).

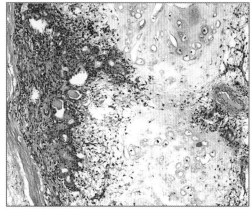

Fig. 11: Benign mixed tumor. The myoepithelial cells are undergoing cartilaginous metaplasia (H&E, 10X).

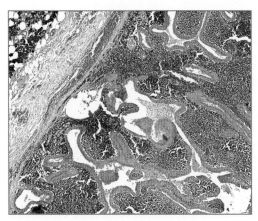

Fig. 12: Warthin tumor. Germinal centers are very prominent (H&E, 10X).

● FURTHER READING

1. Amit M, Binenbaum Y, Sharma K, et al. Incidence of cervical lymph node metastasis and its association with outcomes in patients with adenoid cystic carcinoma. An international collaborative study. Head Neck. 2015;37(7):1032-7.

2. Amit M, Binenbaum Y, Trejo-Leider L, et al. International collaborative validation of intraneural invasion as a prognostic marker in adenoid cystic carcinoma of the head and neck. Head Neck. 2015;37(7):1038-45.

3. Amit M, Na'ara S, Sharma K, et al. Elective neck dissection in patients with head and neck adenoid cystic carcinoma: An international collaborative study. Ann Surg Oncol. 2015;22(4):1353-9.

4. de Araujo VC, Passador-Santos F, Turssi C, et al. Polymorphous low-grade adenocarcinoma: An analysis of epidemiological studies and hints for pathologists. Diagn Pathol. 2013;8:6.

5. Fife TA, Smith B, Sullivan CA, et al. Polymorphous low-grade adenocarcinoma: A 17 patient case series. Am J Otolaryngol. 2013;34(5):445-8.

6. Ilayaraja V, Prasad H, Anuthama K, et al. Acinic cell carcinoma of minor salivary gland showing features of high-grade transformation. J Oral Maxillofac Pathol. 2014;18(1):97-101.

7. Li J, Wang BY, Nelson M, et al. Salivary adenocarcinoma, not otherwise specified: A collection of orphans. Arch Pathol Lab Med. 2004; 128(12):1385-94.

8. Khatib Y, Patel RD, Kane S, et al. Diagnostic dilemma in myoepithelial carcinoma of cheek. Indian J Pathol Microbiol. 2014;57(3):467-9.

9. Kimple AJ, Austin GK, Shah RN, et al. Polymorphous low-grade adenocarcinoma: A case series and determination of recurrence. Laryngoscope. 2014;124(12):2714-9.

10. Politi M, Robiony M, Avellini C, et al. Epithelial-myoepithelial carcinoma of the parotid gland: Clinicopathological aspect, diagnosis and surgical consideration. Ann Maxillofac Surg. 2014; 4(1):99-102.

11. Simpson RH. Salivary duct carcinoma: New developments—Morphological variants including pure in situ high-grade lesions; proposed molecular classification. Head Neck Pathol. 2013;7(Suppl 1):S48-58.

12. Savera AT, Sloman A, Huvos AG, et al. Myoepithelial carcinoma of the salivary glands: A clinicopathologic study of 25 patients. Am J Surg Pathol. 2000;24(6):761-74.

13. Schwarz S, Stiegler C, Müller M, et al. Salivary gland mucoepidermoid carcinoma is a clinically, morphologically and genetically heterogeneous entity: A clinicopathological study of 40 cases with emphasis on grading, histological variants and presence of the t(11;19) translocation. Histopathology. 2011;58(4):557-70.

14. Schwarz S, Zenk J, Müller M, et al. The many faces of acinic cell carcinomas of the salivary glands: A study of 40 cases relating histological and immunohistological subtypes to clinical parameters and prognosis. Histopathology. 2012;61(3):395-408.

CHAPTER 9

Imaging of Salivary Gland Tumors

Sandya CJ, Akshay Kudpaje, Sivakumar Vidhyadharan, Rajsekar CS

• NORMAL ANATOMY

Parotid Gland

The superficial parotid lies below and anterior to the external auditory canal and the mastoid tip, usually extending caudally to about the level of the angle of the mandible. The deep aspect of the parotid gland extends medially through the stylomandibular tunnel and is present between the posterior edge of the mandibular ramus and the anterior borders of the sternocleidomastoid muscle and the posterior belly of the digastric muscle. There is no anatomic division to separate superficial and deep parotid lobes but the nomenclature based on the facial nerve as a reference plane within the gland persists.

Branches of the facial nerve are not visible at ultrasonogram (USG). Parts of the trunk of this nerve may be demonstrated only with high-frequency probes (above 10 MHz). Therefore, the retromandibular vein, which usually lies directly above the trunk of the facial nerve, is used as a USG landmark separating the superficial and deep lobes of the parotid gland **(Fig. 1)**. The retromandibular vein is commonly used as an anatomic landmark in preoperative CT and MR imaging examinations of parotid neoplasms **(Fig. 2)**.

The normal echogenicity of all major salivary glands, including the parotid gland,

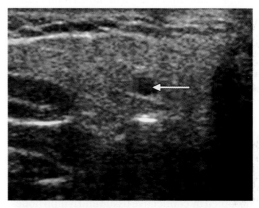

Fig. 1: Normal USG picture of parotid salivary gland. Arrow points to retromandibular vein.

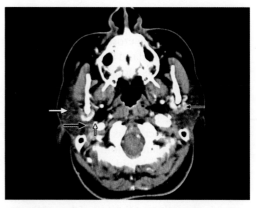

Fig. 2: Normal parotid gland, axial view CT scan: Superficial lobe (White arrow); Deep lobe (Black arrows).

is generally homogeneous, and varies from very bright and markedly hyperechoic to only slightly hyperechoic in comparison to adjacent muscles. The main excretory duct (Stensen duct) lies on the masseter muscle, about 1 cm below the zygomatic arch, then crosses the buccinator muscle, and has its orifice in the parotid papilla at the level of the upper second molar. A nondilated duct normally is not visible during USG. In the parenchyma of the parotid gland, lymph nodes may be found. They are localized mainly in the area of the upper and lower poles of the gland. Normal intraparotid lymph nodes may be oval or have a longitudinal shape. A short axis to long axis ratio greater than 0.5 and presence of a hyperechoic hilum is one of the important criteria for the normality of parotid lymph node.

Submandibular Gland

The submandibular gland lies in the posterior part of the submandibular triangle. The sides of the submandibular triangle are created by the anterior and posterior bellies of the digastric muscle and the body of the mandible. The space anterior to the submandibular gland is occupied by connective tissue and lymph nodes. Generally, the shape of the submandibular gland in longitudinal and transverse sections is close to a triangle. The submandibular gland may be connected with the parotid or sublingual gland by the glandular processes. The facial artery may cross the parenchyma of the submandibular gland in its tortuous course. The facial vein runs along the anterosuperior part of the submandibular gland. Medially to the submandibular gland, run the lingual artery and vein. The submandibular excretory duct (Wharton duct) runs from the area of the submandibular gland hilum at the level of the border of the mylohyoid muscle, then bends around the free part of the mylohyoid muscle and extends to its orifice at the sublingual caruncle along the medial part of the sublingual gland.

Sublingual Gland

The sublingual gland lies between the muscles of the oral cavity floor—the geniohyoid muscle, intrinsic muscles of the tongue and hypoglossal muscle (medially) and the mylohyoid muscle. Its lateral side is adjacent to the mandible. Along its medial part runs the excretory duct of the submandibular gland.

● NEOPLASMS OF SALIVARY GLANDS

The most common benign neoplasms of major salivary glands are pleomorphic adenomas (mixed tumor) and Warthin tumors (adenolymphoma, cystadenolymphoma, and papillary cystadenoma lymphomatosum).

Pleomorphic Adenoma

In USG, pleomorphic adenomas are hypoechoic, well-defined, and lobulated tumors with posterior acoustic enhancement, and may contain calcifications. The features of lobulated shape and homogenicity are being emphasized. Vascularization in pleomorphic adenomas is often poor or absent.

CT features show hyper or hypodense appearance compared with surrounding parotid parenchyma (**Figs. 3 and 4**). Small lesions usually have homogeneous appearance with smooth margins and larger lesions heterogeneous appearance with lobulated borders. Sites of lower attenuation represent areas of necrosis, old hemorrhage, and cystic change. Localized areas of increased attenuation most often represent sites of recent hemorrhage and are associated clinically with a sudden increase in tumor size and localized pain.

On MR imaging, these tumors typically have a low T1-weighted and a high T2-weighted signal intensity. A low signal intensity capsule often is seen on T2-weighted scans and on fat-suppressed, contrast-enhanced, T1-weighted images. Dystrophic calcifications or ossifications can occasionally be seen scattered

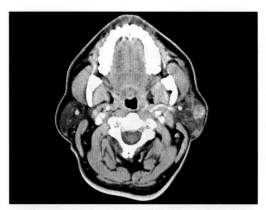

Fig. 3: Axial contrast-enhanced CT scan showing a well-defined enhancing mass in the left superficial lobe, probably a pleomorphic adenoma. A small intra-parotid lymph node is also seen.

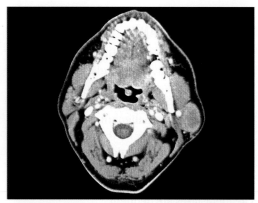

Fig. 4: Pleomorphic adenoma. Axial contrast-enhanced CT scan showing a well-defined enhancing mass superficial to the retromandibular vein, left lobe.

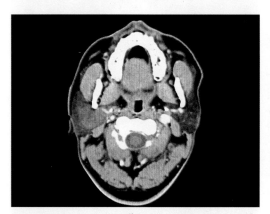

Fig. 5: Warthin tumor. Axial contrast enhanced CT scan showing heterogeneously enhancing cystic mass in the superficial lobe of the right parotid gland.

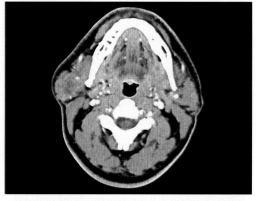

Fig. 6: Facial nerve schwannoma. Axial contrast-enhanced CT scan showing a well-defined mass with minimal enhancement in the superficial lobe extending to the deep lobe.

throughout the tumor, and such densities are highly suggestive of this diagnosis. Areas of hemorrhage appear as regions of high signal intensity on both T1-weighted and T2-weighted images. Regions of necrosis usually have low T1-weighted and high T2-weighted signal intensity.

Warthin Tumor

In USG, they appear as oval, hypoechoic, and well-defined tumors, and often contain multiple anechoic areas. On CT scan, they are often bilateral, usually cystic lesion, relatively well-defined **(Fig. 5)**. Cystic changes appear in the intralesional lower attenuation.

Facial Nerve Schwannoma

They are benign uncommon tumors arising from the facial nerve. CT scan **(Fig. 6)** usually shows homogeneous mass with minimal enhancement. They can extend into the deep lobe and the temporal bone.

• MALIGNANT NEOPLASMS OF PAROTID GLAND

The most common malignant neoplasms occurring in salivary glands are mucoepidermoid carcinoma and adenoid cystic carcinoma. Less than 30% of focal lesions in the parotid gland are malignant, whereas almost 50% of focal lesions in the submandibular gland are malignant. Adenoid cystic carcinoma, which is a slowly growing tumor, shows a particular tendency to nerve infiltration, and late metastases are frequent.

Ultrasound (US) features of malignant salivary neoplasms include the following— an irregular shape, irregular borders, blurred margins, and a hypoechoic inhomogeneous structure. The internal structure of a malignant tumor at US may not only be solid but also cystic or cystic with a mural solid nodule.

Computed tomography (CT) features of malignant salivary neoplasms, especially advanced malignant neoplasm include an irregular shape, irregular borders, blurred margins, and inhomogeneous structure. However, malignant tumors may also be homogeneous and well defined. Well-differentiated tumors may be similar to benign tumors at US or CT (Figs. 7A and B). High vascularization and high systolic peak flow velocity should raise the suspicion of malignancy. But vascularization of malignant tumors is not pathognomonic, and assessment with color Doppler or power Doppler US does not allow reliable differentiation between benign and malignant salivary gland tumors. The presence of metastatic-appearing lymph nodes accompanying a tumor in the salivary gland strongly suggests a malignancy.

Metastasis

Salivary glands are very uncommonly sites of metastases. Primary tumors metastasizing to salivary glands may be located in the head and neck region, as well as in more distant parts of

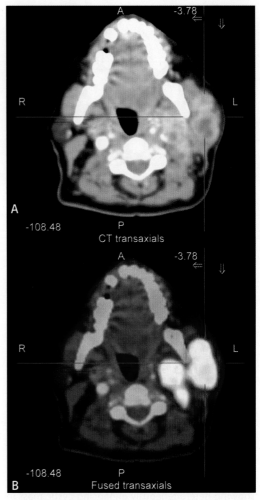

Figs. 7A and B: Malignant parotid tumor. (A) Axial contrast-enhanced CT scan showing heterogeneously enhancing mass in the left parotid involving the superficial and deep lobes with central necrosis; (B) PET–CT scan with FDG uptake in the lesions.

the body like melanoma, spinocellular cancer, breast cancer, and lung cancer.

In USG, metastases may be well-defined and oval. It may be difficult to differentiate multiple metastatic lesions from some patterns of inflammation, Sjögren syndrome, and granulomatous disease.

● FURTHER READING

1. Batsakis JG. Tumor of the head and neck: Clinical and pathological considerations, 2nd edition. Baltimore, MD: Williams and Wilkins; 1979. pp.1-120.
2. Gray H. Anatomy of the human body. In: Goss C (Ed). Philadelphia: Lea and Febiger; 1959. pp. 951-1001.
3. Liyanage SH, Spencer SP, Hogarth KM, et al. Imaging of salivary glands. Imaging. 2007;19:14-27.
4. Mason D, Chisholm D. Salivary glands in health and disease. London: WB Saunders; 1975. pp. 3-18.
5. Som PM, Shugar JM, Sacher M, et al. Benign and malignant parotid pleomorphic adenomas: CT and MR studies. J Comput Assist Tomogr. 1988;12(1):65-9.

CHAPTER 10

Guidelines in the Management of Salivary Gland Malignancies

Mahamaya Prasad Singh, Krishnakumar Thankappan, Subramania Iyer

● INTRODUCTION

Unlike any other head and neck neoplasms, the salivary glands constitute a large collection of highly heterogeneous tumors that exhibit broad spectrum of histology. These tumors have variable biologic behavior ranging from indolent, slow growing to highly aggressive and rapid fatality.

● EPIDEMIOLOGY

Malignant neoplasms of the salivary glands are relatively rare, accounting for approximately 6% of all head and neck malignancies. Approximately, 20% of the parotid gland tumors are malignant. The incidence of malignancy in submandibular and minor salivary gland is approximately 50% and 80%, respectively. The most common type being mucoepidermoid carcinoma (MEC) followed by adenoid cystic, acinic cell, adenocarcinoma, carcinoma ex-pleomorphic. The primary diagnosis of squamous carcinoma of the parotid gland is rare; however, the parotid is the frequent site for metastasis from skin cancer. The histopathologic classification with their description will be dealt in the subsequent chapters.

● CLINICAL PRESENTATION

The clinical presentation of malignant and benign salivary tumors is often indistinguishable. A mobile and painless mass that not rapidly growing is a common presentation for both benign and malignant salivary tumors. Certain features like pain, rapid growth, facial palsy, skin fixation, and cervical lymphadenopathy are highly suggestive of malignancy and should be checked in cases of parotid swelling. The history should also ascertain about potential systemic manifestations such as weight loss, fatigue, pulmonary symptoms, bone pain, and focal neurological deficits. Intraoral examination should be performed to look for any swelling in the parapharyngeal space. Facial nerve function has to be documented.

● IMAGING

Imaging studies are critical for evaluating and planning treatment for salivary gland tumors. Imaging can suggest whether a lesion is benign or malignant. Malignancy should be suspected if the margins are indistinct, enhancing lesion, edema around nerves suggesting perineural invasion, and lymphadenopathy. CT scan is useful in detecting mass as well as its relationship or involvement of bony structures like mandible or the temporal bone. It is also an excellent modality to assess lymph node status. MRI has been preferred over CT because of its better soft tissue delineation and to determine perineural spread **(Tables 1 and 2)**.

Table 1: TNM staging: Major salivary gland tumors (AJCC 8th edition).

T stage	
TX	Primary tumor cannot be assessed
T0	No evidence of primary tumor
Tis	Carcinoma in situ
T1	Tumor 2 cm or smaller in greatest dimension without extraparenchymal extension*
T2	Tumor larger than 2 cm but not larger than 4 cm in greatest dimension without extraparenchymal extension*
T3	Tumor larger than 4 cm and/or tumor having extraparenchymal extension*
T4	Moderately advanced or very advanced disease
T4a	Moderately advanced disease. Tumor invades skin, mandible, ear canal, and/or facial nerve
T4b	Very advanced disease. Tumor invades skull base and/or pterygoid plates and/or encases carotid artery

* Extraparenchymal extension is clinical or macroscopic evidence of invasion of soft tissues. Microscopic evidence alone does not constitute extraparenchymal extension for classification purposes.

Clinical N (cN)	
NX	Regional lymph nodes cannot be assessed
N0	No regional lymph node metastasis
N1	Metastasis in a single ipsilateral lymph node, 3 cm or smaller in greatest dimension and ENE (-)
N2	Metastasis in a single ipsilateral node larger than 3 cm but not larger than 6 cm in greatest dimension and ENE (–); or metastases in multiple ipsilateral lymph nodes, none larger than 6 cm in greatest dimension and ENE (–); or in bilateral or contralateral lymph nodes, none larger than 6 cm in greatest dimension and ENE (–)
N2a	Metastasis in a single ipsilateral node larger than 3 cm but not larger than 6 cm in greatest dimension and ENE (–)
N2b	Metastasis in multiple ipsilateral nodes, none larger than 6 cm in greatest dimension and ENE (–)
N2c	Metastasis in bilateral or contralateral lymph nodes, none larger than 6 cm in greatest dimension and ENE (–)
N3	Metastasis in a lymph node larger than 6 cm in greatest dimension and ENE (–); or metastasis in any node(s) with clinically overt ENE (+)
N3a	Metastasis in a lymph node larger than 6 cm in greatest dimension and ENE (–)
N3b	Metastasis in any node(s) with clinically overt ENE (+)

Pathological N (pN)	
NX	Regional lymph nodes cannot be assessed
N0	No regional lymph node metastasis
N1	Metastasis in a single ipsilateral lymph node, 3 cm or smaller in greatest dimension and ENE (–)
N2	Metastasis in a single ipsilateral node, 3 cm or smaller in greatest dimension and ENE (+); or metastasis in a single ipsilateral node larger than 3 cm but not larger than 6 cm in greatest dimension and ENE (–) or metastases in multiple ipsilateral lymph nodes, none larger than 6 cm in greatest dimension and ENE (–); or in bilateral or contralateral lymph nodes, none larger than 6 cm in greatest dimension and ENE (–)
N2a	Metastasis in a single ipsilateral node, 3 cm or smaller in greatest dimension and ENE (+); or metastasis in a single ipsilateral node larger than 3 cm but not larger than 6 cm in greatest dimension and ENE (–)
N2b	Metastasis in multiple ipsilateral nodes, none larger than 6 cm in greatest dimension and ENE (–)
N2c	Metastasis in bilateral or contralateral lymph nodes, none larger than 6 cm in greatest dimension and ENE (–)

Contd...

Contd...

Pathological N (pN)	
N3	Metastasis in a lymph node larger than 6 cm in greatest dimension and ENE (-); or in a single ipsilateral node larger than 3 cm in greatest dimension and ENE (+); or multiple ipsilateral, contralateral, or bilateral nodes any with ENE (+)
N3a	Metastasis in a lymph node larger than 6 cm in greatest dimension and ENE (–)
N3b	Metastasis in a single ipsilateral node larger than 3 cm in greatest dimension and ENE (+); or multiple ipsilateral, contralateral, or bilateral nodes any with ENE (+)

Note: A designation of "U" or "L" may be used for any N category to indicate metastasis above the lower border of the cricoid (U) or below the lower border of the cricoid (L).
Similarly, clinical and pathological ENE should be recorded as ENE (–) or ENE (+).

Distant metastasis M	
M0	No distant metastasis
M1	Distant metastasis

Table 2: AJCC prognostic stage groups.

When T is ...	And N is ...	And M is ...	Then the stage group is ...
Tis	N0	M0	0
T1	N0	M0	I
T2	N0	M0	II
T3	N0	M0	III
T0, T1, T2, T3	N1	M0	III
T4a	N0, N1	M0	IVA
T0, T1, T2, T3, T4a	N2	M0	IVA
Any T	N3	M0	IVB
T4b	Any N	M0	IVB
Any T	Any N	M1	IVC

● BIOPSY

Acquiring tissue for histopathological examination is a key element in the management as it is needed to confirm the diagnosis of malignancy and also gives us the clue about the histological subtype. Tumors of the salivary glands are quite accessible and fine needle aspiration (FNA) is the preferred method with high accuracy rate of 80–98%. As a general rule, open incisional biopsy of the parotid should be avoided. If FNA fails to yield sufficient diagnosis, then the surgeon should proceed with superficial parotidectomy with in-toto removal of the tumor. Intraoperative frozen section is helpful in determining the extent of tumor spread and assessment of surgical margins.

● TREATMENT

The mainstay of treatment of salivary tumor is surgical resection with or without postoperative radiotherapy. However, the extent of surgery is dependent on the size and site of the tumor. **Flowchart 1** shows the management algorithm for malignant parotid tumors.

Flowchart 1: Management algorithm for malignant parotid tumor.

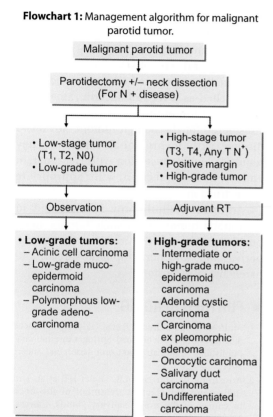

Rest of the histological types will require radiotherapy. Role of adjuvant chemotherapy is controversial.

Management of Neck

All node-positive neck on clinical or radiological examination should undergo neck dissection, usually a comprehensive neck dissection levels I–V, preserving the sternocleidomastoid muscle, accessory nerve, and internal jugular vein if these structures are not involved. Management of node-negative neck is controversial regarding the use of an elective neck irradiation or an elective neck dissection. In addition to clinical examination and radiology, the node-negative status can be confirmed by a USG-guided fine needle aspiration cytology (FNAC) of any suspicious nodes or by an intraoperative frozen section examination of any Level II nodes if found.

The general expert consensus is that the node-negative neck should be addressed in high-grade tumors and high-stage tumors. Since the indications of the adjuvant radiotherapy and that for addressing the node-negative neck are the same, adjuvant radiotherapy may be preferred without an elective neck dissection. At the same time, there is another school of thought that all high-grade tumors should undergo an elective neck dissection prior to adjuvant radiotherapy.

Management of the Facial Nerve in Surgery

The indications for sacrificing the facial nerve intraoperatively are:
- Clinical involvement of the facial nerve preoperatively
- Intraoperative gross encasement and infiltration of the nerve

Management of Recurrences

Locoregional recurrent cases without prior radiotherapy should be evaluated and, if

Surgery

For all parotid malignancies primary surgery is the initial management. There is considerable controversy regarding the extent of surgery in malignant parotid tumors. The tumor has to be excised with adequate clearance. Three dimensional measured margins may not be possible due to the close proximity of the facial nerve in the deeper planes.

Indications of Adjuvant Radiotherapy

Radiotherapy is indicated in high-grade tumors, high-stage (T3, T4) tumors, node-positive status, and positive margins. In general, the low-grade tumors are only acinic cell carcinoma, low-grade mucoepidermoid carcinoma, and polymorphous low-grade adenocarcinoma.

resectable, should undergo complete resection of the tumor followed by adjuvant radiotherapy/chemoradiotherapy. If unresectable, primary radiotherapy/chemoradiotherapy should be considered. Locoregional recurrence or second primary with prior radiotherapy should be evaluated and if resectable, should preferably undergo complete resection of the tumor.

Management of Distant Metastasis

In case of distant metastasis palliative chemotherapy or expectant management or best supportive care should be considered. In case of adenoid cystic carcinoma where the patient may survive long even with distant metastasis, the role of metastasectomy may be considered.

● PROGNOSIS

Prognosis is dependent to a large extent on the stage and grade of the tumor. Good overall survival and local rates have been achieved because of improved surgical techniques and adjuvant therapy.

Management of Submandibular Salivary Gland Tumors

Tumors of the submandibular salivary gland have increased likelihood of malignancy, so requires careful diagnostic evaluation and surgical intervention. Proper history and physical examination should be performed. Suspicious findings like pain, cranial nerve involvement, hard and fixed to adjoining structures, or cervical lymphadenopathy should be accounted. If suspicious, imaging with CT or MRI and FNAC are to be performed.

Mainstay of treatment submandibular salivary gland tumors is surgical resection with clear margins and achieving maximum function and cosmesis. Submandibular gland malignancies are better managed when approached as level I dissection rather than simple excision of the gland which is mainly considered for the benign tumors. Advanced disease with locoregional extension may require adequate resection with clear margin and/or neck dissection with appropriate reconstruction.

Adjuvant radiotherapy is indicated in high-grade tumors, high-stage tumors, node positive status, positive margins, perineural, perivascular and perilymphatic spread, and parenchymal extension.

● FURTHER READING

1. Amin MB, Edge S, Greene F, et al. (Eds). AJCC Cancer Staging Manual (8th edition). Springer International Publishing: American Joint Commission on Cancer; 2017.
2. Armstrong JG, Harrison LB, Thaler HT, et al. The indications for elective treatment of the neck in cancer of the major salivary glands. Cancer. 1992;69(3):6159.
3. Bron LP, Traynor SJ, McNeil EB, et al. Primary and metastatic cancer of the parotid: Comparison of clinical behavior in 232 cases. Laryngoscope. 2003;113(6):10705.
4. Pfister DG, Ang KK, Brizel DM, et al. National Comprehensive Cancer Network. Head and neck cancers, version 2.2013. Featured updates to the NCCN guidelines. J Natl Compr Canc Netw. 2013;11(8):917-23.
5. Spiro RH. Salivary neoplasms: Overview of a 35-year experience with 2,807 patients. Head Neck Surg. 1986;8(3):17784.
6. Weber RS, Byers RM, Petit B, et al. Submandibular gland tumors. Adverse histologic factors and therapeutic implications. Arch Otolaryngol Head Neck Surg. 1990;116(9):105560.

CHAPTER 11

Principles of Salivary Gland Tumor Surgery

Mahamaya Prasad Singh, Krishnakumar Thankappan, Subramania Iyer

• INTRODUCTION

Surgical management remains the mainstay of any treatment algorithm for salivary gland malignancies. Surgical intervention requires careful planning, and execution, particularly in parotid tumor surgery because of the presence of facial nerve within the gland. Most parotid gland tumors are located in the superficial lobe and if the facial nerve is functioning pre-operatively, the nerve can be preserved in most of the cases. Malignant deep lobe tumors are quite rare and require great patience on the part of the operating surgeon to remove the deep lobe and preserve the facial nerve.

• SURGICAL ANATOMY

The exocrine salivary gland system is composed of two distinct classes:

1. Major salivary glands—paired structures which include parotid, submandibular, and sublingual gland.
2. Minor salivary glands—which are dispersed throughout the upper aerodigestive tract consisting between 500 and 1,000 small glands.

Parotid Gland

The parotid gland is the largest of the major salivary glands weighing between 15 g and 30 g each. It lies beneath the skin in front of and below the ear, contained within the deep fascia of the neck, called locally the parotid fascia. The major portion of the gland lies over the ramus of the mandible and the masseter muscle. Superiorly the gland extends up to the zygomatic arch and inferiorly it extends to a variable distance in the neck overlying the sternocleidomastoid (SCM) muscle, referred to as the "tail of the parotid". The gland extends deep behind the mandible through the stylomandibular tunnel to enter the prestyloid component of the parapharyngeal space. From the anterior edge of the gland, the parotid or "Stensen's" duct passes lateral to masseter muscle and turns medial at the anterior margin of the muscle to pierce the buccinator muscle.

The parotid gland is unilobar structure traversed by the extracranial portion of the facial nerve and its branches. After about 1 cm, after entering the gland, it divides into its 5 branches—temporal, zygomatic, buccal, mandibular, and cervical. In most individuals, an initial bifurcation forms an upper temporofacial and a lower cervicofacial branch. The main bulk (80%) of the parotid gland lies lateral to the facial nerve and is known as superficial lobe and much smaller portion lies medially known as the deep lobe. It is, therefore, essential to know the surgical landmarks that facilitate the identification of the facial nerve as well as the anatomic variations of the facial nerve.

Other nerves associated with parotid gland are:

- Auriculotemporal nerve—branch of trigeminal nerve carries sensory innervation to temporal region. It also carries parasympathetic nerve fibers to the parotid gland from the otic ganglion. Cross-innervation may lead to Frey's syndrome.
- Great auricular nerve—formed from rootlets C2 and C3. It courses over the SCM, and divides to form anterior and posterior branch. The anterior branch will course through the gland whereas the posterior branch of the nerve provides sensation to lower half of the auricle. Preservation of the posterior branch is possible through meticulous dissection.

Submandibular Gland

The submandibular gland lies within the submandibular triangle formed by the inferior margin of the mandible and the two bellies of the digastric muscle. Each gland is composed of a large superficial and a small deep lobe. Superficial to the gland is skin, subcutaneous tissue, platysma muscle, and submandibular fascia. Important structures in relation to the gland are facial artery and vein and marginal mandibular, lingual and hypoglossal nerve. The facial artery enters the gland deep to the posterior belly of digastric and is related to posterior and then superior surface of the gland before exiting at the lower border of the mandible. The facial vein courses superficial to the gland on its way to the jugular vein. The marginal mandibular nerve lies superficial to the submandibular fascia and curves superiorly and crosses the lower border of the mandible close to the facial artery. The lingual nerve is connected to the submandibular ganglion and is related to the superior surface of the gland. The hypoglossal nerve lies inferiorly and is deep in the gland and not usually encountered during surgery. The submandibular duct extends forward from the deep portion of the gland and courses beneath the floor of the mouth.

● PAROTIDECTOMY: SURGICAL TECHNIQUE

Preparation

Many surgeons use intraoperative facial nerve monitoring, mainly useful in large tumors, recurrent disease requiring revision surgery where chances of facial nerve injury are high.

Incision

The standard incision is the modified Blair's incision. The incision begins from the pretragal skin crease, extends around the ear lobule towards the mastoid and then gently curving back down to join the neck crease approximately two fingers breadth below the mandible. This incision can be extended forward if neck dissection is indicated.

Flap Elevation

The skin flap should be raised superficial to the parotid fascia and in the neck subplatysmally. The greater auricular nerve is identified, preserved, and tagged for a later use as potential nerve graft. The posterior branch may be preserved depending upon the extent of the tumor.

Identification of the Facial Nerve

The gland is now mobilized anteriorly by releasing the fascial attachments at the digastric muscle and the mastoid which also facilitates exposure of facial nerve trunk. The facial nerve exits from the stylomastoid foramen just superior to the posterior belly of digastric.

The various landmarks used for the facial nerve identification are:

- Tragal pointer—nerve lies 1 cm medial and inferior to tip of pointer.
- Tympanomastoid suture—nerve lies 2–4 mm deep to suture.
- Superior portion of posterior belly of digastric—nerve lies 5–14 mm superior to muscle.

- Posterior auricular artery—nerve lies 2–4 mm deep to its artery.
- Styloid process—nerve will run superficial and inferior to the palpated styloid process.
- Mastoid bone—nerve can be identified through otologic drill out.

If there is inability to identify the main trunk of the facial nerve through antegrade dissection, then retrograde dissection may be carried out by identifying the distal branches of the nerve. Blind clamping of vessels, unipolar electrocautery, traction or stretching of the nerve should be avoided. Despite the facial nerve being anatomically intact at the completion of surgical procedure, a temporary neuropraxia may result. Temporary neuropraxia, either immediate or delayed, results in paresis secondary to traction or thermal injury. This usually resolves in weeks to months and can be managed by supportive care.

Extent of Surgery

The extent of surgery is dependent on the size and site of the tumor and also preoperative functioning of the facial nerve.

- *Superficial parotidectomy*: Once the main trunk of the facial nerve is identified, the overlying parotid tissue is dissected free of the nerve and its branches until the entire superficial lobe is excised.
- *Total parotidectomy*: If total parotidectomy is indicated, the procedure is extended by dissecting the underlying parotid tissue from the facial nerve and its branches in a meticulous way and removing the deep lobe in pieces. Precaution should be taken for minimal handling of the facial nerve so as to avoid traction injury.
- *Extended parotidectomy*: Malignant tumors of the parotid gland can involve the surrounding structures like the masseter muscle, the temporomandibular joint, the external auditory canal or the overlying skin which needs resection for adequate oncologic clearance.

The concept of adequate parotidectomy: Surgical resection of parotid tumor aimed at complete resection with appropriate margin of normal tissue. Three dimensional measured margins may not be possible due to the close proximity of the facial nerve in the deeper planes. Small tumors located at the tail of the parotid may require dissection of only the lower branch of the facial nerve and can be removed with adequate cuff of tissue all around the tumor, thereby avoiding unnecessary dissection to the upper branches.

Management of Facial Nerve

Facial nerve should be identified and every effort should be made to preserve it, if the nerve is functioning normally in the preoperative period. Facial nerve sacrifice should be considered for cases with preoperative facial nerve paralysis or intraoperative gross encasement and infiltration of the nerve.

Reconstruction

Reconstructive efforts should be focused on both function and cosmesis. When facial nerve is sacrificed, primary nerve reconstruction can be considered. Common donor sites include the great auricular nerve, sural nerve, and ansa cervicalis. If nerve grafting is not achievable, then temporalis sling transfer or rehabilitative procedures like eyelid weight implants can be considered. Parotid defects can be reconstructed using SCM muscle rotation flap to free flap transfer. Extensive defects involving skin, mandible, and temporal bone requires free tissue transfer.

Complications of Parotidectomy

- *Facial nerve injury*: It may be temporary or permanent due to the transection of the facial nerve. Temporary weakness or neuropraxia is the most common complication and usually recovers within few weeks. It may result while dissecting over the nerve, traction injury or heat injury secondary to use of cautery.

- Hematoma
- Seroma, saliva, salivary fistula—leakage of serous fluid and saliva from the transected parotid tissue.
- *Frey's syndrome*: Also known as gustatory sweating seen after parotid surgery where the patient develops sweating on the side of the face while eating. Auriculotemporal nerve carries sensory innervation to temporal region. It also carries para-sympathetic nerve fibers to the parotid gland from the otic ganglion, and cross-innervation may lead to Frey's syndrome.
- Ear numbness may result from transection of the greater auricular nerve.
- Duskiness of the postauricular skin flap or necrosis of the skin tip may occur if the flap is large.

● SUBMANDIBULAR GLAND

Treatment of submandibular gland malignancies is significantly managed when approached as Level I dissection rather than simple excision of the gland which is mainly considered for the benign tumors.

● SURGICAL TECHNIQUE

Submandibular Gland Excision

Horizontal skin crease incision placed around 2 finger breadths below the lower border of the mandible. The incision should extend from anterior border of SCM into the submental region overlying the anterior border of digastric muscle. Superior flap is elevated subplatysmally taking care not to injure the marginal mandibular nerve which lies above the submandibular gland fascia, and can be identified crossing the facial vein. The vein is ligated, transected, and retracted upward which displaces the nerve superiorly and protects from getting damaged. The superior dissection proceeds by double ligation and transection of

the facial artery at the base mandible, which frees the superior attachment of the gland. The free (posterior) edge of mylohyoid muscle is retracted anteriorly, while gentle posterior traction on the gland is maintained. This exposes the deep portion of the gland and its duct, the submandibular ganglion and the lingual and hypoglossus muscle. The contribution of the lingual nerve to the submandibular ganglion is transected, and the Warthin's duct is ligated and divided. This delivers the deep portion of the gland. Care should be taken to avoid injury to the lingual and hypoglossal nerves. Finally, the facial artery is divided a second time, deep to the gland, and the gland is removed.

Complications of Submandibular Gland Surgery

- *Nerve injury*: Marginal mandibular nerve may result if care is not taken while raising the flap or during dissection of the gland. Occasionally, there may be injury to the lingual or the hypoglossal nerve.
- Hematoma
- *Seroma or salivary fistula*: Though rare, it may occasionally occur.

● FURTHER READING

1. Malik TH, Kelly G, Ahmed A, et al. A comparison of surgical techniques used in dynamic reanimation of the paralyzed face. Otol Neurotol. 2005;26(2):284-91.
2. Medina JE. Neck dissection in the treatment of cancer of major salivary glands. Otolaryngol Clin North Am. 1998;31(5):815-22.
3. O'Brien CJ. Current management of benign parotid tumors—the role of limited superficial parotidectomy. Head and Neck. 2003;25(11):946-52.
4. Weber RS, Byers RM, Petit B, et al. Submandibular gland tumors. Adverse histologic factors and therapeutic implications. Arch Otolaryngol Head Neck Surg. 1990;116(9):1055-60.
5. Witt RL. Minimally invasive surgery for parotid pleomorphic adenoma. Ear Nose Throat J. 2005;84(5):310-11.
6. Witt RL. The significance of margin in parotid surgery for pleomorphic adenoma. Laryngoscope. 2002;112(12):2141-54.

CHAPTER 12

Imaging in Parapharyngeal Tumors

Sandya CJ, Akshay Kudpaje

• ANATOMY

The parapharyngeal space (PPS) lies on either side of pharynx from the base of skull to styloglossus muscle at the level of angle of mandible. Parapharyngeal space resembles an inverted pyramid with the apex at greater cornu of hyoid bone and base is formed by skull base **(Fig. 1)**. A medial wall is formed by buccopharyngeal fascia covering the outer aspect of pharyngeal constrictor muscles and also buccinator.

Parapharyngeal space is divided into pre- and poststyloid compartment by fascial condensation extending between styloid process and tensor veli palatini. Prestyloid compartment lies on the anterolateral aspect, and poststyloid compartment lies on the posteromedial aspect of tensor veli palatini fascia. Prestyloid compartment contains internal maxillary artery, vein, inferior alveolar nerve, lingual, and auriculotemporal nerve. Medial and lateral pterygoid muscles, deep portion of parotid gland, and numerous lymph nodes also lie in this prestyloid compartment. Poststyloid compartment contains internal carotid artery (ICA), internal jugular vein, last four cranial nerves, sympathetic nerves, and lymph nodes **(Fig. 2)**.

Differentiation of a prestyloid lesion from a poststyloid lesion is critical for guiding the surgeon in both diagnosis and planning the surgical approach.

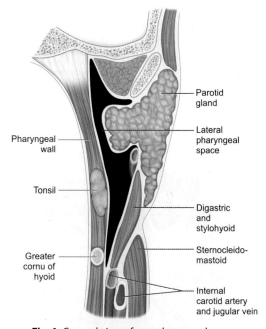

Fig. 1: Coronal view of parapharyngeal space.

• IMAGING ASSESSMENT

Parapharyngeal space lesions being deep seated in location are difficult to assess clinically, and imaging is mandatory for the precise assessment of the size, location, and extent of the tumor which guides the surgical approach **(Fig. 3)**. With the advent of high-resolution computed tomography (CT) and magnetic resonance imaging (MRI) accurate preoperative diagnosis is possible in 90–95% of PPS lesions.

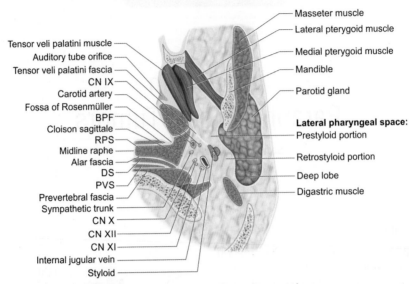

Fig. 2: Axial representation of parapharyngeal space.

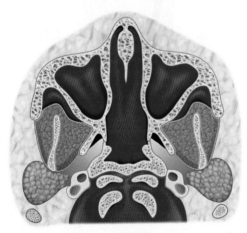

Fig. 3: Parapharyngeal space. Blue area denotes the parapharyngeal space.

Most important landmarks assessed when evaluating a PPS lesion include:

- Deep portion of parotid gland
- Stylomandibular tunnel
- Internal carotid artery
- Direction of displacement of fat of the prestyloid compartment

- Mass effect on the surrounding structures like pharynx, masticator space, mandible, and skull base.

Computed tomography provides information about the internal architecture of the lesion (solid versus cystic), size of the mass, and lymph node status. Dynamic contrast enhancement enables us to distinguish a hypovascular mass (schwannoma/salivary gland tumor) from a hypervascular mass (paraganglioma). Hypervascular tumors have a very rapid early filling phase following a rapid washout due to rich venous drainage, whereas hypovascular tumors tend to retain the contrast in delayed phase.

● PATHOLOGY

Infections/Abscess

Most infections of PPS arise in adjacent spaces and most common sites include palatine tonsils, pharynx or from the tooth structures. CT findings of cellulitis include diffuse swelling of the fat with increase in attenuation.

MRI shows an increase in T2-weighted signal and decrease in T1-weighted signal of the fat due to water logging. Abscess shows a central hypointense signal with an enhancing thick rim in postcontrast T1-weighted images. Differentiation of PPS abscess from cellulitis is important **(Fig. 4)**.

Tumors

Most of the primary tumors of PPS arise from the deep portion of parotid salivary gland in the prestyloid compartment or from neural related elements in retrostyloid compartment.

Salivary Gland Tumors

The most common neoplasm arising in the PPS are of salivary gland origin. These tumors arise from deep lobe of parotid salivary gland; salivary rests within the prestyloid compartment and minor salivary glands of the pharyngeal mucosa. Around 80–90% of these tumors are benign, common, and pleomorphic adenoma. Other malignancies seen are mucoepidermoid carcinoma, adenocystic carcinoma, and acinic cell carcinoma.

Pleomorphic adenomas generally have smooth and noninfiltrating margins but can be lobulated, cystic, and calcified. Occasionally, hemorrhage can also occur resulting in sudden increase in the size of the tumor. MR is the better modality than CT in defining the margins of the lesions. Tumor shows an intermediate signal on T1 and bright signal on T2W images. Bleed shows bright signal on T1-weighted images while cystic changes appear dark on T1 and bright on T2W.

Malignant tumors have infiltrative and irregular margins. Prestyloid lesions like parotid and other extraparotid masses displace the ICA posteriorly when compared with poststyloid lesions like paragangliomas and schwannomas which displace it anteriorly. Vascular tumors show large caliber vessels as signal voids within the lesion. Tumors arising within the prestyloid fat will have fat signal all around the tumor while those from the deep lobe of parotid will have fat signal on the deeper aspect **(Figs. 5 to 7)**.

Neurogenic Tumors

Most of the neurogenic tumors arise from vagus nerve followed by glossopharyngeal and rarely superior sympathetic chain. Schwannomas

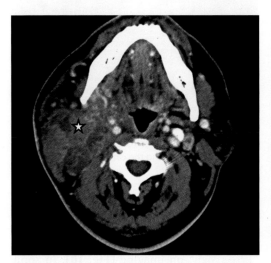

Fig. 4: Axial CT image showing an evolving abscess in right parapharyngeal space.

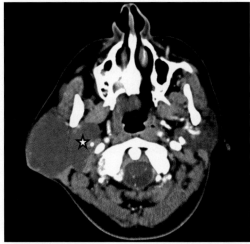

Fig. 5: Axial CT image showing a mass from the deep lobe of right parotid gland protruding into parapharyngeal space.

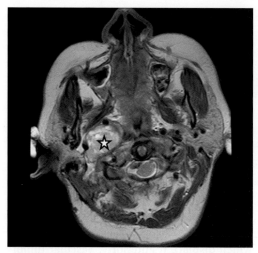

Fig. 6: Axial T2-weighted MR image showing bright lesion in the right PPS displacing the carotid artery anteriorly (Schwannoma).

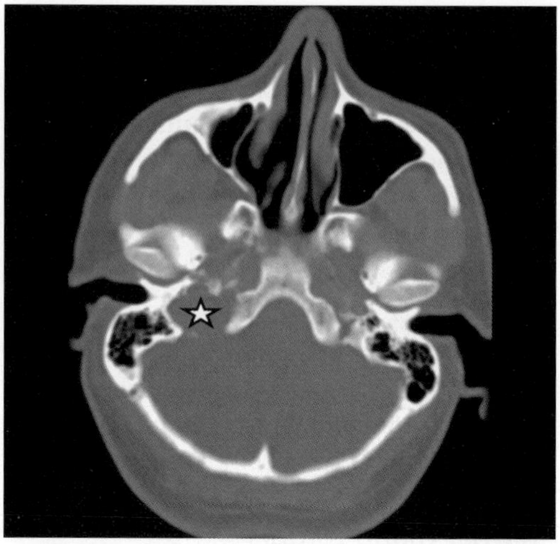

Fig. 7: Axial CT image showing smooth widening of the jugular foramen in a case of schwannoma.

are homogeneous soft tissue masses, areas of necrosis or hemorrhage can occur. These tumors are usually hypovascular and do not enhance in the early phase and imaged using a dynamic CT scan or conventional angiography.

Vagus nerve is situated behind the ICA in carotid sheath and lesions arising in this area displace the carotid anteriorly. Sympathetic chain lies along the posteromedial border of carotid sheath and displace it anteriorly **(Fig. 8)**.

If schwannoma extends through the skull base, foramen will be smoothly enlarged in contrast to malignant lesions where foramen will be ill-defined and shaggy.

Ganglioneuromas and malignant nerve sheath tumors are rarely reported, and on imaging, it is indistinguishable from schwannoma **(Fig. 9)**.

Paragangliomas

Paragangliomas represent 10–15% of all PPS lesions. Depending on the sites of origin, they occur in three different varieties:
1. Carotid body tumor
2. Glomus vagale
3. Glomus jugulare.

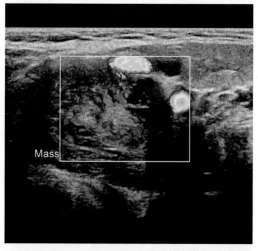

Fig. 8: Duplex Doppler image of parapharyngeal schwannoma displacing the carotid sheath anteriorly.

Carotid body tumor: The carotid body tumor arises from carotid body cells near the carotid bifurcation. This tumor completely fills and splays the carotid bifurcation, exhibiting the "Lyre's sign" on imaging **(Fig. 10)**. In some cases, the tumor may surround the external carotid artery or rarely the internal carotid

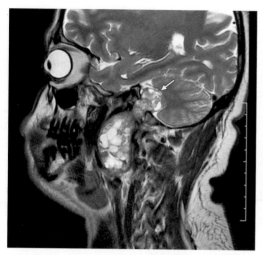

Fig. 9: T2 sagittal MRI showing vagal schwannoma with intracranial extension.

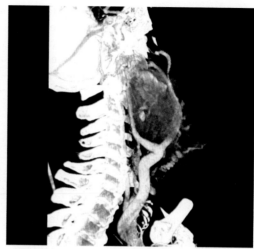

Fig. 10: CT angiogram showing splaying of carotid bifurcation in a carotid body tumor (Lyre sign).

artery. Bilateral carotid body tumor can occur in 5–14% of sporadic tumors. Both right and left carotid arteries should be thoroughly examined in suspected case to rule out multiple lesions.

Dynamic CT scan done shows intense enhancement in the early phase with washout of contrast in delayed phase due to rich tumor blood flow **(Fig. 11)**. This differentiates the carotid body tumor from a hypovascular lesion such as schwannoma which enhances in late phase due to slow extravascular accumulation of contrast in tumor parenchyma.

On MRI, the characteristic "salt and pepper" appearance is seen due to bright tumor parenchyma and dark areas due to signal void from large vascular channels. These are predominantly seen in tumors larger than 2 cm in diameter. CT angiography is routinely being used to demonstrate the blood vessels supplying the tumor.

Conventional angiogram is still the gold standard for evaluating the tumor vascularity. Preoperative embolization is not advisable in carotid body tumors due to risk of embolization after inadvertent material reflux into the internal carotid artery.

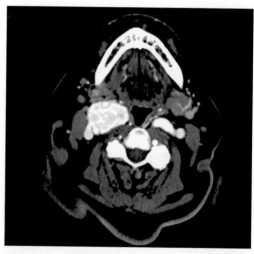

Fig. 11: Axial CT image showing intensely enhancing carotid body tumor with splaying of the vessels.

Glomus vagale: This paraganglioma arises from the nodose ganglion located just below the skull base along the vagus nerve anterior to internal jugular vein. These tumors lie entirely within the PPS and very rarely can extend to the posterior fossa through jugular foramen.

Glomus jugulare: This paraganglioma arises from the paraganglion cells around the jugular ganglion. This ganglion is more cranial and located within jugular foramen. These tumors spread above and below the skull base in equal bulk. Glomus jugulare can erode the skull base and extend into middle ear cleft **(Fig. 12)**.

Glomus vagale and glomus jugulare displace the internal carotid artery anteriorly. Lesion shows a smoothly marginated ovoid mass with vascular flow voids giving a salt and pepper appearance in the T2W MR image. Conventional angiogram is needed for preoperative embolization which can reduce bloodshed during surgery, especially for larger tumors.

Glomus vagale have about 10% incidence of malignancy and glomus jugulare have a 3% incidence of distal metastases.

Benign Soft Tissue Mass/Cysts

Teratoma is a rare tumor and is seen in newborns or infants. CT is useful in the evaluation of these tumors as they can show calcification, cystic areas, and fatty regions **(Fig. 13)**.

Spindle cell neoplasm like solitary fibrous tumors and desmoplastic fibroma (usually pleural based) are also encountered in PPS. MR signal intensity of the tumor will be low in both T1- and T2-weighted MR images.

Branchial cysts of second arch can also be seen in PPS. Second branchial pouch contributes to tonsillar fossa, and cysts are found on the anteromedial aspect of carotid sheath. Cysts have a thin wall and homogeneous fluid attenuation. On MRI, they show bright signal on T2-weighted images and dark signal on T1-weighted images after contrast; only the wall enhances. When the cyst gets infected, the imaging appearance resembles that of an abscess, showing thick enhancing wall and contents show more bright signal on T1-weighted images.

Cystic lymphangioma and cystic hygromas are seen in children below 2 years. They are seen as large cystic mass with thin septae. Lipomas of PPS show high signal on T1- and T2-weighted MR images and fat density on CT scan.

Lymph Nodes

They are the nodes along the upper internal jugular chain. Nodes are either infective or metastatic. Ultrasonography with guided fine

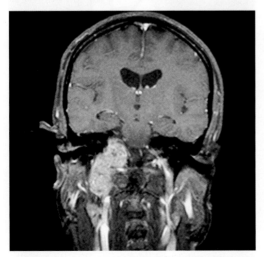

Fig. 12: Coronal MR image showing glomus jugulare.

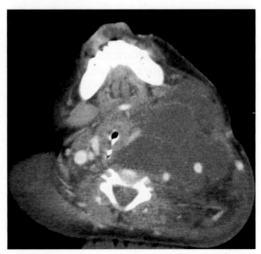

Fig. 13: Axial CT image showing cystic hygroma compressing the airway.

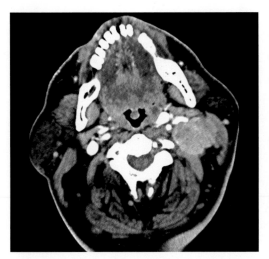

Fig. 14: Axial CT image showing node in the left carotid space.

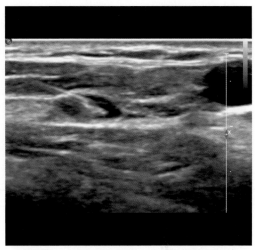

Fig. 15: Ultrasound-guided fine needle aspiration cytology of the node.

needle aspiration cytology is modality of choice for evaluation of these lesions **(Figs. 14 and 15)**.

Diseases/Tumors Arising from the Skull Base

Bony or cartilaginous lesion from skull base can protrude into parapharyngeal space. Tumors include osteoma, osteogenic sarcoma, chondrosarcoma, fibro-osseous lesions, and osteochondroma. These tumors are better diagnosed with CT than MRI.

Diseases or Tumors Arising Intracranially

Intracranial tumors can rarely extend through skull base and project into PPS. Meningioma can extend down rarely and form a bulky neck mass **(Fig. 16)**.

Giant aneurysm of internal carotid artery can present as a vascular mass in PPS. Internal carotid artery dissection, thrombus in the carotid artery, and internal jugular vein can present as a mass in PPS.

Computed tomography and MRI imaging provides a noninvasive means of diagnosing these vascular lesions in neck. Conventional angiography is also reliable.

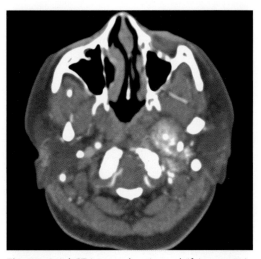

Fig. 16: Axial CT image showing calcifying mass in the left parapharyngeal space (PPS) (meningioma extending into PPS).

Other Tumors

Other rare tumors encountered are rhabdomyosarcoma, lymphoma, infiltrating nasopharyngeal and oropharyngeal carcinoma, hemangiopericytoma and lipoma.

Role of imaging lies mainly in assessing the site and extent of the lesion and to guide in the biopsy of these deep-seated lesions.

● FURTHER READING

1. Bass RM. Approaches to the diagnosis and treatment of tumors of the parapharyngeal space. Head Neck Surg. 1982;4(4):281-9.
2. Biswas S, Saha S, Sadhu A. Pictorial essay - Parapharyngeal space lesion. Indian J Radiol Imaging. 2005;15(1):41-6.
3. Som PM, Curtine HD. Parapharyngeal and masticator space lesions. Head and Neck Imaging, 4th edition. Mosby Publishers; 2003. pp. 1954-87.
4. Shin JH, Lee HK, Kim SY, et al. Imaging of parapharyngeal space lesions: Focus on the prestyloid compartment. AJR Am J Roentgenol. 2001;177(6):1465-70.

CHAPTER 13

Parapharyngeal Space Tumors

Mahamaya Prasad Singh, Krishnakumar Thankappan

• INTRODUCTION

It is a potential space, inverted pyramid shaped, as its name implies, lies laterally on both sides of the upper pharynx. It has many synonyms like pterygomaxillary, pharyngomaxillary, pterygopharyngeal, and lateral pharyngeal space. Detailed understanding of this space is crucial for correct diagnosis and treatment of various tumors of this region. Great advancement in radiology has helped the surgeons to a great extent in this regard.

• ANATOMY

The parapharyngeal space (PPS) is an inverted pyramid in shape and extends from the skull base to the greater cornu of the hyoid bone (Refer to Figs. 1 to 3 of Chapter 12 for anatomy).

• BOUNDARIES

- *Superiorly:* Small area of the temporal and sphenoid bones, including the carotid canal, jugular foramen, and hypoglossal foramen
- *Anteriorly:* Pterygomandibular raphe and pterygoid fascia
- *Posteriorly:* Cervical vertebrae and prevertebral muscles
- *Medially:* The buccopharyngeal fascia covering the superior constrictor muscle
- *Laterally:* Ramus of the mandible, the medial pterygoid muscle, and the deep lobe of the parotid gland; below the level of the mandible by the fascia overlying the posterior belly of the digastric muscle.

The PPS is divided into an anteromedial or prestyloid compartment and a posterolateral or poststyloid compartment by the fascia from the styloid process to the tensor veli palatine. The prestyloid compartment contains the retromandibular portion of the parotid gland, adipose tissue, and lymph nodes. The poststyloid compartment contains the carotid artery, the internal jugular vein, cranial nerves IX–XII, the sympathetic chain, and lymph nodes.

These lymphatics receive afferent drainage from the oral cavity, oropharynx, paranasal sinuses, and thyroid.

• TUMORS OF THE PARAPHARYNGEAL SPACE

Tumors of the PPS are uncommon, comprising less than 1% of all head and neck neoplasms. Both benign and malignant tumors may arise from any of the structures contained within the PPS. Of the tumors, 70–80% is benign, and 20–30% is malignant.

Salivary Tumors

This is the most common neoplasm to involve the PPS, invariably located in the prestyloid compartment and almost always arising from the deep lobe of parotid. A minority of tumors arise from the extraparotid salivary glands in the PPS.

Neurogenic Tumors

This involves the poststyloid compartment. Most commonly are paraganglioma, schwannoma, and neurofibroma. Other tumors are extremely rare. Up to 10% of paragangliomas can be malignant. Schwannomas are the most common neurogenic tumors of the PPS.

Rare Tumors of the PPS

This space contains variety of tissues any of which can potentially become neoplastic. Lipoma, sarcoma, rhabdomyoma, rhabdomyosarcoma, leiomyosarcoma, hemangiopericytoma, intravascular papillary endothelial hyperplasia or Masson's tumor, and extracranial meningioma are few of the rare tumors of the PPS.

Metastasis to PPS

From nasopharyngeal carcinoma, 30% of undifferentiated carcinoma metastasizes to PPS in 5 years. Maxillary carcinoma and occult thyroid cancer can give metastasis to PPS. Regions outside head and neck like breast cancer can also metastasize to PPS.

● CLINICAL PRESENTATION

Neck swelling is the most common presentation, accounting for about half of the cases. Tumors more than 2 cm of size may medially displace the oropharyngeal wall or the lateral pharyngeal wall leading to symptoms of obstructive sleep apnea, dyspnea, and dysphagia. Often, a PPS lesion is discovered incidentally on routine physical examination. High poststyloid lesion can compress the eustachian tube and present with middle ear effusion.

Tumors in this space can involve the cranial nerves resulting in symptoms of hoarseness, dysarthria, and dysphagia. Horner syndrome may result from pressure on the cervical sympathetic chain.

Pain may be found in 10–20% of cases. Pain is often indicative of malignancy with infiltration of the skull base. But, it may be associated with benign lesions, because of compression and hemorrhage.

Syncope can be a presenting symptom for primary or secondary malignancy involving the glossopharyngeal nerve, and in particular, the carotid sinus or may be associated with benign lesion pressing over carotid sinus. Tumors like neuroblastoma, small cell neuroendocrine carcinoma, adenoid cystic carcinoma, undifferentiated carcinoma, though rare in PPS, can present with syndrome of inappropriate antidiuretic hormone secretion.

Fine Needle Aspiration Cytology

Fine needle aspiration is an important tool with high accuracy rate. When the tumor is inaccessible it may be combined with computed tomography (CT); in some cases, ultrasonography is sufficient. An idea of the preoperative histopathology helps the surgeon to plan and explain the patient.

Radiology

Imaging studies should be done to know whether the mass is prestyloid or poststyloid, relationship of the tumor to parotid gland and great vessels, to ascertain the soft tissue characteristics of the tumor. MRI, particularly useful in PPS as the soft tissue resolution is better compared to CT scan and it can accurately distinguish between vascular and nonvascular tumor. There are characteristic appearances of different tumors on MRI. Pleomorphic adenomas have low intensity signal in T1 images and high on T2 images, and displace carotid posteriorly. Schwannomas have higher signal intensity at T2 images but displaces carotid anteriorly. Paragangliomas have characteristic "salt and pepper" appearance on T2-weighted images because of flow voids. CT allows deep soft tissue planes to be evaluated and also provides excellent bony details. Positron emission tomography (PET) scan is better in detecting recurrences.

Shamblin's classification is commonly used to stage carotid body tumors and though this is based on intraoperative findings, it can be applied to radiologic findings prior to treatment.

- *Type I*: Relatively small tumor with minimal attachment to the carotid vessels.
- *Type II*: Larger tumor with moderate attachment but carotid vessels can be preserved.
- *Type III*: Tumor encases the carotid vessel requiring arterial sacrifice with reconstruction.

Angiography

Angiography is recommended in the workup of most vascular lesions and also useful in the evaluation of poststyloid lesions to demonstrate their relationship to the great vessels. Findings on angiography may be diagnostic of neurogenic lesions. Carotid body tumors are usually located at the bifurcation and cause splaying of the carotid bifurcation, called the "Lyre sign".

Please refer to the Chapter 12 on radiology for the details on imaging in parapharyngeal space tumors.

Balloon Occlusion Test

The balloon occlusion test measures the effect of internal carotid artery occlusion on cerebral blood flow and the adequacy of the contralateral circulation. It is indicated when carotid resection is planned for tumor clearance.

MIBG Scan

If screening for a functional paraganglioma by urinary vanillylmandelic acid and metanephrine levels is positive, then we need to obtain an MIBG (metaiodobenzylguanidine) scan. This radioisotope has a similar molecular structure to norepinephrine and is used to trace catecholamine uptake and storage.

Metastatic Workup

If a metastatic lesion is suspected, the primary tumor should be sought by performing a full clinical evaluation, panendoscopy, and a full metastatic workup as directed by the clinical examination findings.

● TREATMENT

Wait and watch policy can be applied to lipoma or carotid body tumor in an elderly patient without any symptoms.

Surgical Treatment

Surgical excision is the treatment of choice. Malignant tumors may require adjuvant radiotherapy.

● APPROACHES TO THE PARAPHARYNGEAL SPACE

Transoral Approach

The transoral approach has been described for the removal of small and benign neoplasms that originate in the prestyloid PPS and manifest as an oropharyngeal mass. The limitations of this approach are limited exposure, inability to visualize the great vessels, and an increased risk of facial nerve injury and increased risk of tumor spillage.

Transcervical Approach

Most authors recommend this approach as the method for removal of most poststyloid PPS tumors. A transverse incision at the level of the hyoid bone or 2 finger breadths below the mandible is performed, with submandibular gland either retracted anteriorly or removed, if necessary. The carotid artery and internal jugular vein are identified. The digastric, stylohyoid and styloglossus muscles are retracted to allow access to the PPS. Most of the benign tumors except the high vascular tumors can be removed with this approach.

Transcervical–Transparotid Approach

The transcervical approach can be combined with a transparotid approach by extending the incision superiorly for tumors arising from the deep lobe of the parotid. The facial nerve is identified and dissected, superficial parotidectomy is performed, and the deep lobe portion of the tumor is identified. The cervical incision allows access to the PPS component of the tumor.

Transcervical–Transmandibular Approach

For very large tumors, vascular tumors with superior PPS extension, malignancies in which better exposure facilitates oncologic resection, and cases in which distal control of the carotid at the skull base is required, the transcervical approach may be combined with mandibulotomy for better exposure. A lip-splitting incision is used to expose the mandible and after mandibulotomy, incision given intraorally along the floor of the mouth and the mandible is retracted laterally.

Infratemporal Fossa Approach

A preauricular infratemporal fossa approach, as described by Fisch, can be used for tumors involving the skull base or jugular foramen. This approach can be combined with frontotemporal craniotomy for removal of tumors with significant intracranial extension.

Transoral Robotic Surgery

Transoral robotic surgery (TORS) is latest tool for resection of PPS tumor but is highly expensive and not readily available.

Complications of Parapharyngeal Tumor Surgery

- *Vascular injury*: Advancement in diagnostic methods, preoperative planning, and microsurgical techniques has reduced the risk of internal carotid artery (ICA) injury and sacrifice. But large tumors may require resection with a stroke rate of 0–2%.
- *Baroreflex failure*: Resection of bilateral carotid body tumors leads to loss of baroreceptor reflex which results in labile refractory hypertension, tachycardia, headache, etc.
- *Cranial nerve injury*: Risk of injury to lower cranial nerves depends on the histology, size, and location of the tumor. Single nerve injury may result in temporary swallowing difficulty, dysphonia, tongue movement problems, and/or aspiration problems from which the patients recover gradually but multiple nerve injuries have additive effects and are poorly tolerated by the patients. Sympathetic chain injury leads to Horner's syndrome. Denervation hypersensitivity of the myoepithelial cells of the parotid gland can lead to first bite syndrome, which is intense pain with first bite and it improves gradually after that.

● CONCLUSION

Understanding the anatomy and pathology of the tumors of this space is crucial for correct diagnosis and planning of treatment. Radiology has helped the surgeons to a great extent in this regard. Preoperative counseling to be done regarding the surgical morbidity.

● FURTHER READING

1. Andrews JC, Valavanis A, Fisch U. Management of the internal carotid artery in surgery of the skull base. Laryngoscope. 1989;99(12):1224-9.
2. Carrau RL, Meyers EN, Johnson JT. Management of tumors arising in the parapharyngeal space. Laryngoscope. 1990;100(6):583-9.

3. Cross RR, Shapiro MD, Som PM. MRI of the parapharyngeal space. Radiol Clin North Am. 1989;27(2):353-78.

4. Hinerman RW, Mendenhall WM, Amdur RJ, et al. Definitive radiotherapy in the management of chemodectomas arising in the temporal bone, carotid body, and glomus vagale. Head Neck. 2001;23(5):363-71.

5. Netterville JL, Jackson CG, Miller FR, et al. Vagal paraganglioma: A review of 46 patients treated during a 20-year period. Arch Otolaryngol Head Neck Surg. 1998;124(10):1133-40.

6. Oslen KD. Tumors and surgery of the parapharyngeal space. Laryngoscope. 1994;104(5 Pt 2 Suppl 63):1-28.

CHAPTER 14

Tumors of Infratemporal Fossa: Approaches and Management

Divya GM

● INTRODUCTION

The infratemporal fossa (ITF) is a deeply situated area having a complex anatomy with communications to many surrounding areas. This area can give rise to a range of benign and malignant tumors. Lesions in this area, with the exception of those with an inherent rapid growth pattern, may continue to grow unnoticed for a considerable period and delay the diagnosis. This delay in diagnosis, extensive disease, and the course of critical neurovascular structures through ITF in intimate association with one another pose a challenging scenario.

● SURGICAL ANATOMY

Infratemporal fossa is roughly quadrangular in shape **(Fig. 1)**. It is bounded superiorly by the greater wing of the sphenoid medially and a part of the squama of the temporal bone laterally. The anterior boundary is formed by the posterior surface of the maxilla and posteriorly it is related to styloid apparatus, carotid sheath, and deep part of the parotid gland. The lateral boundary is formed by the zygomatic arch, masseter, and temporalis muscles, and the ascending ramus of the mandible and medial boundary is by the lateral surface of the lateral pterygoid plate, and the superior constrictor muscle of the pharynx. The bony boundaries are depicted in **Figure 2**. The ITF has no anatomical floor; it is limited anteriorly by the attachment of the medial pterygoid muscle and communicates with the parapharyngeal space anterior to the internal carotid artery.

The contents of the ITF are the medial and lateral pterygoid muscles, the mandibular division of the trigeminal nerve (V3), chorda tympani branch of facial nerve, otic ganglion, internal maxillary artery, and pterygoid venous plexus. The lateral pterygoid muscle arising from the infratemporal surface of the skull and the lateral aspect of the lateral pterygoid plate inserting into the mandibular condyle, crosses the entire ITF in an anterior-posterior direction and effectively divides the ITF into superior and inferior compartments.

The ITF communicates with the temporal fossa deep to the zygomatic arch. It communicates with the pterygopalatine fossa through the pterygomaxillary fissure and orbit via the inferior orbital fissure. It is connected to the middle cranial fossa via the foramen ovale and foramen spinosum. Because of these communications, tumors of ITF can easily spread to various surrounding areas.

● CLASSIFICATION OF TUMORS OF INFRATEMPORAL FOSSA

The ITF encounters various types of pathologies. A systematic classification of tumors of the ITF was first put forward by Conley and according to him they are classified as primary, contiguous,

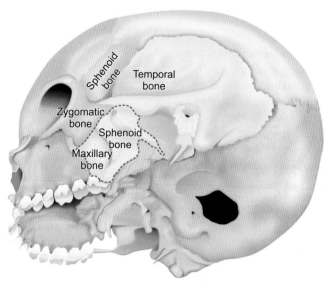

Fig. 1: Infratemporal fossa in quadrangular shape.

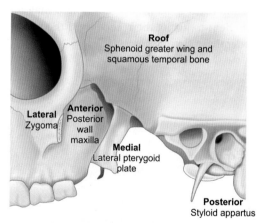

Fig. 2: Bony boundaries.

and metastatic. Extension of tumors from adjoining anatomical areas such as the maxilla, nasal cavity, nasopharynx, sphenoid, mandible, parotid gland, external acoustic meatus, and the cranial cavity are termed contiguous. This is the largest group and comprises both benign and malignant tumors. Approach to the ITF is then combined with the approach to the location of the primary pathology to obtain en

bloc excision. This group of tumors is diagnosed relatively early because they usually present with symptoms pertaining to the site of their origin.

Primary tumors of the ITF are mesodermal in origin and comprise 25–30% of all the tumors seen in the area. Both benign and malignant tumors are encountered and they may remain undiagnosed for long periods of time. The symptoms are few and insidious and often referred to other areas. Conductive hearing loss, trismus, and sensory disturbances of the face are often present, but their onset may be so gradual that the patient may not have taken them seriously for a long time before seeking medical attention. The primary ITF tumors include meningioma, schwannoma, neurofibroma, malignant lymphoma, hemangioma, rhabdomyosarcoma, fibrosarcoma, and histocytosis X.

Metastatic tumors to the ITF by the hematogenous route are rare, but there are reports on metastases to ITF from lung, ovary, and breast carcinoma.

● DIAGNOSIS

The essential prerequisites in the management of ITF tumors are histopathology and assessment of tumor extension. Radiographic imaging is the vital component for knowing the exact extent of the tumor, owing to the inaccessibility of the ITF to physical examination. Both computed tomography (CT) and magnetic resonance imaging (MRI) provide valuable information and are obtained using standard skull base protocols. CT is superior to MRI in showing the remodeling or erosion of neurovascular foramina or other bones of the skull base. MRI better delineates the soft tissue planes, the tumor–soft tissue interface, and the presence of tumor along neural and vascular structures **(Figs. 3A and B)**. It may also help to identify the tissue of origin of the tumor to some extent, but is difficult in large tumors and those with multiple extensions CT and MRI are often complementary.

The relationship of the tumor to the ICA is a crucial issue and this information can be obtained noninvasively by magnetic resonance angiography (MRA) and computed tomography angiography (CTA). Angiography is preferred, if preoperative embolization of the tumor is indicated. If the risk for injury or sacrifice of the ICA is high, the collateral cerebral blood flow may be evaluated using angiography balloon occlusion with xenon CT.

In majority of cases, a histologic diagnosis can be obtained by aspiration cytology, but in deep-seated lesions, a CT-guided and fine needle aspiration may be needed. If cytology is not conclusive or in suspected cases of soft-tissue sarcomas, biopsy is indicated. The transantral and transoral route via the gingivolabial sulcus are the most frequently used routes for obtaining a biopsy. Rarely, a histologic diagnosis cannot be obtained before the approach. A frozen section analysis, obtained via a skull base approach, may be sufficient to justify the resection of the tumor under these circumstances.

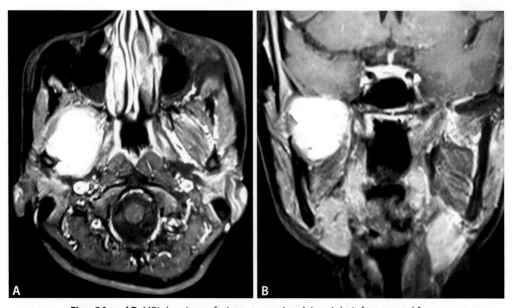

Figs. 3A and B: MRI showing soft tissue tumor involving right infratemporal fossa.

● PATIENT SELECTION

For the therapeutic-surgical plan, assessment of the nature, origin, and extension of the tumor is crucial. The selection of the surgical approach is also affected by other factors as patient needs and demands the biologic behavior of the tumor, other coexistent diseases, and the training and experience of the surgeon. A multidisciplinary approach is needed in most pathologies affecting the ITF to stage, diagnose, and extirpate the tumor, and at the same time to provide an acceptable cosmetic and functional reconstruction.

● APPROACHES TO INFRATEMPORAL FOSSA

The advances in imaging, surgical techniques developed in the fields of head and neck, craniofacial, orthognathic, and skull base surgery, and an improved understanding of the anatomy of the skull base have improved and modified the surgical approaches to the ITF.

The approach to ITF may be anterior, lateral or combinations.

- *Anterior*:
  - Transmandibular
  - Transfacial
  - Intraoral.
- *Lateral*:
  - Transmandibular
  - Transzygomatic
  - Subtemporal preauricular approach
  - Lateral Fisch approaches.
- *Combinations*: These approaches may be combined with a (fronto) temporal craniotomy as necessary.

Anterior Approaches

Transmandibular: Mandibular or Extended Mandibular Swing

This approach provides good control of the vessels and nerves and en bloc resection of nasopharynx, posterior maxilla, ITF structures, mandibular ramus, and parotid gland. Here the lower lip is divided in the midline **(Fig. 4A)**, the mandible is sectioned anterior to the mental foramen, and the hemimandible swung laterally, providing the exposure **(Fig. 4B)**. The procedure has been modified by Attia et al. by a second osteotomy of the mandibular ramus above the lingula to allow the ascending ramus to be retracted further laterally and superiorly for improved access.

Transfacial Approaches

Facial translocation: Janecka described this approach which combined facial soft tissue translocation and craniofacial osteotomies. The facial incision resembles a Weber–Ferguson incision. Craniofacial osteotomies include the maxilla with floor of the orbit and complete zygoma as separate units. The coronoid process is also removed giving an excellent exposure. At the end of the procedure the removed bones are replaced and fixed by miniplates.

Pedicled bone cheek flaps: The basic concept of the transfacial approaches is the mobilization of pedicled bone cheek flaps (PBCF) in which the midfacial bone segment remains pedicled to the soft tissues of the cheek thereby retaining their blood supply. According to the classification system proposed by Clauser **(Table 1)**, there are four levels of transfacial approaches with the aim of simplifying surgical planning. The approach is determined by the anatomical site of the lesion.

The transfacial approach providing maximum access to the ITF is the Maxillo-Cheek Flap (MCF) combined with the mandibular cheek flap. By taking the maxilla laterally out of the operative field, the MCF removes the anterior boundary of the ITF. The inclusion of the zygoma and/or the mandible from either an anterior or lateral approach then removes its lateral boundary. The addition of a (fronto) temporal craniotomy allows the

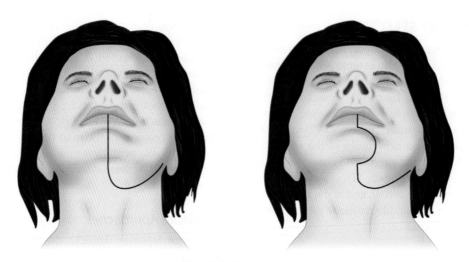

Fig. 4A: Midline lip-split.

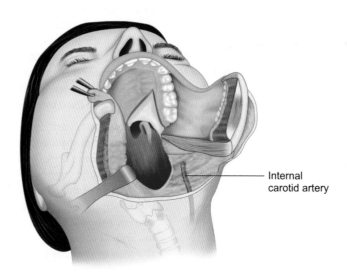

Internal
carotid artery

Fig. 4B: Left paramedian mandibulotomy.

roof to be removed under direct vision. These combination approaches give a wide exposure to ITF.

Maxillary swing: Wei, et al. described this technique. Here the maxilla is separated from the facial skeleton, but remains attached anteriorly to the cheek flap and is known to offer excellent exposure to midline structures. The major limitation of the maxillary swing

is limited exposure of tumors involving the petrotemporal compartment of the skull base, as well as extension into the middle cranial fossa.

Intraoral Approaches

These approaches provide limited access that cannot be easily extended peroperatively. The superior gingivolabial sulcus posteriorly is close to the tuberosity of the maxilla and provides

Table 1: Transfacial approaches.

Levels	Extent of lesions	Approach
Level 1	Lesions of the ethmoid, sphenoid, upper nasopharynx, and anterior cranial base	Nasal cheek flap + Le Fort I Optional: Nasal Maxillo-cheek Flap (NMCF)
Level 2	Lesions involving the retropharynx and clivus	NMCF ± Contralateral Maxillo-cheek Flap (MCF)
Level 3	Lesions of the retromaxilla or pterygomaxillary space	MCF
Level 4	Lesions of the parapharyngeal space or infratemporal fossa	MCF or mandibular cheek flap or combination of the two

access to the lower part of the ITF. They can provide access for biopsy purposes and very occasionally can be employed for the removal of small, benign, and well-circumscribed lesions.

Le Fort I approach: After down-fracturing the maxilla, removal of the posterolateral wall of the maxilla provides limited exposure to the ITF, by removing its anterior boundary.

Transantral approach: The anterior, lateral, medial, and posterior walls of the maxilla are removed leaving the alveolus and the orbital floor intact. This will give minimal access to the ITF and nasopharynx.

Transpalatine approach: Limited exposure of the inferomedial aspect of the ITF can be achieved with this approach.

Lateral Approaches

Lateral Transmandibular Approaches

The exposure of the ITF obtained from a lateral approach via the mandible is variable. An osteotomy of the mandibular ramus with separation/distraction of the bone ends can provide limited exposure. More extensive exposure similar to that achieved with the extended mandibular swing may be achieved by elevation of the ascending ramus and masseter muscle out of the operative field with a simple osteotomy at the junction of the body and ascending ramus. By resection of the ascending ramus of the mandible, wide lateral exposure of the ITF and adjacent areas may be obtained.

Lateral Transzygomatic Approach

The lateral transzygomatic approaches to the ITF and adjacent areas involve the disarticulation and inferior displacement of the zygoma, usually pedicled to the masseter muscle, as well as the displacement of the temporalis muscle. The temporalis muscle may be displaced in either a superior or inferior direction. These techniques improve access to the superior compartment of the ITF by removing its lateral boundary.

Subtemporal Preauricular Approach

This approach uses a preauricular incision. It involves dividing the zygomatic arch and displacing it inferiorly, dividing the malar eminence (zygoma) and displacing it anteriorly, and cutting the coronoid process and retracting it superiorly with the attached temporalis muscle. Reconstruction is accomplished by using the temporalis muscle or a pericranial flap to cover the dura, a free fat graft to fill the space left by tumor excision, and by wiring the zygomatic arch and malar eminence into their original positions. It can be combined with intradural approaches to provide additional exposure to the anterior and middle cranial fossa, cavernous sinus, and sella turcica. Extradurally, the orbit, pterygopalatine fossa, and nasopharynx can also be addressed using this approach.

Lateral Fisch Approaches

Access to the ITF and adjacent areas using the lateral approach was described by Fisch et al. Fisch has offered three basic approaches. The type A approach consists of radical mastoidectomy, anterior transposition of the facial nerve, and exploration of the posterior ITF. The Fisch type B and C approaches are designed to approach more anterior pathology involving the petrous apex, clivus, and superior ITF. The type C approach is an extension of the type B approach, and is used for lesions of the anterior ITF, sella, and nasopharynx. These approaches are by postauricular incision.

The type D approach is a preauricular ITF approach that uses orbitozygomatic osteotomies and resection of the floor of the middle fossa to expose the medial middle cranial fossa without a lateral temporal craniotomy. Subtype D1 addresses tumors of the anterior ITF, while the subtype D2 is designed for lateral orbital wall lesions and high pterygopalatine fossa tumors. Although these preauricular approaches do not include a temporal craniotomy, the floor of the skull base can be drilled away to allow full access to the ITF.

There is no one correct/ideal approach to the ITF. The only requirements are that the approach adopted should provide adequate access for the lesion, and the morbidity of the approach is considered acceptable.

Endoscopic Approach to the Infratemporal Fossa

The endoscopic endonasal approach provides an alternative to open surgical approaches. A transmaxillary corridor with transpterygoid dissection is used to expose the pterygopalatine fossa. Further removal of the posterior wall of the maxillary sinus transgresses the pterygomaxillary fossa to provide access to the ITF.

● **FURTHER READING**

1. Givi B, Liu J, Bilsky M, et al. Outcome of resection of infratemporal fossa tumors. Head Neck. 2013;35(11):1567-72.
2. Janecka IP, Sen CN, Sekhar LN, et al. Facial translocation: A new approach to the cranial base. Otolaryngol Head Neck Surg. 1990;103(3):413-9.
3. McCoul ED, Schwartz TH, Anand VK. Endoscopic approach to the infratemporal fossa. Operative Techniques in Otolaryngology. 2011;22(4):285-90.
4. Sekhar LN, Schramm VL Jr, Jones NF. Subtemporal-preauricular infratemporal fossa approach to large lateral and posterior cranial base neoplasms. J Neurosurg. 1987;67(4):488-99.
5. Taylor RJ, Patel MR, Wheless SA, et al. Endoscopic endonasal approaches to infratemporal fossa tumors: A classification system and case series. Laryngoscope. 2014;124(11):2443-50.

CHAPTER 15

Malignant Tumors of the Temporal Bone

Deepak Balasubramanian

• INTRODUCTION

Tumors of the temporal bone are a rare group of malignancies in the head and neck. They usually are epithelial tumors which can occur primarily in the skin of the external auditory canal (EAC). Tumors can also arise from the lining of the middle ear and the mastoid. The temporal bone can be secondarily involved from tumors of the salivary gland and superior extension from the infratemporal fossa. The close relation of the hearing apparatus, facial nerve, the structures traversing the jugular foramen, and the carotid artery make managing these tumors challenging.

• ETIOLOGY

As with a majority of the epithelial tumors, ultraviolet exposure has been implicated in the development of these tumors. Chronic ear infections have also been linked to development of these tumors. A prior history of radiation has also been identified as a risk factor; however, due to the rarity of these tumors, the causative factors have not yet been fully explained.

• SPECTRUM OF MALIGNANCIES IN THE TEMPORAL BONE

The temporal bone forms part of the lateral skull base. The pinna and the EAC are skin lined and have with them the adnexal structures. Most commonly, squamous cell carcinomas occur in the skin lined portion. Other skin tumors like basal cell carcinoma can arise from the EAC. Malignant melanomas, adenocarcinomas, adenoid cystic carcinomas, and tumors arising from the adnexal structures can also occur. The pinna and the EAC also have a cartilaginous scaffold and hence tumors of the cartilage can also arise from these areas. Bone tumors can arise from any part of the temporal bone. More commonly in clinical practice, advanced salivary gland malignancies, tumors of the skull base, and skin tumors can secondarily invade the temporal bone. So, a wide variety of tumors can affect the temporal bone. The biological behavior and more importantly the extent of the tumor dictate the management.

• PATHWAYS OF TUMOR SPREAD IN THE TEMPORAL BONE

From a practical point of view, the tumors of the temporal bone can be divided as those arising from the external ear, middle ear—mastoid, and temporal bone involvement from extension of tumor from extratemporal sites. The pinna and the EAC form a contiguous structure, being separated from the middle ear by the tympanic membrane. Tumors affecting the pinna tend to involve the cartilage of the pinna and by contiguous spread involve the EAC. The tympanic membrane offers little resistance to tumor spread. Through the foramina in the bone, the tumor can spread to the periparotid tissue inferiorly. Medial extension beyond the middle ear puts at risk the neurovascular structures at the skull base. Intracranial extension could result in temporal lobe invasion by the tumor. Invasion of the mastoid cavity also puts the sigmoid sinus at risk.

CLINICAL PRESENTATION

A majority of these tumors present between the 4th and 6th decades of life with the exception of rhabdomyosarcoma which have a younger age of presentation. The common symptom is pain with otorrhea and mass in the EAC. This must be differentiated from aural granulations and polyps. The diagnosis of malignancy becomes more apparent once adjacent structures are involved with bone destruction with or without cranial nerve involvement. However long-standing middle ear infections can produce a similar picture. Extensive tumors can present with periauricular swelling, cavernous sinus involvement, and temporomandibular joint infiltration, with or without neck nodes.

CLINICAL EVALUATION

Clinical evaluation begins with the examination of an otoscopic examination. A mass in the EAC or growth in the pinna needs to be biopsied. Special consideration is to be given to assess hearing; however, a majority of these patients do have conductive hearing loss. The cranial nerves need to be examined to rule out extension to the mastoid, cavernous sinus, or the jugular foramen. Temporal lobe signs also have to be excluded to rule out intraparenchymal extension.

Imaging techniques should encompass modalities which can adequately delineate the bony and soft tissue extent of the tumor. CT scan with contrast depicts bone erosions and sclerosis whereas contrast enhanced

MRI is helpful in delineating the soft tissue extent, dural involvement, cavernous invasion, perineural invasion, and the intracranial extension. In advanced disease, the neck needs to be evaluated for nodal metastasis. Attention should be paid to the peri- and intraparotid lymph nodes, the postauricular lymph nodes, and the retropharyngeal lymph nodes.

A special area of interest while imaging these patients is to study the internal carotid artery. When surgical management is contemplated, the petrous carotid needs to be assessed for tumor invasion or encasement. While carotid artery sacrifice is not performed in malignancies with poor outcomes, a more selective approach to carotid sacrifice can be made based on patient factors, tumor factors, and adequacy of cerebral cross circulation. The adequacy of cerebral perfusion can be ascertained by a balloon occlusion test or a cerebral xenon perfusion scan.

STAGING

The commonly used staging system is the Pittsburg staging system which divides tumors between T1 and T4 **(Table 1)**.

Table 1: Modified Pittsburgh staging system for temporal bone carcinomas.

T1	Tumor limited to the EAC without bone erosion, or soft tissue involvement
T2	Tumor with bone erosion limited to the EAC (without involving the entire thickness) or limited involvement (<0.5 cm) of soft tissues
T3	Tumor with bone erosion throughout the EAC thickness with limited involvement (<0.5 cm) of soft tissues, or tumor involving the middle ear/mastoid
T4	Tumor with erosion of the cochlea, petrous apex, medial wall of the middle ear, carotid canal, jugular foramen or dura, or large involvement (>0.5 cm) of soft tissues (e.g. involvement of the temporomandibular joint, styloid apophysis) or evidence of peripheral facial paralysis

(EAC: External auditory canal)

• TREATMENT

Surgery is the primary modality of choice in managing these tumors. Resection of the temporal bone along with the required soft tissue margins forms the mainstay. Temporal bone resections are divided into:

- *Lateral temporal bone resection* wherein the structures lateral to the stapes are removed. The resection can include the pinna if it is involved, otherwise the pinna can be preserved and the EAC blind sacked. The goal of the operation is to remove the EAC en bloc including the tympanic membrane, malleus, and incus. A cortical mastoidectomy is done and the middle ear cut is entered through a posterior tympanotomy. The zygoma, capsule of the TMJ, the tegmen, cochlea, and the sigmoid sinus form the boundaries for the resection. This is usually indicated for T1–T2 tumors which have not involved the middle ear.
- *Subtotal temporal bone resection* wherein the medial extent of resection is up to the petrous apex but does not include it. This is indicated for tumors involving the middle ear. The operation involves securing margins along the middle cranial fossa floor, posterior fossa, internal auditory meatus, and bone along the jugular foramen and carotid canal. The operation may be combined with a middle fossa approach for facilitating the superior bony osteotomy. A part of the petrous apex is preserved. This approach is for more advanced tumors and can be individualized as per the tumor extent. A piecemeal approach may be used when an en bloc resection cannot be achieved especially at the dural margins. Facial nerve rerouting may be considered if the nerve is not involved and functional at the end of the operation.
- *Total temporal bone resection* wherein the whole temporal bone is excised with or without sacrifice of the internal carotid

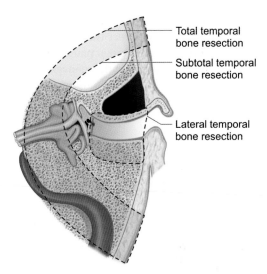

Fig. 1: Temporal bone resections.

artery. This is seldom practiced now due to its morbidity.

The above operations **(Fig. 1)** can be combined with varying degrees of skin excision, parotidectomy and condyle resections. A neck dissection is also frequently performed. In cases of skin loss during resection of tumor, a soft tissue flap can be used to close the defect. Facial nerve reconstruction can be performed with cable grafting or nerve substitution.

Adjuvant Treatment

A majority of the cases usually present in advanced stages thereby requiring combined modality treatment. Postoperative adjuvant radiation is usually given at a dose of 66–70 Gy over 30 fractions.

• PROGNOSIS

These tumors by virtue of their delayed presentations have guarded outcomes. Literature is varied on the survival, but early lesions have a 50–80% 5-year survival whereas advanced lesions have a less than 50% long-term survival. Positive margins, nodal metastasis, dural, and parenchymal invasion and invasion of the periparotid tissue including the facial nerve also adversely affect the outcomes. In unresectable tumors, there is paucity of data, but principles employed in the management of unresectable tumors may be employed in this context as well.

● **FURTHER READING**

1. Beyea JA, Moberly AC. Squamous cell carcinoma of the temporal bone. Otolaryngol Clin North Am. 2015;48(2):281-92.
2. Gidley PW, DeMonte F. Temporal bone malignancies. Neurosurg Clin N Am. 2013;24(1):97-110.

CHAPTER 16

Facial Nerve

Salima Rema Windsor

● INTRODUCTION

The facial nerve dysfunction can dramatically affect quality of life of the patients. Human face forms the principal focus of expression and communication. Motor movements of the facial nerve contribute to eye protection, speech articulation, chewing and swallowing, and emotional expression. Patients with facial palsy suffer not only the functional consequences of impaired facial movement but also psychological impact of skewed facial appearance.

● ANATOMY

Facial nerve is the nerve of second branchial arch and is a mixed nerve. It has motor, sensory (*nervus intermedius*), and autonomic fibers. Course of the nerve can be divided into six named segments **(Table 1)**.

Intracranial (Cisternal)

The facial nerve nucleus is situated in the pons. It receives the corticobulbar fibers from the precentral gyrus. From the nucleus, the facial nerve loops around the abducent nucleus and emerges from the ventral surface of pons anteroinferior to the vestibulocochlear nerve. Here it is joined by *nervus intermedius* (nerve of Wrisberg). They together travel through the cerebellopontine angle to reach the internal acoustic meatus. This segment has no branches.

Table 1: Segments of the facial nerve.

Segment	Length
Intracranial (cisternal)	23–24 mm
Meatal	8 mm
Labyrinthine	3–4 mm
Tympanic	8–11 mm
Mastoid	10–14 mm
Extratemporal	15–20 mm

Meatal

The nerve travels from the porus to the fundus of the internal acoustic meatus. It is located in the anterosuperior quadrant of the internal acoustic meatus above the falciform crest anterior to Bill's bar. Meatal segment also has no branches.

Labyrinthine

From the anterosuperior part of the internal acoustic meatus, this segment runs anterolaterally into the fallopian canal up to first genu where it takes a sharp turn posteriorly. Here it lies between the cochlea and the ampulla of horizontal and superior semicircular canal. This is the narrowest segment of facial nerve and is susceptible to compression and vascular insults. Geniculate ganglion is situated at the first genu. This forms the sensory ganglion of the facial nerve receiving taste fibers from the anterior two-thirds of tongue through the chordae tympani and from the palate through the greater superficial petrosal nerve. The greater superficial petrosal nerve is a branch of geniculate ganglion which joins the deep petrosal nerve to form the nerve of pterygoid canal and synapse in the pterygopalatine ganglion. The postganglionic parasympathetic secretomotor fibers supply the lacrimal gland and the mucus glands of oral and nasal cavity **(Figs. 1 and 2)**.

Tympanic

This segment passes from the geniculate ganglion to the second genu behind processus cochleariformis. The nerve lies against the medial wall of the middle ear above and posterior to the oval window and below the lateral semicircular canal. The canal may be deficient in up to 50% of cases.

Mastoid

The second genu marks the beginning of this segment. It runs vertically down in the anterior wall of the mastoid to the stylomastoid foramen. This segment gives rise to three branches—the nerve to stapedius, chordae tympani, and a communicating branch to auricular branch of vagus.

Extratemporal

The facial nerve exits the stylomastoid foramen, passes inferiorly and laterally around the styloid

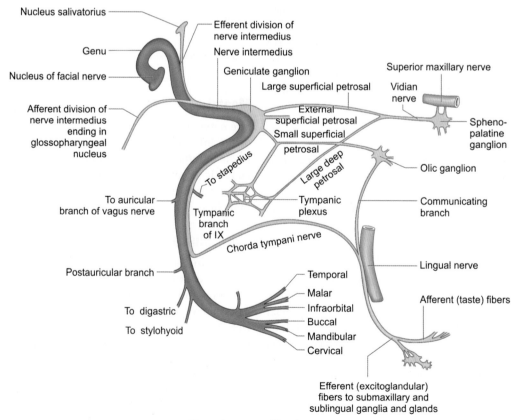

Fig. 1: Anatomy of facial nerve.

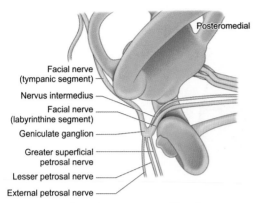

Fig. 2: Labyrinthine segment of facial nerve.

process, and enters the parotid gland. It gives off a postauricular sensory branch, branches to stylohyoid and posterior belly of digastric. Within the gland, it divides into temporofacial and cervicofacial divisions. They divide five major branches forming the pes anserinus:
1. Temporal
2. Zygomatic
3. Buccal
4. Marginal mandibular
5. Cervical.

Variations may exist where division occurs before it exits the stylomastoid foramen. Also there can be variations in the branching patterns.

Davis et al. has described six basic branching patterns:

Type I: No anastomose between branches

Type II: Anastomosis between branches of temporofacial division only

Type III: Anastomosis between branches of temporofacial division and cervicofacial division

Type IV: Combination of II and III

Type V: Double anastomoses between branches of temporofacial division and cervicofacial division

Type VI: Complex multiple anastomoses between two divisions. In this the buccal branch may receive anastomosis from cervical division or marginal mandibular nerve.

● SURGICAL LANDMARKS FOR FACIAL NERVE

For Mastoid and Middle Ear Surgeries

Processus Cochleariformis

The nerve lies posterior and superior to the processus cochleariformis.

Oval Window and Horizontal Semicircular Canal

Facial nerve lies below the horizontal semicircular canal above the oval window.

Short Process of Incus

Facial nerve lies medial to the short process of incus at the level of aditus.

Pyramid

The nerve runs behind the pyramid and posterior tympanic sulcus.

Digastric Ridge

The nerve leaves the mastoid at the anterior edge of digastric ridge.

For Parotid Surgery

Tympanomastoid Suture Line

The nerve lies 6–8 mm deep to this suture line.

Tragal Pointer

The nerve can be located 1–1.25 cm inferomedial to the triangular cartilaginous pointer.

Posterior Belly of Digastric

If the posterior belly of digastric is traced backward along its upper border to its attachment to the digastric groove, the nerve lies between this and the styloid process.

Styloid Process

The nerve crosses lateral to the styloid process.

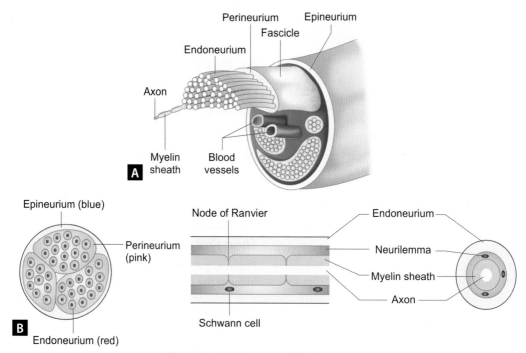

Figs. 3A and B: Structure of the facial nerve.

● PATHOPHYSIOLOGY

The nerve from inside out consists of axons, myelin sheath, neurilemma, and endoneurium. A group of nerve fibers is enclosed in perineurium to form a fascicle, and fascicles are bound together by perineurium **(Figs. 3A and B)**. The degree of nerve injury determines the regeneration of nerve and its function. Both the Sunderland and Seddons classifications of nerve injury are commonly used to determine the severity of injury and better understanding of electrophysiological studies **(Table 2)**.

The topodiagnostic tests like taste, salivary flow, Schirmer's test, and stapedial reflex are of historical significance and are not routinely employed as they have no prognostic value and provide limited clinical correlation.

Electrophysiology tests evaluate the degree of facial nerve dysfunction and potential for recovery and guide the management, specifically, the timing of surgical decompression and facial reanimation. Currently most commonly used tests are:

- Electroneuronography (ENoG)
- Electromyography (EMG).

Electroneuronography

This is a sort of evoked electromyography. The facial nerve at the stylomastoid foramen is stimulated by supramaximal stimulation. The compound action potentials are picked up by the surface electrodes at the nasolabial fold. The response of action potential on the paralyzed side is compared with the results of stimulation on the normal side. More than 90% degeneration occurring within 3–21 days of insult indicates a poor prognosis. It takes 3 days for Wallerian degeneration to occur and after 21 days due to simultaneous degeneration and regeneration. ENoG is of less value.

Table 2: Classifications of nerve injury.

Pathology	Sunderland	Seddon	Prognosis
Conduction block; no anatomical disruption	First degree	Neuropraxia	Reversible with full recovery
Division of axon	Second degree	Axonotmesis	Reasonable recovery
Division of axon and endoneurium	Third degree	Axonotmesis/neurotmesis	Incomplete recovery
Transection of nerve with intact epineurium	Fourth degree	Neurotmesis	Poor recovery
Complete transection of nerve	Fifth degree	Neurotmesis	No recovery

Table 3: The House–Brackmann score for grading facial weakness.

Grade	Gross	Resting tone	Forehead	Eye closure	Mouth
I		Normal function			
II	Slight weakness, very slight synkinesis	Normal	Moderate to good function	Complete closure with minimal effort	Slight asymmetry
III	Obvious weakness, noticeable but not severe synkinesis, contracture, and/or hemifacial spasm	Normal	Slight to moderate function	Complete closure with full effort	Slight weakness with maximum effort
IV	Disfiguring	Normal	None	Incomplete closure	Asymmetric with maximum effort
V	Barely perceptible motion	Normal	None	Incomplete closure	Slight movement
VI		Total paralysis			

Electromyography

This is employed in delayed paralysis as well as cases of bilateral facial palsy and is used in conjunction with ENoG. This measures the voluntary motor unit action potential by inserting needle into the orbicularis oris and orbicularis oculi muscles. The recordings are made during rest and voluntary contraction of muscles.

Three types of potentials are recorded:
1. Biphasic and triphasic—seen in normal resting muscle, every 30–60 milliseconds
2. Fibrillation potential—suggests Wallerian degeneration and arises 2–3 weeks following injury

3. Polyphasic potential—indicates early signs of reinnervation which can precede clinical recovery signs by 3 months.

Electrical silence is a poor prognostic indicator and argues against the attempt of facial reanimation using native facial musculature.

The House-Brackmann score (HB score), first described in 1985 is widely used in grading the facial motor weakness **(Table 3)**.

● ETIOLOGY OF FACIAL NERVE PARALYSIS

The various causes of facial nerve paralysis are listed in **Table 4**.

Table 4: Etiology of facial nerve paralysis.

Idiopathic	Bell's palsy
Infection	• Acute otitis media • Cholesteatoma • Skull base osteomyelitis • Herpes zoster oticus • Lyme disease • Mastoiditis • Tuberculous otitis media
Traumatic	• Basilar skull fracture • Penetrating temporal bone trauma • Birth injury • Parotid injury • Iatrogenic
Neoplastic	• Facial nerve Schwannoma • Vestibular schwannoma • Meningioma • Hemangioma • Carcinoma (primary of metastatic intra- or extratemporal) • Glomus jugulare • Rhabdomyosarcoma • Parotid malignancy
Neurological	• Lacunar/brainstem infarct • Guillain–Barré syndrome
Congenital	Mobius syndrome
Others	• Sarcoidosis • Wegener's granulomatosis

• MANAGEMENT OF FACIAL NERVE PARALYSIS

History and Clinical Examination

The proper diagnosis is the cornerstone in the proper management of facial nerve paralysis. This is based on (1) identification of site of lesion, (2) probable etiology, and (3) clinical staging with House–Brackmann stage.

Careful delineation of history includes onset of symptoms, quality of other associated symptoms, and prior systemic and infectious diseases. Thorough physical examination is of paramount importance to assess the pattern and degree of involvement of facial musculature. It also involves use of tests for salivation, lacrimation, and taste.

Tests of facial musculature include:
- Wrinkling of forehead (frontalis)
- Closing of eyes (orbicularis oculi)
- Blowing of cheek (orbicularis oris, zygomaticus, buccinator)
- Whistling (buccinator).

The general status of other musculature like latissimus dorsi and rectus abdominis is assessed for eventual reconstruction. The nerve involvement is graded using House–Brackmann scale.

Imaging

Imaging of facial nerve should be tailored to both the suspected pathology and clinical localization of the lesion. Typically, if facial palsy is localized to the cisternal or meatal segment or the pontine nuclei, contrast-enhanced MRI is indicated. A high-resolution temporal bone CT is recommended for the evaluation of fallopian canal (mastoid, tympanic, and labyrinthine segment). Contrast-enhanced MRI should be performed first in cases where the palsy cannot be definitely localized clinically. Both high-resolution temporal bone CT and MRI should be typically performed for evaluation of tumors involving the facial nerve.

Role of Ultrasound

In a recent study, ultrasound has been utilized to predict the facial nerve outcome in Bell's palsy. The average facial nerve diameter was calculated from the ultrasonographic measurement of facial nerve at three points (proximally at stylomastoid foramen, proximal to pes anserinus, midway between these two) between 2–7 days after onset of paralysis. A normal ultrasound measurement of facial nerve had 100% positive predictive value for normal facial nerve function recovery at 3 months.

Diffusion Tensor Tractography

In case of a large vestibular schwannoma, it is difficult to differentiate between the facial nerve and tumor on MRI because they have similar signal intensities, extreme thinning of the nerve by large tumors, and absence of intervening cerebrospinal fluid between the nerve and the tumor. In these cases, diffusion tensor (DT) tractography is useful in evaluation of facial nerve course and displacement. DT tractography successfully delineated the nerve from pons to porus acusticus. But, currently it is not automated requiring highly skilled personnel in image reconstruction. Further advances in automation techniques will likely lead to its greater use.

Electrophysiological Tests

As mentioned earlier these tests are useful to determine the extent of nerve disruption, possible outcome, and treatment options.

● TREATMENT OF FACIAL PARALYSIS

The various treatment options in facial paralysis include:
- Medical management with steroids
- Physiotherapy
- Eye care
- Surgery.

Further discussions will be confined to the management of facial nerve in tumors and will be focused on facial reanimation. Facial nerve management in tumors depends on weighing the balance between the risk of facial weakness that may result with primary surgical resection and slow-growing nature of the tumors. Schwannomas form the majority of intrinsic facial nerve tumors. This can occur anywhere along the course of the facial nerve. Hemangiomas are extremely rare tumors that tend to arise around the geniculate ganglion and internal acoustic meatus. Malignant involvement includes direct perineural spread of mucoepidermoid carcinoma, adenoid cystic carcinoma, and squamous cell carcinoma.

Benign intrinsic tumors with good facial motor function shall be managed conservatively.

Schwannomas reach relatively large size before they become symptomatic. Hemangiomas may cause severe neurological defect while they are still small and hence early resection offers a good chance of recovery of facial nerve function.

Tumor location, size, and level of residual hearing dictate the surgical approach. A middle fossa approach is preferred for small lesions up to geniculate ganglion in patients with good hearing. Large tumors or patient's poor hearing requires a translabyrinthine approach. Transmastoid approach is used for horizontal and vertical segments of facial nerve.

● FACIAL REANIMATION

Facial paralysis results in both evident deformity and functional problems of eyelid closure, oral incontinence, and speech. Patient with persistent weakness should be offered treatment to improve cosmesis and function. The main factor that determines the reconstruction is the status of facial musculature. Evaluation of patients with complete facial nerve paralysis includes determination of:
- Nerve continuity
- Viability of cell bodies in facial nucleus
- Presence of an intact proximal segment
- Presence of distal segment with endoneural tubes that can accept and transmit regenerating axons to facial muscles
- Presence of viable facial muscles with intact endplate.

The various reanimation techniques employed depend on the availability of the proximal and distal segments as well as viability of facial muscles. The various options are described here.

Viable Facial Musculature

The proximal and distal segment of nerve available:
- Direct coaptation (primary neurorrhaphy)
- Interposition grafting.

The proximal segment of nerve unavailable:
- Cranial nerve substitution
- Hypoglossal to facial substitution
- Facial to facial substitution [cross-facial nerve grafting (CFNG]
- Masseteric nerve substitution.

Nonviable Facial Musculature

- Pedicle muscle transfer
- Neuromuscular free flap transfer with nerve substitution
- Static reanimation.

Direct Coaptation (Primary Neurorrhaphy)

Tension-free primary reattachment of the transacted nerve gives the best chance of recovery. The goal of the procedure is to unite the perineural fascicles to permit axonal regeneration. The best results are seen with early repair. Options for primary repair include suture neurorrhaphy or utilization of fibrin glue. The technique of suturing is usually perineural technique for the proximal nerve and epineural technique for distal nerve (distal to pes anserinus). The oblique preparation of nerve provides a greater surface area for coaptation. The fewest number of sutures should be used. Suturing is done with 10.0 monofilament suture with atraumatic tapered needle with 1 mm bite. Three to four interrupted sutures are employed.

Interposition Grafting

When the tension-free primary repair is not possible, the next best option is interposition (cable) grafting. Cable graft uses an autogenous donor graft as a conduit to permit axonal regeneration to span the distance. Due to the low morbidity associated with loss of sensation at the donor site, the following nerves are preferred as graft.
- Greater auricular nerve
- Sural nerve
- Lateral femoral cutaneous nerve
- Medial antebrachial cutaneous nerve.

Cranial Nerve Substitution

A nerve substitution is considered in facial nerve injury when proximal segment is not available. This implies redirection of motor axons of the donor nerve to the distal facial nerve. This can be employed up to 2 years beyond which there are high chances of nerve fibrosis and muscle atrophy. The choice of donor nerve is limited by axonal density, proximity, and donor site morbidity. The donor nerves chosen are:

Hypoglossal nerve: This nerve has got acceptable relationship with the facial kinetics. Learned elevation of tongue in the mouth brings some smile and voluntary movements of facial expression. But some involuntary movements can happen during eating and talking. To minimize the complete hypoglossal sacrifice, split graft and interposition jump graft can be used. The mass movement of face can be avoided using coaptation of lower division alone.

Masseteric nerve: The close proximity, well-matched axonal load, and negligible donor site morbidity matched the masseteric division of trigeminal nerve a good choice for nerve substitution. Anatomically, it is much related to the facial nerve and this adds to the ease of cortical adaptation.

Cross-facial nerve grafting (CFNG): The use of CFNG is based on the principle that the emotional expressions are guided naturally by the same muscle groups of the normal side. The best outcome is associated with early CFNG within 6 months. CFNG requires a cable graft to bridge the long distance across the face.

Babysitter procedure: If CFNG is used, more time is needed because the graft and therefore the distance to be reinnervated are much longer. To overcome this situation, the facial nerve on the lesion side can be additionally reanimated by a hypoglossal facial jump graft. Recently masseteric nerve has also been used for baby-sitter procedure.

Regional Muscle Transfer

Indications for regional muscle transfer are facial nerve interruption of at least 3 years, electrical silence on EMG, and congenital facial paralysis. This involves the temporalis muscle and masseteric muscle transposition powered by the trigeminal nerve in smile reanimation. The middle third of the muscle is dissected and tunneled below the zygomatic arch and is secured to the medial border of orbicularis oris. Slips of masseteric muscle can also be attached to the lips and oral commissure. Anterior belly of digastric muscle and tendon can also be used for this purpose.

Neuromuscular Free Flap Transfer

The other option for dynamic reanimation in the presence of electrical silence in EMG includes two-stage procedure utilizing CFNG with a microvascular muscle free flap transfer. The gracilis is the most commonly used muscle for free flap muscle transfer. The other muscles include latissimus dorsi, serratus anterior, pectoralis minor and inferior rectus abdominis.

Static Rehabilitation

Indications include:
- Debilitated individuals
- To achieve symmetry at rest
- When nerve or muscle not available for dynamic procedures
- As an adjuvant to dynamic procedures for immediate restoration of symmetry.

Elevation and positioning of soft tissue of oral commissure or nasal ala is done along with procedures to correct eye closure. The various procedures involve face, eye, nose, and oral rehabilitation.

Face rehabilitation: Suspension of nasolabial fold or the perioral muscles achieves good resting symmetry.
- Fascia lata sling
- Palmaris tendon sling

- Gore-Tex or Alloderm
- Face lift.

Eye rehabilitation:
- Platinum or gold weight implant and suture tarsorrhaphy for lagophthalmos
- Median and lateral canthoplasty to correct lower lid ectropion
- Brow lift for brow ptosis
- Blepharoplasty for supratarsal fold sagging.

Nose rehabilitation: Alar suspension with fascia lata

Oral rehabilitation:
- Oral commissuroplasty (Z-plasty) for drooping mouth
- Lateral wedge resection with digastric tendon transfer for oral incompetence.

Botulinum Toxin Therapy

Management of synkinesis and hyperkinesis include botulinum toxin injection. Botox injection into the nonparalyzed side plays a role to reduce asymmetry in selected cases.

● FURTHER READING

1. Byrne PJ, Kim M, Boahene K, et al. Temporalis tendon transfer as a part of a comprehensive approach to facial reanimation. Arch Facial Plast Surg. 2007;9(4);234-41.
2. Hardy A, Muzaffar J, Kumar R, et al. The surgical management of bilateral facial paralysis: Case report. The Laryngol Otol. 2018;132(9):842-5.
3. Ramakrishnan Y, Alam S, Kotecha A, et al. Reanimation following facial palsy: Present and future directions. J Laryngol Otol. 2010;124(11):1146-52.
4. Sataloff RT. Sataloff's Comprehensive Textbook of Otolaryngology: Head and Neck Surgery: Otology/Neurotology/Skull Base Surgery. New Delhi: JP Medical Ltd; 2015. pp. 1-750.
5. Terzis JK, Tzafetta K. The "babysitter" procedure: Minihypoglossal to facial nerve transfer and cross-facial nerve grafting. Plast Reconstr Surg. 2009;123(3):865-76.
6. Volk GF, Pantel M, Guntinas-Lichius O. Modern concepts in facial nerve reconstruction. Head Face Med. 2010;6:25.

Neck

Chapters

CHAPTER 17

Neck Nodal Levels and Classification of Neck Dissection

Shashikant Vishnubhai Limbachiya, Deepak Balasubramanian

● INTRODUCTION

Head and neck carcinoma is commonly associated with neck nodal metastasis. Because the presence of such metastasis has a significant negative impact on prognosis, regardless of the anatomic subsite of the primary tumor, the appropriate management of neck metastasis is most important factor in the overall management of the head and neck cancer. Before starting management of the neck, one should know the detail anatomy of the neck.

● ANATOMY OF THE FASCIAL SPACES OF THE NECK

The anatomic structures of the neck are invested in loose connective tissue fascia, the layers of which define surgical planes for separation and dissection of tissues. Utilization of these tissue planes forms the basis of the en bloc removal of lymphatic tissue in neck dissection. For practical reasons we will consider two distinct fascial layers in the neck, the superficial cervical fascia and the deep cervical fascia. The deep cervical fascia is composed of a—(1) superficial layer which invests the sternocleidomastoid, trapezius, and strap muscles; (2) middle or visceral layer which invests the thyroid gland, trachea, and esophagus; and (3) Deep layer (also prevertebral fascia) which invests the vertebral muscles and the phrenic nerve.

● NECK LYMPHATICS

Thirty percent of the lymph nodes in the body are located in the neck. The cervical lymph nodes are arranged anatomically as follows:

- *The outer circle of superficial nodes* includes submental, submandibular, facial, preauricular, postauricular, and anterior cervical nodes.
- *The inner circle surrounding larynx, trachea, and pharynx* includes pretracheal, para tracheal and retropharyngeal nodes.
- The deep cervical nodes surrounding internal jugular vein (IJV), lies in between the outer and inner circles, and drain them. These are grouped into antero-superior (jugulodigastric), anteroinferior, posterosuperior, and posteroinferior (jugulo-omohyoid, supraclavicular) nodes.

● CLASSIFICATION OF NECK NODAL LEVELS

The Memorial Sloan Kettering Cancer Center had given classification describing the patterns of metastatic dissemination observed in more than 1,000 patients who were treated at the center with radical neck dissection (RND). Lymph nodes in the neck are grouped into six levels corresponding with the submandibular and submental nodes (level I); upper, middle, and lower jugular nodes (levels II, III, IV); posterior triangle nodes (level V), and central;

prelaryngeal, pretracheal, and paratracheal nodes (level VI). The superior mediastinal nodes are denoted as level VII which is paratracheal below the sternal notch **(Tables 1 and 2)**.

Thus, the first echelon lymph nodes of various sites are:

- *Oral cavity*: Levels I, II ,III
- *Larynx, pharynx*: II, III, IV
- *Thyroid*: VI, VII, IV
- *Parotid*: Parotid, preauricular, II, III, VA

Evaluation

Clinical Examination

Clinical examination is an important initial method of assessing regional lymph nodes with accuracy of 75%. More than 1 cm node can be easily palpable in most cases. Sensitivity is of 74% and specificity of 81%. It is difficult to examine accurately in short necks. Retropharyngeal area is inaccessible to clinical examination.

Table 1: Neck levels as given by the American Academy of Otolaryngology: Head and neck surgery **(Figs. 1 and 2)**.

Level	Clinical location	Surgical boundaries	
Ia	Submental triangle	Superior	Symphysis of mandible
		Inferior	Hyoid bone
		Anterior (medial)	Left anterior belly of digastric
		Posterior (lateral)	Right anterior belly of digastrics
Ib	Submandibular triangle	Superior	Body of mandible
		Inferior	Posterior belly of digastric
		Anterior (medial)	Anterior belly of digastric
		Posterior (lateral)	Stylohyoid muscle
IIa	Upper jugular	Superior	Lower level of bony margin of jugular fossa
		Inferior	Level of lower body of hyoid bone
		Anterior (medial)	Stylohyoid muscle
		Posterior (lateral)	Vertical plane defined by accessory nerve
IIb	Upper jugular	Superior	Lower level of bony margin of jugular fossa
		Inferior	Level of lower body of hyoid bone
		Anterior (medial)	Vertical plane defined by accessory nerve
		Posterior (lateral)	Posterior border of sternomastoid muscle
III	Midjugular	Superior	Level of lower body of hyoid bone
		Inferior	Horizontal plane along inferior border of anterior cricoid arch
		Anterior (medial)	Lateral border of sternohyoid muscle
		Posterior (lateral)	Posterior border of sternocleidomastoid muscle or sensory branches of the cervical plexus
IV	Lower jugular	Superior	Horizontal plane along inferior border of anterior cricoid arch
		Inferior	Clavicle
		Anterior (medial)	Lateral border of sternohyoid muscle
		Posterior (lateral)	Posterior border of sternocleidomastoid muscle or sensory branches of the cervical plexus

Contd...

Contd...

Level	Clinical location	Surgical boundaries	
Va	Posterior triangle	Superior Inferior	Convergence of sternocleidomastoid (SCM) and trapezius muscles Horizontal plane along inferior border of anterior cricoid arch
		Anterior (medial)	Posterior border of sternocleidomastoid muscle or sensory branches of the cervical plexus
		Posterior (lateral)	Anterior border of trapezius muscle
Vb	Posterior triangle (supraclavicular)	Superior Inferior Anterior (medial)	Horizontal plane along inferior border of anterior cricoid arch clavicle Posterior border of sternocleidomastoid muscle or sensory branches of the cervical plexus
		Posterior (lateral)	Anterior border of trapezius muscle
VI	Anterior compartment	Superior Inferior	Hyoid bone Sternal notch
		Anterior (medial)	Common carotid artery
		Posterior (lateral)	Common carotid artery
VII	Superior mediastinum	Superior Inferior	Sternal notch Innominate artery
		Anterior (medial)	Common carotid artery
		Posterior (lateral)	Common carotid artery

Table 2: The predictable patterns of lymph node metastases (Lindberg and Jatin Shah).

Level I	Oral cavity, anterior nose, maxillary sinus and mid-face
Level II	Oral cavity, nasal cavity, nasopharynx, oropharynx, hypopharynx, larynx, and parotid
Level III	Oral cavity, nasopharynx, oropharynx, hypopharynx, and larynx
Level IV	Hypopharynx, larynx and cervical esophagus
Level V	Nasopharynx and oropharynx
Level VI	Thyroid, larynx (glottis, subglottis) and cervical esophagus

Fine Needle Aspiration Cytology

It is the gold standard in establishing the diagnosis of a mass in the neck. Fine needle aspiration (FNA) has a sensitivity and specificity of 99% for squamous cell carcinoma. For a mass in the thyroid, accuracy of FNA is 95%. Open biopsy is used primarily in patients when suspected of having lymphoma or if two fine needle aspiration cytology (FNACs) (at least one image guided) are inconclusive.

Imaging

In clinically N0 neck, imaging is used to evaluate the subclinical disease and to verify the absence of contralateral disease. Imaging should be considered to assess the resectability in advanced nodal disease, to assist in the detection of primary tumors not identified on physical examination and also help in planning nonsurgical therapy like radiation. Imaging should be used to evaluate the carotid artery invasion, retropharyngeal and paratracheal involvement. Most commonly used imaging modalities are USG, CT,

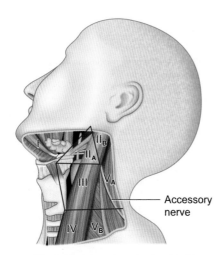

Fig. 1: Neck lymph nodes levels I–V.

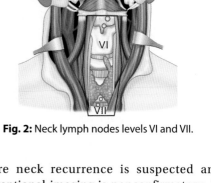

Fig. 2: Neck lymph nodes levels VI and VII.

and MRI. New modalities like PET-CT scan and lymphoscintigraphy are emerging.

Ultrasound scan: It is noninvasive, fast, and inexpensive imaging modality. It can be used to guide FNAC. Operator dependency is considered to disadvantage. Absent fatty hilum and increases in short axis length are features of metastatic neck nodes. Sensitivity is 87% and specificity is 86%.

Computed tomography: It is the most commonly used imaging modality in evaluation of lymphatics in the neck. It is noninvasive and easy to interpret. Rim enhancement of the node may be present. Nodes >1 cm in size may contain metastatic disease. Drawbacks include exposing patient to ionizing radiation. The patient may be allergic to intravenous contrast; contrast cannot be given in altered renal function. Sensitivity is 81% and specificity is 76%.

Magnetic resonance imaging: Noninvasive with no radiation exposure. Better for evaluating perineural invasion and soft tissue delineation. It may be difficult in claustrophobic patients. Sensitivity is 81% and specificity is 63%.

Computed tomography: Positron emission tomography fusion imaging: It is performed

where neck recurrence is suspected and conventional imaging is nonconfirmatory. In pretreatment setting, sensitivity of 90–95% and specificity of 95–99% have been noted. In post-treatment neck setting, sensitivity of 100% and specificity of 98–100% have been observed.

Predictors of Neck Metastasis

Several factors contribute to the incidence of neck metastasis like characteristics of the primary tumor, the location of the primary tumor, the size, the T stage, and histological differentiation. Lymph node metastases at levels IV and V are generally considered to have the worst prognosis, a high incidence of local recurrence, and a high incidence of distant metastasis.

Lesions of the tonsil and base of the tongue have a very high incidence of nodal metastasis, whereas tumors of the hypopharynx universally have metastatic disease in the neck nodes. Interestingly, the free border of the vocal cord has sparse lymphatics, and generally early stage laryngeal cancer has no neck node metastasis. In the oral cavity, the tongue has the highest incidence of nodal metastasis due to its physiological function while chewing, whereas the hard palate and the lip rarely present primarily with metastatic disease.

Following histological characteristics of the primary tumor are predictors of node metastasis:

- Depth of the tumor (the most important prognostic factor)
- Endophytic versus exophytic differentiation
- Pushing margins
- Presence of tumor emboli
- Perivascular and perineural infiltration of the tumor
- Presence of extranodal spread/extracapsular spread
- Nodal infiltration into the subdermal area or platysma.

Most important factor for high incidence of both local neck recurrence and distant metastasis is extracapsular spread of disease.

● TERMINOLOGY OF NECK DISSECTION

The terminology for describing neck dissections was standardized by the American Academy of Otolaryngology: Head and Neck Surgery in 1991, and modified in 2002.

The classification, as currently endorsed by both the AAO–HNS and the American Society for Head and Neck Surgery, has accepted the terms RND and modified RND (MRND) when all five levels are removed.

Comprehensive Neck Dissection

It denotes when all the five levels of neck nodes are removed. It can be either RND or MRND.

Radical Neck Dissection

This is the standard basic procedure. All other procedures represent one or more modifications to this procedure. It involves removal of levels I–V, spinal accessory nerve, internal jugular vein, sternocleidomastoid muscle (SCM).

Modified Radical Neck Dissection

Involves preservation of one or more nonlymphatic structures (spinal accessory nerve—IX, IJV—SCM). All lymph node groups (I to V) are removed.

- *Type I*: Preserves XI.
- *Type II*: Preserves XI and SCM, sacrifices IJV (Jatin Shah's Cancer of the Head and Neck): Preserves XI, IJV (Stell and Maran's Head and Neck Surgery, 5th edition, Eugene M Myers Cancer of Head and Neck, 4th edition.)
- *Type III*: Preserves XI, SCM, IJV. To prevent confusion, the current practice is that the preserved structure should be named; for example: MRND with preservation of nerve XI.

Selective Neck Dissection

Selective neck dissection (SND) involves preservation of one or more of the nodal levels removed in RND or MRND while preserving the nonlymphatic structures removed in RND.

Types of Selective Neck Dissection (Figs. 3A to E)

- *Supraomohyoid neck dissection (SOHND)*: Levels I, II, III are removed.
- *Extended SOHND*: Level IV is also removed. Recommended for oral tongue lesions for "skip metastases" (Byers et al.), not accepted by some others.
- *Lateral ND (jugular neck dissection)*: Lymph node levels II, III, IV are removed. This is recommended for lesions of hypopharynx and larynx.
- *Anterolateral ND*: Lymph node levels I, II, III, IV, and V are removed. This is recommended for oropharyngeal lesions when surgery is used for treatment of the primary.
- *Posterolateral ND*: Levels II, III, IV, and V are removed. This is recommended for posterior scalp lesions.

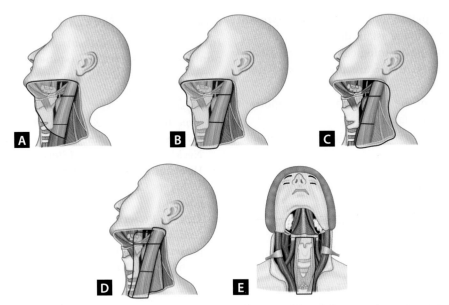

Figs. 3A to E: Selective neck dissection. (A) Levels I–III (supraomohyoid); (B) Levels I–IV (extended supraomohyoid); (C) Level II–IV (lateral); (D) Level II–V (posterolateral); (E) Level VI–VII (anterior/paratracheal).

- *Central compartment ND*: Lymph node level VI is removed (i.e. lymphatics from hyoid to suprasternal notch and laterally up to carotid arteries). It is recommended in thyroid, subglottic and postcricoid carcinoma.

• STAGING OF THE NECK

American Joint Committee on Cancer (AJCC) 8th edition has introduced major changes in the neck staging. Appropriate staging tables are given in the chapters separately.

The major changes are:

- Separate N staging approaches have been described for human papillomavirus (HPV)-related and HPV-unrelated cancers (for oropharyngeal cancers).
- Separate N category approaches have been described for patients treated without cervical lymph node dissection (clinical N) and patients treated with cervical lymph node dissection (pathological N).

- Extranodal extension (ENE) is introduced as a descriptor in all HPV unrelated cancers.
- *ENE in HPV-negative cancers:* Only clinically and radiographically overt ENE should be used for cN.

  Any pathologically detected ENE is considered ENE (+) and is used for pN.

  Presence of ENE is designated pN2a for a single ipsilateral node <3 cm and pN3b for all other node(s).

- *Classification of ENE:* Clinically overt ENE is classified as ENEC and is considered ENE (+) for cN. Pathologically detected ENE is classified as either ENEmi (≤2 mm) or ENE_{ma}, (>2 mm) for data collection purposes only but both are considered ENE(+) for definition of pN.

Note: Metastasis at level VII are considered to be regional lymph node metastasis and central compartment nodes VI considered to be ipsilateral.

The history of neck management has evolved paradoxically, from an era in which the most radical neck surgeries were performed for minimal or nonexistent disease to the present era in which functional neck dissection is efficient enough. Radiation, chemotherapy strategies are often employed in advanced metastatic disease. At present, the management of cervical lymphatics in squamous cell carcinoma of the head and neck has been either elective (when the neck is clinically N0) or therapeutic (when the neck is N+).

● FURTHER READING

1. de Bondt RB, Nelemans PJ, Hofman PA, et al. Detection of lymph node metastases in head and neck cancer: A meta-analysis comparing US, USgFNAC, CT and MR imaging. Eur J Radiol. 2007;64(2):266-72.
2. D'Cruz AK, Chaukar D, Gupta T. Guidelines for Head and Neck Cancers, Vol. XI(A). Mumbai: Tata Memorial Centre; 2012.
3. Fasunla AJ, Grene BH, Timmesfeld N, et al. A meta-analysis of the randomized controlled trials on elective neck dissection versus therapeutic neck dissection in oral cavity cancers with clinically node-negative neck. Oral Oncol. 2011;47(5):320-4.
4. Frank DK, Sessions RB. Management of the neck surgery. In: Harrison LB, Sessions RB, Hong WK (Eds). Head and Cancer: A Multidisciplinary Approach, 3rd edition. Philadelphia: Lippincott Williams and Wilkins, A Wolters Kluwer Business; 2009. pp. 181-200.
5. Medina JE. A rationale classification of neck dissections. Otolaryngol Head Neck Surg. 1989; 100(3):169-76.
6. Robbins KT, Clayman G, Levine PA, et al.; American Head and Neck Society; American Academy of Otolaryngology—Head and Neck Surgery. Neck Dissection Classification update: Revisions proposed by the American Head and Neck Society and the American Academy of Otolaryngology-Head and Neck Surgery. Arch Otolaryngol Head Neck Surg. 2002;128(7):751-8.
7. Robbins KT, Medina JE, Wolfe GT, et al. Standardizing neck dissection terminology. Official report of the Academy's Committee for Head and Neck Surgery and Oncology. Arch Otolaryngol Head Neck Surg. 1991;117(6):601-5.
8. Shaha AR. Radical neck dissection. Operative techniques in general surgery. 2004;6(2):72-82.
9. Shah JP, Strong E, Spiro RH, et al. Surgical grand rounds. Neck dissection: Current status and future possibilities. Clin Bull. 1981;11(1):25-33.

CHAPTER 18

Management of the Node Negative Neck

Shashikant Vishnubhai Limbachiya, Deepak Balasubramanian

● INTRODUCTION

Treatment of the node negative (N0) neck has been a controversial issue in head and neck cancers. The rationale for elective treatment of the node negative neck has been due to presence of subclinical "occult" metastasis, especially from oral cancers. The presence of lymph node metastasis reduces the survival by 50%. There have been numerous trials in the past comparing elective neck dissection versus observation with varying results. Currently elective neck treatment is advocated in scenarios where the risk of lymph node metastasis is more than 20%.

● TREATMENT OPTIONS

- Elective neck dissection
- Elective radiotherapy
- Observation **(Flowchart 1)**.

Elective Neck Dissection

It is performed when primary tumor is treated with surgery. Selective neck dissection (SND) is the type of neck dissection usually performed. For patients with oral cavity cancer, SND of at least levels I–III should be carried out, with the addition of level IV for tongue cancers. Levels II–IV need to be cleared for laryngeal and hypopharyngeal cancer. Levels II–IV are recommended for oropharyngeal cancers. There

appears to be little advantage in dissecting level V for any of the mucosal primaries electively. Excellent local control rates can be obtained with SND.

Factors Favoring Elective Neck Dissection

- Allows for adequate staging of the neck especially with regards to number of nodes involved and extracapsular. These are important for planning adjuvant treatment.
- Treatment of occult metastatic disease.
- Selective neck dissection as compared to radical or modified radical neck dissection has a low morbidity and mortality.
- Evidence from randomized trials and a recent meta-analysis show a benefit of elective neck dissection versus observation.
- The control rate for neck dissection is decreased if gland enlargement occurs or multiple nodes appear.

Factors Opposing Elective Neck Dissection

- Close clinical follow up combined with imaging is required to identify early nodal metastasis.
- The neck control of a therapeutic neck dissection for nodal recurrence is inferior.

Flowchart 1: Management algorithm for treating N0 neck.

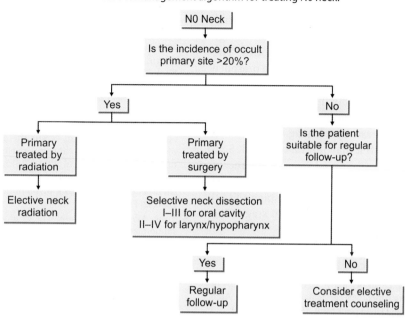

Elective versus therapeutic neck dissection (observation and neck dissection if any nodal recurrence occurs) in node-negative oral cancer: Whether patients with early-stage oral cancers should be treated with elective neck dissection at the time of the primary surgery or with therapeutic neck dissection after nodal relapse has been a matter of debate. A prospective, randomized, controlled trial by D'Cruz et al., evaluated the effect on survival of elective node dissection (ipsilateral neck dissection at the time of the primary surgery) versus therapeutic node dissection (watchful waiting followed by neck dissection for nodal relapse) in patients with lateralized stage T1 or T2 oral squamous cell carcinomas. The trial showed that elective neck dissection resulted in higher rates of overall and disease-free survival than therapeutic neck dissection.

Elective Neck Irradiation

It is performed when the primary tumor is treated by radiotherapy.

If primary is treated with brachytherapy then neck should be either treated with radiation or surgery. The recommended dose for N0 neck is 50–54 Gy in 20–30 fractions. A radiation dose of 50 Gy or more can eradicate 99% of subclinical carcinoma in the lymph nodes.

Disadvantage of elective neck irradiation is that important prognostic factors, such as nodal specimen for histopathological examination and information regarding pathological staging of the neck are not available. With regard to recurrence in the neck after radiation therapy, salvage, surgery is more difficult in an irradiated neck than in a previously untreated neck.

Observation

It can be adopted for patients with low-risk for nodal metastases (e.g. very superficial T1 lesions of subsites of oral cavity and glottis) in patients who are reliable for regular follow up (3 monthly clinical examination and ultrasonography of neck).

Sentinel Node Biopsy

Sentinel node biopsy (SNB) with lympho-scintigraphy is emerging as a new tool to stage patients with clinically N0 neck nodes. The status of the sentinel node predicts the presence of metastasis in the rest of the nodes within the nodal basin. This forms the basis of SNB. The purpose of SNB is to accurately stage the neck without unnecessarily causing morbidity in patients in which it may not be required. SNB is still in the investigational stage. Some recent guidelines recommended it only in patients with previously untreated early stage (T1/2) oral cavity cancer with clinical N0 stage. The procedure is technique sensitive.

● FURTHER READING

1. Chow JM, Levin BC, Krivit JS, et al. Radiotherapy or surgery for subclinical cervical node metastases. Arch Otolaryngol Head Neck Surg. 1989;115(8):981-4.

2. D'Cruz AK, Siddachari RC, Walvekar RR, et al. Elective neck dissection for the management of the N0 neck in early cancer of the oral tongue: Need for a randomized controlled trial. Head Neck. 2009;31(5):618-24.

3. D'Cruz AK, Vaish R, Kapre N, et al.; Head and Neck Disease Management Group. Elective versus Therapeutic Neck Dissection in Node-Negative Oral Cancer. N Engl J Med. 2015;373(6):521-9.

4. Fasunla AJ, Grene BH, Timmesfeld N, et al. A meta-analysis of the randomized controlled trials on elective neck dissection versus therapeutic neck dissection in oral cavity cancers with clinically node-negative neck. Oral Oncol. 2011;47(5):320-4.

5. Ferlito A, Rinaldo A, Silver CE, et al. Elective and therapeutic selective neck dissection. Oral Oncol. 2006;42(1):14-25.

6. Yuen AP, Ho CM, Chow TL, et al. Prospective randomized study of selective neck dissection versus observation for N0 neck of early tongue carcinoma. Head Neck. 2009;31(6):765-72.

7. Yuen AP, Wei WI, Wong YM, et al. Elective neck dissection versus observation in the treatment of early oral tongue carcinoma. Head Neck. 1997;19(7):583-8.

CHAPTER 19

Management of the Node Positive Neck

Shashikant Vishnubhai Limbachiya, Deepak Balasubramanian

• INTRODUCTION

The treatment offered to the neck often depends on the modality used to treat the primary site. Studies have shown that survival is decreased approximately by 50% when cervical nodes are involved. This is due to the innate ability of carcinoma to spread to regional and distant sites, which makes curative intent treatment more difficult. Several treatment options are available including surgery, radiation, chemoradiation and combined treatment. Generally, the treatment modality selected for primary cancer determines treatment approach for neck metastasis. The standard treatment approach for metastatic lymphadenopathy is surgery with postoperative radiotherapy. However, carcinomas from certain anatomic sites, such as nasopharynx and oropharynx respond well to irradiation and can be treated either by radiation therapy or concurrent chemoradiation.

• TREATMENT FOR N+ NECK

Generally, treatment of N+ neck is a comprehensive neck dissection. It is usually a modified radical neck dissection. However, in cases of advanced nodal disease, N3 with involvement of adjacent structures, radical neck dissection should be considered. Adjuvant radiation therapy is usually recommended if multiple positive nodes (two or more nodes)

or nodes more than 3 cm in size are present. If extracapsular spread is present, studies have found that, adjuvant chemoradiation has shown both improved locoregional control and disease-free survival. Postoperative neck irradiation requires a dose of 60–63 Gy over 6–6.5 weeks **(Flowchart 1)**.

Management of Post-chemoradiotherapy N+ Neck

In the post-chemoradiotherapy situation with a N+ neck, a "salvage" neck dissection is performed. The extent depends on the level of the node and the structures involved. The term "planned neck dissection" is used when neck dissection is performed within 6 weeks of completion of definitive chemoradiotherapy for squamous cell carcinoma of head and neck. This strategy employs lower doses of radiation (during chemoradiotherapy) to the neck in anticipation of neck dissection **(Flowchart 2)**.

• RADICAL NECK DISSECTION

Indications

Classical radical neck dissection, although not practiced commonly today, has the following important indications:

- Advanced nodal disease (N2b, N2c, and N3) with involvement of spinal accessory nerve, internal jugular vein (IJV) or sternocleidomastoid (SCM) muscle.

Flowchart 1: Treatment algorithm for patients undergoing primary surgery.

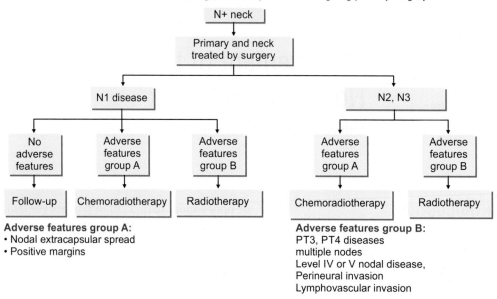

Adverse features group A:
• Nodal extracapsular spread
• Positive margins

Adverse features group B:
PT3, PT4 diseases
multiple nodes
Level IV or V nodal disease,
Perineural invasion
Lymphovascular invasion

Flowchart 2: Treatment algorithm for patients undergoing primary chemoradiation.

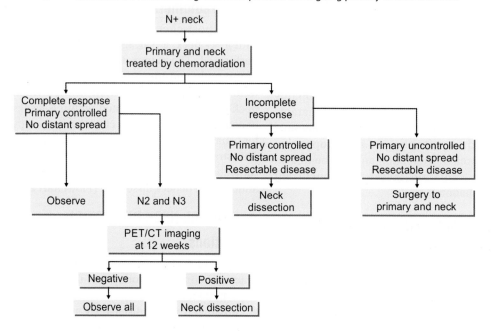

- Recurrent metastatic tumor after previous treatment in a salvage setting.
- Involvement of the platysma or skin, requiring sacrifice of a portion of skin in the upper neck.
- Clinical signs of obvious extranodal disease.

Contraindications

Tumors that involve the skull base or those tumors with massive extension to prevertebral fascia, more than 270° encasement of the common carotid artery, and brachial plexus may be considered to be inoperable.

Techniques

Anesthesia

It is performed under general anesthesia with an endotracheal tube in place.

Position of the Patient

The patient is placed supine and with neck extended and with a lateral tilt of the neck on the contralateral side of the neck dissection. Neck extension is achieved by putting sand bag under shoulders and head ring to stabilize the head.

Incisions

Kocher Incision or Double Trifurcate

This is the standard incision until the middle of last century. Unfortunately, both the trifurcation angles were invariably on the carotid artery. Hence, it is rarely used today.

Modified Schobinger or Modified Conley Incision

It is "Y" shaped incision which creates a long anteromedial flap, the tip of which may necrose as a result of the limited ascending blood supply. Care must be taken to place the descending limb of this incision approximately 2–3 cm

behind the carotid. A more posterior placement of this incision jeopardizes the viability of the lateral and superior portion of the flap. It has the advantage of adequate exposure and the incision can be easily extended anteriorly as lip splitting incision in order to expose the primary oral cavity tumor. This is the standard incision used for radical neck dissection.

McFee Incision

Horizontal double-parallel incision is also rarely used today except in young women, thyroid cancer, and especially in patients who have had prior radiotherapy.

J-shaped or Apron Incision

This is used mainly for thyroid cancer. Once again, it is rarely used today. However, even for patients with thyroid cancer and neck dissection, an extended necklace incision is commonly used in place of the J extension.

Transverse Neck Skin Crease Incision

This is preferred incision for selective neck dissections. Begins just below the tip of the mastoid process in a curvilinear fashion two finger breadths below the angle of the mandible and extends onto the tip of the hyoid bone and medially to the midline of the chin area. This incision can be extended through the midline of the chin and lip for exposure of tumors of the oral cavity or for a cheek flap in composite resections. This incision can be extended to the opposite neck along the hyoid when contralateral neck dissection is necessary.

Steps

- Incision should be marked with marking pen.
- Skin is infiltrated with 1% lidocaine and epinephrine to avoid excess bleeding from the skin.

- Standard painting and draping is done. Keep the ear lobule open on the side of neck dissection while draping.
- The horizontal neck skin crease incision is made. A vertical limb is dropped from the posterior aspect of the incision behind the carotid artery and extending inferiorly to the clavicle in a lazy S fashion. Then, the skin and subcutaneous tissue are incised.
- The platysma is incised. Dissection is performed between the platysma and the deeper structures in the avascular plane beneath the platysma.
- The posterior flaps are elevated in the continuation of subplatysmal plane. The dissection is performed posteriorly up to the trapezius muscle, with good exposure of the SCM muscle.
- The greater auricular nerve is identified posteriorly at Erb's point.
- The spinal accessory nerve can be located about 1 cm above Erb's point behind the SCM muscle; anteriorly it is crossing the IJV.
- Superiorly, dissection begins near the mastoid area with transection of the origin of the sternomastoid muscle and exposure of the splenius capitis muscle.
- Inferiorly, the dissection is extended along the anterior border of trapezius muscle up to the clavicle.
- The inferior belly of the omohyoid muscle is cut near the clavicle which serves as a good landmark to avoid injury to the brachial plexus, as the brachial plexus lies behind the inferior belly of the omohyoid muscle.
- The dissection is then extended anteriorly behind the sternomastoid muscle and effort is made to avoid injury to both the brachial plexus and to the phrenic nerve.
- The external jugular vein entering deep to the clavicle into the subclavian system is identified and ligated.
- The dissection is continued medially, up to the submental area. The anterior flap is raised up to the midline, and the superior flap is raised up to the free border of the mandible, avoiding any injury to the marginal mandibular branch of facial nerve (can be identified on the surface of the fascia covering the submandibular salivary gland and by elevating the fascia deep to common facial vein after dividing it).
- Internal jugular vein is exposed and dissected from the carotid sheath; the vagus nerve is identified and carefully preserved. Inferiorly, the IJV is clamped, divided, and doubly ligated.
- While doing on the left side lower neck, it is important to avoid any injury to the thoracic duct which can cause chyle leak.
- The dissection is continued superiorly behind the IJV; the middle thyroid vein may be identified and ligated.
- As the dissection is continued superiorly, the superior belly of the omohyoid is transected near the hyoid and the dissection is performed near the carotid bulb. It is important to inform the anesthesiologist to check the blood pressure and the pulse rate.
- The hypoglossal nerve is identified approximately 1.5 cm above the carotid bifurcation. The posterior belly of digastric also helps identify hypoglossal in the floor of mouth. Just above this level, the entire sternomastoid is transected superiorly and the dissection is performed medial to the sternomastoid muscle.
- The contents of the submental triangle are cleared between the anterior bellies of the two-sided digastric muscle. The mylohyoid muscle is exposed medial to the digastric; it is pulled medially, exposing the deeper portion of the submandibular salivary gland.
- The dissection is extended along the free border of the mandible, exposing the submandibular salivary gland.
- The facial artery and facial vein are identified in front of the posterior belly of

the digastric. This needs to be clamped and ligated carefully. A double ligature is performed to avoid any unexpected slipping of the ligature.

- The lingual nerve is exposed superior to the submandibular salivary gland, and the hypoglossal nerve is exposed inferiorly. The branch of the lingual nerve supplying the parasympathetic fibers to the submandibular salivary gland is transected, and the submandibular salivary gland is retracted posteriorly. Ligate Wharton's duct and pull the entire submandibular salivary gland laterally.
- There may be a group of prefacial lymph nodes in this area that may be removed carefully, without causing any injury to the marginal mandibular nerve.
- The superior portion of the IJV is exposed just behind the posterior belly of the digastric. The IJV is clamped and ligated after separating the vagus and the hypoglossal nerves from it.
- The spinal accessory nerve is transected in this area along with the branch entering the sternomastoid muscle. The entire neck specimen is mobilized and separated from the remaining portion of the levator scapulae muscle.
- After removal of the entire neck specimen, the wound is irrigated and any bleeding spots on the surface of the muscles are cauterized. The wound is irrigated copiously with warm distilled water, and the lower neck area is once again visualized for any lymphatic leak by requesting the anesthesiologist to do Valsalva maneuver.
- Two suction drains are commonly inserted and secured with silk sutures, one in the anterior portion and another in the posterior portion extending superiorly up to the skull base. It is important to avoid placing the suction drains across the carotid vessels.
- The neck extension is reduced. The platysma is closed with vicryl sutures; platysma is closed tightly to hold the suction drains; and the skin is approximated generally with nylon sutures. Patient is then extubated and shifted to the recovery room.

- Ideally the surgeon should take the specimen personally to the pathology department and identifying various levels of the lymph nodes. Alternatively, the specimen may be pinned to cardboard or a template for better localization of the various levels of the neck lymph nodes.

● MODIFIED RADICAL NECK DISSECTION

Patients with gross nodal metastasis to the neck that does not directly infiltrate or adhere to the nonlymphatic structures previously mentioned. The technique of anesthesia, position of the patient, and incision are the same as explained in the technique of radical neck dissection.

Steps

- Skin flaps are elevated in subplatysmal plane; superiorly to the inferior border of mandible, inferiorly to the clavicle, anteriorly to the lateral border of the strap muscles and the anterior belly of the contralateral digastric muscle, and posteriorly to the anterior border of trapezius.
- Marginal mandibular nerve is preserved by elevating the submandibular fascia or elevating the fascia deep to facial vein after dividing and ligating it.
- The nodes in level IA are dissected off from submental triangle; the inferior border of the mandible and the opposite digastric muscle, leaving the underlying mylohyoid muscle intact.
- The mylohyoid muscle is retracted anteromedially and the submandibular duct is identified, ligated and divided. The parasympathetic contributions of lingual nerve to the gland are divided inferior to the submandibular ganglion. The dissected

nodal tissues in level IB and submandibular gland are then elevated from the digastric muscle, in continuity with the nondissected portion of the neck. The hypoglossal nerve coursing superior to the digastric muscle identified and preserved.

- Anterior border of SCM muscle is skeletonized till posterior border hugging close to the muscle to avoid injury to IJV.
- Spinal accessory nerve is identified in the posterior triangle, about 1 cm above the Erb's point. The nerve is delineated. It separates the level II in IIA (anterior) and IIB (posterior). The surgeon has to be aware of the relationship of the SAN to the IJV. Tandler-Parsons and Keith suggested the relationship of the SAN to the IJV at the base of the skull: anterior (70%), posterior (27%), and through the IJV (3%).
- Dissection is then continued posterocaudally till the trapezius muscle. The cN XI must be carefully dissected by identifying the nerve both anterior and posterior to the SCM muscle. The branches to the muscle must carefully be divided, atraumatically dissecting the spinal accessory nerve from the SCM muscle.
- Commencing at the anterior border of the trapezius muscle, a posterior to anterior dissection is performed. The posterior triangle contents are elevated in an en bloc fashion off the fascia of the deep cervical musculature, preserving the phrenic nerve and the brachial plexus, located deep to this fascia.
- The posterior triangle contents which posterosuperior to the nerve (level VA) are passed inferiorly below the nerve. The contents are then dissected from the posterior border and the undersurface of the SCM.
- The contents of levels IIB, IIA, III, and IV are dissected above the plane of cervical roots after division of the omohyoid muscle. The specimen is then dissected from the IJV,

taking care to avoid injury to the carotid artery and vagus nerve.

- The neck dissection specimen is then removed and oriented for lymph node levels for specific histopathologic evaluation and pathologic staging purposes. Suction drains are strategically placed and a two-layered closure with platysma and skin is done.

● COMPLICATIONS OF NECK DISSECTION

Intraoperative Complications

- *Excessive bleeding*: It occurs from slipping of ligatures from the blood vessels (IJV) or inadvertent injury to the carotid artery.
- *Air embolism*: Slipping of the jugular vein in the inferior portion may lead to air embolism. Air embolism may be related to inadvertent suction of air into the venous system; effectively, air enters the cardiac system.
- *Pneumothorax*: It may occur due to injury to the apical pleura during dissection of either levels IV or VI.
- *Carotid sinus syndrome*: Bradycardia and hypotension may occur during dissection near the carotid body.
- *Chylous leak*: Meticulous identification and ligation of the branches of the thoracic duct are important for preventing a chyle leak.
- *Nerve injury*: Injury to the marginal mandibular, lingual, hypoglossal, vagus, and phrenic nerves. Neuropraxia should recover in few months.

Postoperative Complications

- *Shoulder dysfunction*: It is a functional morbidity due to sacrifice or stretching of the spinal accessory nerve.
- *Indentation in the neck*: It is a cosmetic deformity related to resection of SCM muscle.
- Persistent chyle leak or fistula.

- *Cutaneous fistula*: It is common in irradiated necks.
- *Facial/cerebral edema*: It can arise in synchronous bilateral radical neck dissections, in which both IJVs are ligated. It is managed conservatively.
- Postsurgical fibrosis of the neck.

● FURTHER READING

1. Ambrosch P, Kron M, Pradier O, et al. Efficacy of selective neck dissection: A review of 503 cases of elective and therapeutic treatment of the neck in squamous cell carcinoma of the upper aerodigestive tract. Otolaryngol Head Neck Surg. 2001;124(2):180-7.
2. Andersen PE, Shah JP, Cambronero E, et al. The role of comprehensive neck dissection with preservation of the spinal accessory nerve in the clinically positive neck. Am J Surg. 1994;168(5):499-502.
3. Andersen PE, Warren F, Spiro J, et al. Results of selective neck dissection in management of the node-positive neck. Arch Otolaryngol Head Neck Surg. 2002;128(10):1180-4.
4. Bernier J, Domenge C, Ozsahin M, et al.; European Organization for Research and Treatment of Cancer Trial 22931. Postoperative irradiation with or without concomitant chemotherapy for locally advanced head and neck cancer. N Engl J Med. 2004;350(19):1945-52.
5. Brizel DM, Prosnitz RG, Hunter S, et al. Necessity for adjuvant neck dissection in setting of concurrent chemoradiation for advanced head-and-neck cancer. Int J Radiat Oncol Biol Phys. 2004;58(5):1418-23.
6. Byers RM, Clayman GL, McGill D, et al. Selective neck dissections for squamous carcinoma of the upper aerodigestive tract: Patterns of regional failure. Head Neck. 1999;21(6):499-505.
7. Cağli S, Yüce I, Yiğitbaşi OG, et al. Is routine bilateral neck dissection absolutely necessary in the management of N0 neck in patients with supraglottic carcinoma? Eur Arch Otorhinolaryngol. 2007;264(12):1453-7.
8. Chan SW, Mukesh BN, Sizeland A. Treatment outcome of N3 nodal head and neck squamous cell carcinoma. Otolaryngol Head Neck Surg. 2003;129(1):55-60.
9. Chepeha DB, Hoff PT, Taylor RJ, et al. Selective neck dissection for the treatment of neck metastasis from squamous cell carcinoma of the head and neck. Laryngoscope. 2002;112(3):434-8.
10. Cooper JS, Pajak TF, Forastiere AA, et al.; Radiation Therapy Oncology Group 9501/Intergroup. Postoperative concurrent radiotherapy and chemotherapy for high-risk squamous-cell carcinoma of the head and neck. N Engl J Med. 2004;350(19):1937-44.
11. Jones AS, Goodyear PW, Ghosh S, et al. Extensive neck node metastases (n3) in head and neck squamous carcinoma: Is radical treatment warranted? Otolaryngol Head Neck Surg. 2011;144(1):29-35.
12. Kao J, Lavaf A, Teng MS, et al. Adjuvant radiotherapy and survival for patients with node-positive head and neck cancer: An analysis by primary site and nodal stage. Int J Radiat Oncol Biol Phys. 2008;71(2):362-70.
13. Kolli VR, Datta RV, Orner JB, et al. The role of supraomohyoid neck dissection in patients with positive nodes. Arch Otolaryngol Head Neck Surg. 2000;126(3):413-6.
14. Lavaf A, Genden EM, Cesaretti JA, et al. Adjuvant radiotherapy improves overall survival for patients with lymph node-positive head and neck squamous cell carcinoma. Cancer. 2008;112(3):535-43.
15. Mendenhall WM, Cassisi NJ, Stringer SP, Tannehill SP. Therapeutic principles in the management of head and neck tumors. In: Souhami RL, Tannock I, Hohenberger P, Horiot JC (Eds). Oxford Textbook of Oncology. New York: Oxford University Press; 2002. pp. 1322-43.
16. Moore MG, Bhattacharyya N. Effectiveness of chemotherapy and radiotherapy in sterilizing cervical nodal disease in squamous cell carcinoma of the head and neck. Laryngoscope. 2005;115(4):570-3.
17. Muzaffar K. Therapeutic selective neck dissection: A 25-year review. Laryngoscope. 2003;113(9):1460-5.
18. Richards BL, Spiro JD. Controlling advanced neck disease: Efficacy of neck dissection and radiotherapy. Laryngoscope. 2000;110(7):1124-7.
19. Simental AA Jr, Duvuri U, Johnson JT, et al. Selective neck dissection in patients with upper aerodigestive tract cancer with clinically positive nodal disease. Ann Otol Rhinol Laryngol. 2006;115(11):846-9.
20. Watkinson JC, Owen C, Thompson S, et al. Conservation surgery in the management of T1 and T2 oropharyngeal squamous cell carcinoma: The Birmingham UK experience. Clin Otolaryngol Allied Sci. 2002;27(6):541-8

CHAPTER 20

Nodal Metastasis from an Unknown Primary Origin

Krishnakumar Thankappan

● INTRODUCTION

The incidence of a neck node with unknown primary origin in the head and neck region is about 3%. Squamous cell carcinoma accounts for about two-thirds of this. Carcinoma of unknown primary (CUP) is defined as the histological confirmation of at least one cervical lymph node metastasis in the absence of a primary tumor, as determined by the diagnostic modalities that includes careful physical and endoscopic examinations of the aerodigestive tract and imaging. There is no prospective randomized data to guide the management of this condition. Management strategies are based on retrospective studies, few prospective studies, and experience from treating patients with known primary cancers. In literature, the entity is being described in different names like "Head and Neck Cancer with Occult Primary",

"Carcinoma of Unknown Primary", "Squamous Cell Carcinoma of Unknown Primary (SCCUP)", and "Occult Primary".

● THEORIES OF OCCURRENCE

Various proposed theories are:
- Squamous elements of branchial remnants in lymph nodes turning malignant
- Small primary hidden in tonsil/base tongue crypts with aggressive nodal metastasis
- Primary regressing due to immune hyperactivity
- Subclinical primary with nodal metastasis; either due to faster growth rate of the nodal metastasis or sloughing of necrotic carcinoma.

● EVALUATION

Evaluation consists of evaluation of the neck nodes and evaluation for the occult primary.

Evaluation of the Neck Node

Neck node/(s) has to be evaluated with reference to the site in the neck, size, extent, fixation to surrounding structures, and skin and any cranial nerve deficits. Site of the node can give clue to the primary. Levels I to III nodes can have primary usually in the lip and oral cavity, Levels II to IV or level VI can have primary in the oropharynx, hypopharynx, larynx, or thyroid. Level IV and/or supraclavicular nodes may have a primary arising below the clavicle (lung, breast, gastrointestinal tract, kidney, or ovary). Level V nodes may arise from the nasopharynx primary. Level II is the most common site with head and neck primary; majority of the cases are N2a or N2b. They may be bilateral in up to 10%. Nasopharynx, base of tongue, tonsil, hypopharynx, or supraglottis are the potential sites of the occult primary.

Evaluation for the Occult Primary

Clinical examination of the head and neck areas including oral cavity and oropharynx, palpation of the base of tongue and tonsils, flexible or rigid office endoscopy to see nasopharynx, larynx and hypopharynx, is essential.

The first investigation usually is a fine needle aspiration cytology (FNAC) or core biopsy to find the pathology. Open biopsy is usually not recommended. It may have a role when repeated FNACs followed by a core needle biopsy are nondiagnostic or in masses clinically and cytologically suspicious for lymphoma. Immunohistochemistry may be helpful. Cytokeratins (CK) suggest carcinoma, lymphoma by CLA, CD30, CD43; melanoma by S100, HMB45; sarcoma by vimentin, actin and desmin, squamous cell carcinoma by CK5/6; thyroid by TTF1 and thyroglobulin.

Imaging

The traditional investigations were computed tomography (CT) scan and magnetic resonance imaging (MRI). Contrast-enhanced CT scan from the base of the skull to the level of the thoracic inlet and CT thorax are done. This helped to search for the occult primary site, evaluate the extent of the nodal disease, check for any obvious extracapsular spread, soft tissue involvement, and suspicious nodes in the contralateral neck. Literature finds 9–23% detection of the occult primary and the rates rising to 60% when the suspicious radiological findings direct subsequent endoscopic biopsies.

Role of Positron Emission Tomography–CT

A meta-analysis by Rusthoven et al. showed that positron emission tomography (PET) had a detection rate of 24% (sensitivity 88% and specificity 75%). A recent meta-analysis by Kwee, et al. showed PET–CT had a detection rate of 37% (sensitivity 84% and specificity

84%). False-positivity rates are up to 15%. The drawbacks of the PET–CT scan are the possibility of false-positive findings when performed after a biopsy, in the oropharynx, by the secretion of FDG from the salivary glands. The chances of false-negativity in the base of the tongue when the primary is small, is less than 5 mm in size. Limited availability, costs, and radiation exposure are other disadvantages. PET–CT can lead to targeted biopsies.

Tonsillectomy and Random Biopsies

Ipsilateral tonsillectomy has about 18–44% detection rate. The evidence for bilateral tonsillectomy is less. The rate of detection of the primary in the contralateral tonsil is up to 10%. Some guidelines also suggest panendoscopy and random mucosal biopsies from the sites of predilection for a primary tumor like the ipsilateral tonsil, base of tongue, naso- and hypopharynx. Current recommendations are more favoring PET–CT scan direct biopsies. Transoral robotic surgery (TORS) has led to the concept of base of tongue mucosal resection to find the primary.

Molecular studies for human papilloma virus (HPV) may show a positive causal relationship between HPV in the node and oropharynx primary site. Similarly, Epstein–Barr virus (EBV) markers may point to undifferentiated carcinoma of the nasopharynx. If HPV positive, it suggests a better prognosis and a possibility of treatment de-escalation. The evaluation for unknown primary is shown in **Flowchart 1**.

● AJCC 8TH EDITION: CHANGES IN RELATION TO CERVICAL METASTASIS WITH UNKNOWN PRIMARY

These patients are categorized as T0 but cannot be assigned to a specific anatomic site. Currently, greater than 90% of these T0 (unknown primary) designations (lymph

Flowchart 1: Evaluation and management of neck node with unknown primary.

(FNAC: Fine needle aspiration cytology; IHC: Immunohistochemistry;
PET–CT: Positron emission tomography–computed tomography)

nodes in patients with no detectable primary) reflect HPV-associated cancers (in HPV prevalent geographic areas). A large majority of nasopharyngeal cancers are positive for EBV by Epstein-Barr—encoded RNA (EBER) on ISH. Consequently, in the proper clinical context, demonstrating the presence of either EBV or HPV can establish an anatomic site of origin. HPV–ISH, p16 immunohistochemistry, and EBER–ISH are recommended for all cervical lymph nodes with carcinoma of unknown primary site. Thus, one key change from prior editions of the TNM system is the elimination of the T0 category in sites other than the nasopharynx, HPV-associated OPC, and salivary gland cancers (which can be identified by their unique histology). If no primary lesion can be identified, then the lymph node may have emanated from any mucosal site; so there is no rationale to support retaining the T0 designation outside of the virally associated cancers of the oropharynx and nasopharynx.

Key Changes: p16 and EBER are Required for Staging

- p16+ will be staged as T0 N-appropriate in HPV-mediated p16+ oropharynx.
- EBER+ will be staged T0 N-appropriate in nasopharynx chapter
- EBER–, p16–squamous cell carcinoma will be staged in the cervical node as T0 N-appropriate and will need extranodal extension (ENE) designation.
- T0 eliminated from all other chapters except EBV-related nasopharynx, HPV-related oropharynx, and salivary gland based on histology of lymph node **(Tables 1 and 2)**.

● TREATMENT

Treatment includes treatment of the neck and the prophylactic treatment of the primary site. Long-term disease-free survival rates are about 50–60%. The chances of appearance of a subsequent primary is about 10%.

Early-stage Neck Disease (cN1 or pN1 without Extracapsular Spread)

The treatment options are single-modality treatment with neck dissection alone or involved field-limited radiation alone. The advantage of neck dissection is the ability to detect extranodal spread which, if positive, will have impact on the further treatment and prognosis. Some authors advocate combined modality treatment

because the nodal metastasis upstages it to stage III disease and that the possible primary cannot be left alone. Radiation with salvage surgery if required and surgery with adjuvant radiotherapy (RT) are the options. No strong evidence support either single- or combined-modality treatment.

Advanced-stage Disease (pN1 with Extranodal Spread, N2, N3 Disease)

Combined modality is usually recommended. It can be either surgery followed by RT or chemoradiotherapy, initial chemoradiotherapy followed by salvage neck dissection, in case of no complete response either clinical or metabolic (PET–CT after 12 weeks). No high-level evidence supports either. In N2 disease, either N2a or N2b, initial chemoradiotherapy is favored because most primary are in the radio-curable sites like oropharynx, hypopharynx, nasopharynx or larynx. In N3 disease, surgery followed by RT or chemoradiotherapy is favored because anyway surgery will have to be incorporated and surgery in the nonirradiated neck is less morbid.

Limited Radiotherapy versus Extensive Radiotherapy

There is a controversy as to whether the RT should be unilateral or bilateral, involved field versus whole mucosal. Most single institutional retrospective data shows comparable results. There is no high level of evidence favoring either. The points in favor of limited RT are that the emergence rates of the primary are comparable. The emergence rates of mucosal primary tumors (10%) after unilateral neck irradiation are similar to the risk of occurrence of metachronous second primary tumors in patients cured of a known head and neck squamous cell carcinoma primary. The risk of missing a curable occult primary after a

Table 1: TNM staging (AJCC, 8th edition) for EBER-negative and p16-negative nodal metastasis with unknown primary.

T staging	
T0	No evidence of primary tumor
Clinical N (cN)	
NX	Regional lymph nodes cannot be assessed
N0	No regional lymph node metastasis
N1	Metastasis in a single ipsilateral lymph node, 3 cm or smaller in greatest dimension and ENE (–)
N2	Metastasis in a single ipsilateral node larger than 3 cm but not larger than 6 cm in greatest dimension and ENE (–); or metastases in multiple ipsilateral lymph nodes, none larger than 6 cm in greatest dimension and ENE (–); or in bilateral or contralateral lymph nodes, none larger than 6 cm in greatest dimension and ENE (–)
N2a	Metastasis in a single ipsilateral node larger than 3 cm but not larger than 6 cm in greatest dimension and ENE (–)
N2b	Metastasis in multiple ipsilateral nodes, none larger than 6 cm in greatest dimension and ENE (–)
N2c	Metastasis in bilateral or contralateral lymph nodes, none larger than 6 cm in greatest dimension and ENE (–)
N3	Metastasis in a lymph node larger than 6 cm in greatest dimension and ENE (–); or metastasis in any node(s) with clinically overt ENE (+)
N3a	Metastasis in a lymph node larger than 6 cm in greatest dimension and ENE (–)
N3b	Metastasis in any node (s) with clinically overt ENE (+)
Pathological N (pN)	
NX	Regional lymph nodes cannot be assessed
N0	No regional lymph node metastasis
N1	Metastasis in a single ipsilateral lymph node, 3 cm or smaller in greatest dimension and ENE (–)
N2	Metastasis in a single ipsilateral node, 3 cm or smaller in greatest dimension and ENE (+); or metastasis in a single ipsilateral node larger than 3 cm but not larger than 6 cm in greatest dimension and ENE (–) or metastases in multiple ipsilateral lymph nodes, none larger than 6 cm in greatest dimension and ENE (–); or in bilateral or contralateral lymph nodes, none larger than 6 cm in greatest dimension and ENE (–)
N2a	Metastasis in a single ipsilateral node, 3 cm or smaller in greatest dimension and ENE (+); or metastasis in a single ipsilateral node larger than 3 cm but not larger than 6 cm in greatest dimension and ENE (–)
N2b	Metastasis in multiple ipsilateral nodes, none larger than 6 cm in greatest dimension and ENE (–)
N2c	Metastasis in bilateral or contralateral lymph nodes, none larger than 6 cm in greatest dimension and ENE (–)
N3	Metastasis in a lymph node larger than 6 cm in greatest dimension and ENE (–); or in a single ipsilateral node larger than 3 cm in greatest dimension and ENE (+); or multiple ipsilateral, contralateral, or bilateral nodes any with ENE (+)
N3a	Metastasis in a lymph node larger than 6 cm in greatest dimension and ENE (–)
N3b	Metastasis in a single ipsilateral node larger than 3 cm in greatest dimension and ENE (+); or multiple ipsilateral, contralateral, or bilateral nodes any with ENE (+)
Note: A designation of "U" or "L" may be used for any N category to indicate metastasis above the lower border of the cricoid (U) or below the lower border of the cricoid (L) Similarly, clinical and pathological ENE should be recorded as ENE (–) or ENE (+)	
Distant metastasis M	
M0	No distant metastasis
M1	Distant metastasis

(AJCC: American Joint Committee on Cancer; EBER: Epstein–Barr—encoded RNA); ENE: Extranodal extension

Table 2: AJCC, 8th edition, prognostic staging.

When T is ...	and N is ...	and M is ...	Then the stage group is ...
T0	N1	M0	III
T0	N2	M0	IVA
T0	N3	M0	IVB
T0	Any N	M1	IVC

(AJCC: American Joint Committee on Cancer)

thorough initial work-up is too small to justify the morbidity of elective irradiation of the potential primary sites. The survival rates are not related to the appearance of the primary tumor. Potential complexity of adding re-irradiation for the primary site if and when a primary cancer emerges and limitations of salvage surgery after extensive RT are further points favoring limited RT.

● FURTHER READING

1. Strojan P, Ferlito A, Langendijk JA, et al. Contemporary management of lymph node metastases from an unknown primary to the neck: II. A review of therapeutic options. Head Neck 2013;35(2):286-93.
2. Strojan P, Ferlito A, Medina JE, et al. Contemporary management of lymph node metastases from an unknown primary to the neck: I. A review of diagnostic approaches. Head Neck. 2013;35(1):123-32.

Paranasal Sinuses

Chapters

- Pathology of Tumors of the Nose and Paranasal Sinuses
- Imaging of the Paranasal Sinus Tumors
- Guidelines in the Management of Malignancies in Maxillo-ethmoid Complex
- Principles of Surgery in the Management of Tumors of Maxillo-ethmoid Complex

CHAPTER 21

Pathology of Tumors of the Nose and Paranasal Sinuses

Chaya Prasad

● INTRODUCTION

The nasal cavity and paranasal sinuses occupy a relatively small anatomical space. They are the sites of origin of some of the more complex and histologically diverse group of tumors in the entire human body. These include neoplasms derived from mucosal epithelium, seromucinous glands, soft tissues, bone, cartilage, neural or neuroectodermal tissue, hematolymphoid cells, and the odontogenic apparatus.

● WHO HISTOLOGICAL CLASSIFICATION

- *Malignant epithelial tumors*:
  - Squamous cell carcinoma
  - Verrucous carcinoma
  - Papillary squamous cell carcinoma
  - Basaloid squamous cell carcinoma
  - Spindle cell carcinoma
  - Adenosquamous carcinoma
  - Acantholytic squamous cell carcinoma
  - Lymphoepithelial carcinoma
  - Sinonasal undifferentiated carcinoma
  - Adenocarcinoma
  - Intestinal-type adenocarcinoma
  - Nonintestinal-type adenocarcinoma
  - Salivary gland-type carcinoma
  - Adenoid cystic carcinoma
  - Acinic cell carcinoma
  - Mucoepidermoid carcinoma
  - Epithelial–myoepithelial carcinoma
  - Clear cell carcinoma not otherwise specified (NOS)
  - Myoepithelial carcinoma
  - Carcinoma expleomorphic adenoma
  - Polymorphous low-grade adeno-carcinoma
  - Neuroendocrine tumors
  - Typical carcinoid
  - Atypical carcinoid
  - Small cell carcinoma, neuroendocrine type
- *Benign epithelial tumors*:
  - Sinonasal papillomas
  - Inverted papilloma (Schneiderian papilloma, inverted type)
  - Oncocytic papilloma (Schneiderian papilloma, oncocytic type)
  - Exophytic papilloma (Schneiderian papilloma, exophytic type)
  - Salivary gland-type adenomas
  - Pleomorphic adenoma
  - Myoepithelioma
  - Oncocytoma
- *Soft tissue tumors*:
  - Malignant tumors:
    - Fibrosarcoma
    - Malignant fibrous histiocytoma
    - Leiomyosarcoma
    - Rhabdomyosarcoma

- ◆ Angiosarcoma
- ◆ Malignant peripheral nerve sheath tumor
- ◆ Borderline and low malignant potential tumors
- ◆ Desmoid-type fibromatosis
- ◆ Inflammatory myofibroblastic tumor
- ◆ Glomangiopericytoma (Sinonasal-type hemangiopericytoma)
- ◆ Extrapleural solitary fibrous tumor
- Benign tumors:
  - ◆ Myxoma
  - ◆ Leiomyoma
  - ◆ Hemangioma
  - ◆ Schwannoma
  - ◆ Neurofibroma
  - ◆ Meningioma
- ▪ Tumors of bone and cartilage
- ▪ Hematolymphoid tumors
- ▪ *Neuroectodermal*:
  - • Ewing sarcoma
  - • Primitive neuroectodermal tumor
  - • Olfactory neuroblastoma
  - • Melanotic neuroectodermal tumor of infancy
  - • Mucosal malignant melanoma
- ▪ Germ cell tumors:
  - • Secondary tumors.

Sinonasal Carcinoma

It is an unusual tumor with marked left-sided preponderance. Occupational groups known to be at an increased risk are nickel refiners and woodworkers.

Location and Spread

Intranasal carcinomas occur more commonly in the vestibule and lateral wall and only rarely in the septum. Sinonasal carcinomas are diagnosed late in their course, when extensive bone destruction is already present. Intranasal tumors may extend into the medial wall of the antrum, ethmoid sinuses, orbit, anterior skull bone, and upper lip. Tumors of the infrastructure of the maxillary sinus spread inferiorly into the alveolar process or gingivobuccal sulcus, anteriorly into the soft tissues of the cheek beneath the zygoma, or medially into the nasal cavity and hard palate. Those of the suprastructure may extend superiorly and medially into the orbit, ethmoid sinus, and cribriform plate; posterolaterally into the pterygoid space, sphenoid sinus, or base of the skull; anterolaterally into the zygoma; or posterolaterally into the infratemporal fossa.

Microscopic Features

Squamous cell carcinoma: A malignant epithelial neoplasm originating from the mucosal epithelium of the nasal cavities or paranasal sinuses, which includes a keratinizing and a nonkeratinizing type **(Fig. 1)**.

Variants

Verrucous carcinoma, basaloid squamous cell carcinoma **(Fig. 2)**, and sarcomatoid carcinoma (spindle cell carcinoma, carcinosarcoma) are the three types of malignant tumor that are rare in the sinonasal region. They are similar to their more common counterparts in the upper digestive tract and larynx.

Adenocarcinoma without a specific salivary gland pattern usually arises on the middle turbinate or in the ethmoid sinus and from there extends laterally into the orbit, and upward into the anterior cranial fossa. These tumors may arise from the surface epithelium (the majority) or from the subjacent seromucous glands.

Microscopically, two main categories are recognized—(1) intestinal-type adenocarcinoma and (2) nonintestinal-type adenocarcinoma, which can be further divided into low-grade and high-grade subtypes. Adenocarcinomas are locally aggressive tumors, with a propensity for local recurrence. Lymph node metastases are rare.

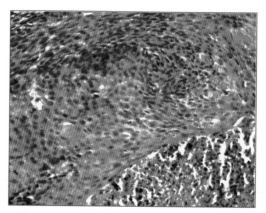

Fig. 1: Nonkeratinizing squamous cell carcinoma.

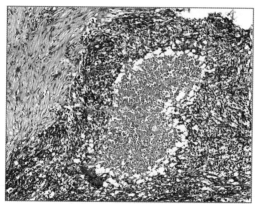

Fig. 2: Basaloid squamous cell carcinoma.

The most important prognostic factor is tumor stage. Histology-wise, it would seem that adenocarcinoma carries a slightly better prognosis than squamous cell carcinoma. Among the adenocarcinomas, there is a relationship between degree of differentiation and prognosis. Tubulopapillary tumors showing minimal atypia run an indolent clinical course. Cylindrical cell (transitional; nonkeratinizing) carcinoma is closely related to squamous cell carcinoma. In most instances, the microscopic diagnosis is obvious because of the atypicality and stromal infiltration. In others, the identification is more difficult because the growth pattern is similar to that of a papilloma in the sense that stromal invasion is not immediately apparent. The differential diagnosis includes olfactory neuroblastomas or neuroendocrine carcinomas.

Small cell neuroendocrine carcinoma has a morphologic, immunohistochemical, and ultrastructural appearance similar to that of its pulmonary homolog. The main differential diagnosis is with undifferentiated (anaplastic) carcinoma and with olfactory neuroblastoma. Undifferentiated (anaplastic) carcinoma is a highly aggressive and clinicopathologically distinctive carcinoma of uncertain histogenesis that typically presents with locally extensive disease. It is composed of pleomorphic tumor cells with frequent necrosis, and should be differentiated from lymphoepithelial carcinoma. Despite aggressive management, the prognosis is poor, with median survival of less than 18 months and 5-year survival of less than 20%.

NUT midline carcinoma accounts for a proportion of cases conventionally diagnosed as sinonasal undifferentiated carcinomas; the diagnosis has to be confirmed by immunostaining with an NUT-specific antibody or by molecular techniques. Strong immunoreactivity for p16 seems to correlate with the cylindrical cell carcinoma subtype, whereas (keratinizing) squamous cell carcinoma and small cell undifferentiated carcinoma are more likely to show reactivity for p53.

Salivary Gland Tumors

Tumors of minor salivary gland origin occur in the nasal cavity as well as in the sinuses especially in the antrum. Most tumors of the paranasal sinuses are malignant; adenoid cystic carcinoma is the most common variety. In the nasal cavity, there is a relatively high proportion of benign neoplasms in the form of benign mixed tumor (pleomorphic adenoma). Other types of salivary gland tumors include mucoepidermoid carcinoma, acinic cell carcinoma, and myoepithelioma.

Respiratory Epithelial Adenomatoid Hamartomas

They are benign nonneoplastic overgrowth of indigenous glands of the nasal cavity, paranasal sinuses and nasopharynx associated with the surface epithelium, and devoid of ectodermal neuroectodermal, and/or mesodermal elements. Conservative, but complete surgical excision is curative **(Figs. 3A and B)**.

Neurogenous and Related Tumors and Tumor-like Conditions

Meningiomas can also present as primary intranasal or paranasal masses. Astrocytomas and other glial tumors can also extend into the root of the nasal cavity from their initial intracranial location.

Olfactory Neuroblastoma (Esthesioneuroblastoma)

A malignant neuroectodermal tumor thought to originate from the olfactory membrane of the sinonasal tract.

Epidemiology: It is an uncommon neoplasm representing approximately 2–3% of sinonasal tract tumors. Patients range in age from as young as 2 years to 90 years, and a bimodal age distribution has been noted in the 2nd and 6th decades of life. Both genders are affected equally. No racial predilection has been noted.

Localization: The most common site of origin is in the upper nasal cavity in the region of the cribriform plate. Included in the areas of the proposed origin are Jacobson's organ (vomeronasal organ), sphenopalatine (pterygoid palatine) ganglion, olfactory placode, and the ganglion of loci (nervus terminalis). "Ectopic" origin in lower nasal cavity or within one of the paranasal sinuses (e.g. maxillary sinus) may occur.

Macroscopy: The tumor appears as a reddish gray, highly vascular polypoid mass of generally soft consistency located in the roof of the nasal fossa.

*Microscopy **(Fig. 4)**:* It is a cellular tumor composed of uniform small cells with round nuclei, scanty cytoplasm, indistinct nuclear membrane, and a prominent fibrillary or reticular background, similar to that seen in other neurogenic tumors (such as ganglioneuroblastoma). Rosettes of the Homer Wright type may be present, but differentiation into mature ganglion cells takes place only in rare cases. Fibrovascular stroma and vascular proliferation can be present. The differential

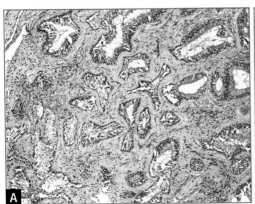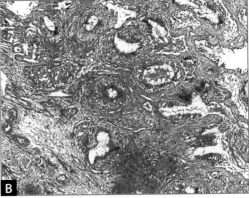

Figs. 3A and B: (A) Respiratory epithelial adenomatoid hamartoma; (B) PAS stain highlighting the mucus cells.

diagnosis of tumors with this appearance is with malignant lymphoma, plasmacytoma, embryonal or alveolar rhabdomyosarcoma, and the Ewing sarcoma/primitive neuroectodermal tumor family, undifferentiated carcinoma, and small cell neuroendocrine carcinoma.

Grading

Grading of olfactory neuroblastoma is done using Hyams histological grading system **(Table 1)**.

Immunoprofile *(Fig. 5)*

It includes synaptophysin, neurofilament protein S-100 staining limited to the sustentacular

cell. In addition, immunoreactivity may be present for chromogranin, GFAP, and Leu-7. Cytokeratin is usually negative, but some cases can show some positive cells. EMA, CEA, LCA, HMB-45, desmin and CD99 are absent. Ki-67 shows a high proliferative index of 10–50%.

Electron Microscopy

Presence of neurofilaments, neurotubules, and dense-core neurosecretory cytoplasmic granules.

Prognosis and Predictive Factors

The tumor shows local invasiveness into the paranasal sinuses, nasopharynx, palate, orbit,

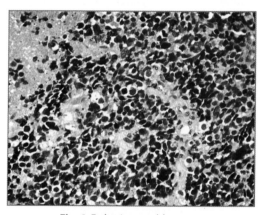

Fig. 4: Esthesioneuroblastoma.
Nesting pattern of growth.

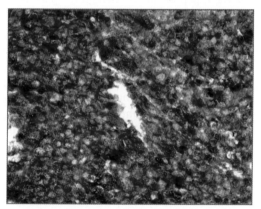

Fig. 5: Esthesioneuroblastoma. Tumor cells are positive for synaptophysin.

Table 1: Grading: Hyams' histologic grading system for olfactory neuroblastoma.

Microscopy	Grade 1	Grade 2	Grade 3	Grade 4
Architecture	Lobular	Lobular	±Lobular	±Lobular
Pleomorphism	Absent to slight	Present	Prominent	Marked
Neurofibrillary matrix	Prominent	Present	May be present	Absent
Rosettes	Present*	Present*	May be present**	May be present**
Mitoses	Absent	Present	Prominent	Marked
Necrosis	Absent	Absent	Present	Prominent
Glands	May be present	May be present	May be present	May be present
Calcification	Variable	Variable	Absent	Absent

*Homer Wright rosettes (pseudorosettes)
**Rexner–Wintersteiner rosettes (True rosettes)

base of skull, and brain. Distant metastases occur in about one-fifth of cases, the most common sites being the cervical lymph nodes and lungs. Late recurrence is common. This tumor has been shown to be radiosensitive, and a combination of surgery and radiation therapy offers the best chances of cure. From the surgical standpoint, endoscopic removal results in outcomes comparable to those obtained with open surgery. Systemic spread is more common in the small cell neuroendocrine carcinoma-like tumors than among the neuroblastoma-type neoplasms.

Sinonasal Papilloma

Sinonasal papillomas are benign neoplasms of the respiratory mucosa presenting with nasal stuffiness, nasal obstruction, or epistaxis. The ectodermally derived Schneiderian membrane, gives rise to three morphologically distinct types of papillomas—inverted, oncocytic, and exophytic papillomas or, collectively, as Schneiderian papillomas. Microscopically, papillomas are composed of proliferating columnar and/or squamous epithelial cells, with an admixture of mucin-containing cells and numerous microcysts **(Figs. 6 and 7)**.

Carcinoid tumor has been found in rare cases to present as an intranasal tumor.

Pituitary adenoma can present as a primary lesion of the nasopharynx or nasal cavity.

Paragangliomas have been reported both intranasally and in the nasopharynx.

Peripheral nerve tumors of the sinonasal region are extremely rare. The most common type is the schwannoma and neurofibromas.

Tumors of Melanocytes

Primary sinonasal malignant melanomas usually present as solid polypoid growths. Their most common location is the nasal cavity, followed by antrum, ethmoid, and frontal sinuses. They arise from melanocytes located in the epithelium and stroma of the respiratory mucosa. Most sinonasal melanomas are easily recognizable microscopically, but some can be missed because of their lack of pigmentation, pleomorphic features, pseudopapillary configuration, or prominent spindle cell appearance. Occasional examples have shown prominent myxoid features and others have been accompanied by metaplastic bone formation. The epithelial basal layer should be searched for the presence of

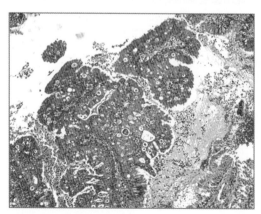

Fig. 6: Oncocytic papilloma. Stratified columnar epithelium with oncocytic features and small neutrophilic microabscesses are characteristic (H&E x 10X).

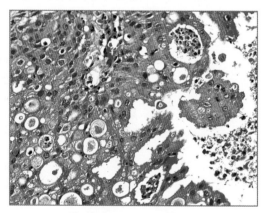

Fig. 7: Oncocytic papilloma. High power view (H&E x 40X).

theque-like growth or 'junctional' activity. Immunohistochemically, these tumors are reactive for vimentin, S-100 protein, Melan-A (Mart-1), and HMB-45, i.e. they have a profile similar to that of their cutaneous counterparts. The prognosis is extremely poor, with most patients dying of metastatic tumor in less than 5 years.

Lymphoid Tumors and Tumor-like Conditions

Malignant lymphoma can present initially as a mass in the sinonasal region or nasopharynx. Nearly all cases are of non-Hodgkin type and the large majority falls into one of three categories: (1) natural killer (NK)/T-cell type; (2) B-cell type; and (3) peripheral T-cell type.

Extranodal NK/T-cell lymphoma is highly associated with EBV.

B-cell lymphoma of the sinonasal region usually presents as a large cell lymphoma with a diffuse pattern of growth and a relatively monomorphic appearance. It is much more common in the paranasal sinuses than in the nasal Burkitt lymphoma.

Peripheral T-cell lymphoma does not express CD56 and usually lacks the necrotizing and angiocentric features of NK/T-cell lymphoma. In contrast to the latter, it usually shows rearrangement of the T-cell receptor gene.

Plasmacytoma (extramedullary plasma-cytoma) arising in the nasal cavity or nasopharynx may present primarily as a soft bleeding mass. Microscopic examination shows a monomorphic infiltration by plasma cells which can range in appearance from mature to immature and anaplastic. Amyloid deposition among the neoplastic cells is sometimes present.

Angiotropic (Intravascular) Lymphoma

It is not to be confused with angiocentric (NK/T-cell) lymphoma. In this condition, the neoplastic lymphocytes are predominantly within the lumen of the vessels rather than infiltrating the vessel wall, and are usually of B lineage. This unusual type of lymphoma can present initially as an intranasal lesion.

Hodgkin lymphoma: A primary disease in this region is exceptional.

Myeloid sarcoma has been seen limited to the sinonasal region.

True teratomas have been reported in the sinuses and nasopharynx of infants and children. The large majority are benign.

Vascular Tumors

Lobular capillary hemangioma is a common tumor of the nasal cavity. Hemangiopericytoma-like tumor (glomangiopericytoma; sinonasal-type hemangiopericytoma) is a vascular mesenchymal neoplasm that may arise either in a paranasal sinus or in the nasal cavity. Other vascular tumors of the region include hemangioma, lymphangioma, conventional glomus tumor, Masson hemangioma (papillary endothelial hyperplasia), angioleiomyoma (vascular leiomyoma), Kaposi sarcoma, and the exceptionally rare angiosarcoma.

Ameloblastoma

It has microscopic appearance indistinguishable from that of its more common counterpart in the jaw and can present as a primary tumor in the sinonasal tract.

Rhabdomyosarcoma of the embryonal type is one of the three most common types of nasopharyngeal malignancy in children, the other two being lymphoepithelioma and malignant lymphoma. Both embryonal and alveolar rhabdomyosarcoma can also develop in this region in adults.

Teratoid carcinosarcoma (teratocarcino-sarcoma) is a unique sinonasal tract neoplasm that combines features of carcinosarcoma and teratoma. The patients are adults, and the prognosis is poor, with 60% of the patients not surviving beyond 3 years.

Soft tissue tumors of this region include osseous and fibro-osseous lesions, cartilaginous tumors, smooth muscle tumors, benign skeletal muscle tumors, fibroblastic and myofibroblastic tumors (fibromatosis, "fibromas", and fibrosarcomas), myxomas, adipose tissue tumors, monotypic angiomyolipoma, fibrous histiocytomas, synovial sarcomas, extraskeletal Ewing sarcoma/primitive neuroectodermal tumor (PNET), phosphaturic mesenchymal tumor, and desmoplastic small cell tumor.

Follicular dendritic cell tumor/sarcoma is a malignant neoplasm arising from the follicular subset of the dendritic/reticulum cells family.

Choriocarcinoma presenting as a primary sinonasal lesion has been recently described.

Metastatic tumors to this region renal cell carcinoma, malignant melanoma, and breast carcinoma head the list.

● **FURTHER READING**

1. Lewis JT, Oliveira AM, Nascimento AG, et al. Low-grade sinonasal sarcoma with neural and myogenic features: A clinicopathologic analysis of 28 cases. Am J Surg Pathol. 2012;36(4):517-25.

2. Slootweg PJ, Ferlito A, Cardesa A, et al. Sinonasal tumors: A clinicopathologic update of selected tumors. Eur Arch Otorhinolaryngol. 2013;270(1):5-20.

CHAPTER 22

Imaging of the Paranasal Sinus Tumors

Sandya CJ, Akshay Kudpaje, Sivakumar Vidhyadharan, Chinmay Kulkarni

● SINONASAL NEOPLASMS

Imaging is performed before surgical intervention to best determine the extent of the disease, neck nodal involvement, and to rule out any distant disease. Orbital and intracranial or skull base involvement has to be assessed. It also helps see the resectability and assess the potential risk for intraoperative complications. Imaging is also essential for adjuvant therapy planning.

● IMAGING MODALITIES

Computed tomography (CT) and magnetic resonance imaging (MRI) offer complementary information, and sinonasal masses, and anterior skull base lesions may be evaluated with both techniques. CT demonstrates osseous involvement and erosion allowing surgical mapping. MRI helps differentiate between inflammatory disease and sinonasal masses, and also shows the tumor boundaries and extent **(Figs. 1A and B)**.

Magnetic resonance imaging has multiplanar capability and can be performed with or without contrast using axial and coronal planes of imaging. Standard protocol MRI of the paranasal sinuses using thin-slice technique (e.g. 3 mm) should also include the orbits, skull base, and adjacent intracranial structures. T1- and T2-weighted sequencing is done because of the variability of signal intensity of sinonasal secretions resulting from protein concentration **(Fig. 2)**.

T2-weighted sequences can usually differentiate between the tumor mass and postobstructive mucosal secretions based on differential signal intensities. The tumor usually has T2 intermediate to low signal intensity, whereas the sinus secretions are commonly of higher T2 signal. Evaluation on both T1- and T2-weighted sequences is important for this differentiation. As sinonasal mucosa has higher water content than tumors, higher T2 signal intensity with smooth, peripheral, and linear mucosal enhancement is seen; mucosal enhancement is typically also more avid than tumoral enhancement. Sinonasal malignancies, by contrast, have intermediate to low T2 signal intensity secondary to tumor cellularity and show solid tumor enhancement, with nonenhancement and signal heterogeneity in regions of necrosis. Sinonasal secretions have variable T1 and T2 signal intensities, but there is no associated postcontrast enhancement.

● LYMPHATIC SPREAD

Lymphadenopathy is present in approximately 15% of patients at presentation and is associated with a poor prognosis. Maxillary sinus malignancies typically drain to submandibular

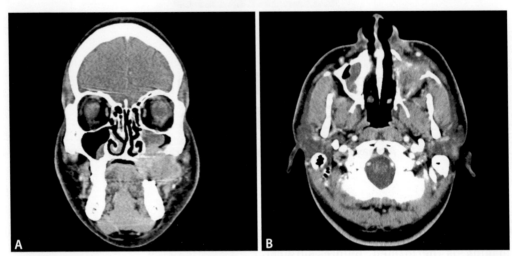

Figs. 1A and B: (A) Coronal contrast enhanced CT image showing mass in the left maxillary sinus eroding the floor, lateral wall, extending to oral cavity, and infratemporal fossa; (B) Axial CECT image showing mass in the left maxillary sinus eroding the anterior, medial, and posterior wall.

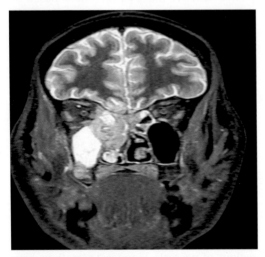

Fig. 2: Coronal STIR (short tau inversion recovery) MR image sequence showing tumor in right ethmoid sinus showing an intermediate signal. Bright signal in the right maxillary sinus is due to pooled secretions.

lymph nodes. Retropharyngeal drainage is inconsistent. Retropharyngeal lymph nodes are not readily detected clinically, and close attention should be paid to this region on both MRI and CT.

● PERINEURAL SPREAD

Owing to its higher occurrence, squamous cell carcinoma is the most common cause of perineural spread; adenoid cystic carcinoma, however, is the sinonasal malignancy with the highest predilection for neurotrophic extension **(Fig. 3)**.

An important site to evaluate when assessing for perineural spread is the pterygopalatine fossa. Once the pterygopalatine fossa is involved, the tumor can extend into the orbit, intracranial compartment, infratemporal fossa, skull base, and oral cavity. The tumor can also directly extend from the nasal cavity through the sphenopalatine fossa, which communicates with the medial aspect of the pterygopalatine fossa **(Fig. 4)**.

Extension of tumor laterally from the pterygopalatine fossa through the pterygomaxillary fissure leads to the infratemporal space. Further extension of tumor through the inferior orbital fissure leads to the orbit. Tumor can extend posteriorly through the foramen rotundum along the second division of the trigeminal nerve (cN V2) or along the vidian canal into the intracranial compartment.

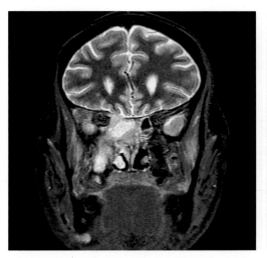

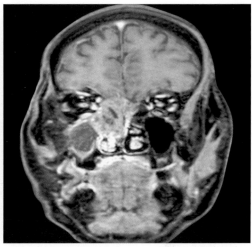

Fig. 3: Coronal STIR (short tau inversion recovery) MR image sequence showing a breach in the roof of the ethmoid sinus, by the tumor.

Fig. 4: Postcontrast T1 MR image, coronal section showing enhancement of tumor in the right ethmoidal sinus. The secretion in the right maxillary sinus is not enhancing.

On CT, imaging findings that support the presence of perineural spread include enlargement and erosion of the affected skull base foramina, loss of the normal hypo-attenuating perineural fat, and soft tissue attenuation within the pterygopalatine fossa and/or Meckel's cave depending on the pattern of tumor involvement. MRI is more sensitive for perineural tumor spread. While high-resolution fat-suppressed T1 postcontrast images are necessary for neurotrophic spread evaluation, evaluation of the perineural fat planes on nonfat-saturated T1 precontrast sequence is also helpful. Findings include enlargement and enhancement of the affected cranial nerve, loss of the normal T1 hyper intense fat in the pterygopalatine fossa, loss of the normal cerebrospinal fluid signal intensity and enlargement of Meckel's cave and the cavernous sinus **(Figs. 5A and B)**.

● ORBITAL INVOLVEMENT

CT and MRI are both used to evaluate orbital invasion. Orbital fat stranding, when present, is a strong predictor for orbital invasion; however,

this finding is inconsistent with sensitivity for orbital involvement of 40% on MRI and 60% on CT. Other characteristics such as the relationship between the tumor and periorbital (abutment, displacement), nodularity at the tumor—periorbital interface, extraocular muscle changes (enlargement, signal abnormality, distortion, or displacement), and the integrity of the orbital walls adjacent to tumor have all been studied. CT has been shown to be slightly more accurate than MRI in the evaluation of orbital invasion, mostly because of its ability to evaluate both fat and bone involvement. MRI is limited because differentiation between bone and periorbital is difficult, as both are hypointense on all sequences **(Figs. 6A and B)**.

● BRAIN AND DURAL INVOLVEMENT

Dural involvement is ideally assessed by MRI scan. T2-weighted MR sequence shows absence of normal dark dural line at the skull base at the site of the lesion. Brain infiltration is suggested by the obliteration of the cerebrospinal fluid space and the irregular intervening margins between the tumor and brain parenchyma.

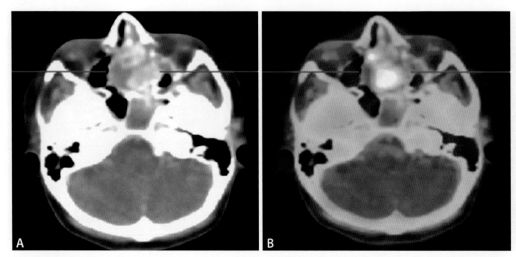

Figs. 5A and B: (A) Axial CT, showing a contrast enhanced lesion in the nasal cavity; (B) Same patient, positron-emission tomography (PET) image showing fluorodeoxyglucose (FDG) uptake. The secretions in the sphenoid sinus is not showing uptake.

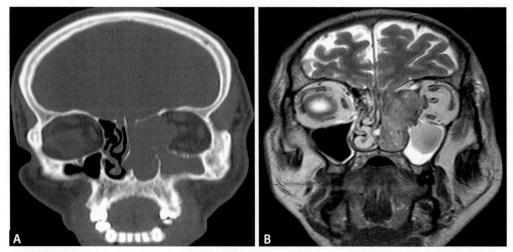

Figs. 6A and B: (A) Coronal CT image (bone window) showing erosion of the medial wall of left orbit by a tumor in left ethmoid sinus; (B) Coronal T2-weighted MR image of the same patient showing intermediate signal tumor in the left ethmoid sinus, nasal cavity, and maxillary sinus, extending to extraconal space of the left orbit. Pooled secretions seen in the left maxillary sinus.

Associated mass effects on the ventricles and brain edema are also noted. Brain edema is seen as a bright signal in the white matter on T2-weighted MR images **(Figs. 7 and 8)**.

● **SOFT TISSUE INVOLVEMENT**

MRI scan is better for soft tissue delineation **(Figs. 9A and B)**.

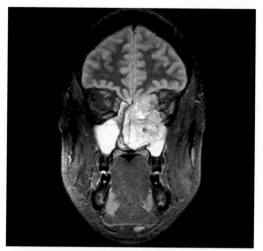

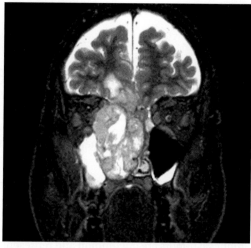

Fig. 7: Magnetic resonance STIR (short tau inversion recovery) coronal image showing mass in the left ethmoid, nasal cavity extending to the left ethmoid, nasal cavity extending to left orbit, and maxillary sinus. Note the breach in the roof of the ethmoid sinus, with loss of dark dural line suggestive of dural involvement.

Fig. 8: Coronal T2 image showing intermediate signal tumor in the ethmoid sinus, nasal cavity infiltrating the frontal lobe, with edema in the adjacent white matter.

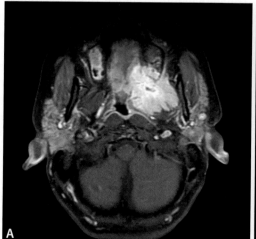

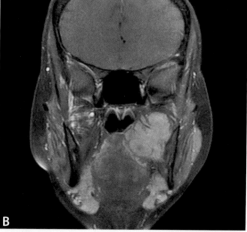

Figs. 9A and B: (A) Axial T1 postcontrast MR image showing mass in the left maxilla, hard palate and upper alveolus extending to parapharyngeal space and masticator space; (B) Coronal postcontrast T1 MR image of the same patient.

● FURTHER READING

1. Dym RJ, Masri D, Shifteh K. Imaging of the paranasal sinuses. Oral Maxillofac Surg Clin North Am. 2012;24(2):175-89, vii.

2. Parmar H, Gujar S, Shah G, et al. Imaging of the anterior skull base. Neuroimaging Clin N Am. 2009;19(3):427-39.

3. Singh N, Eskander A, Huang SH, et al. Imaging and resectability issues of sinonasal tumors. Expert Rev Anticancer Ther. 2013;13(3):297-312.

CHAPTER 23

Guidelines in the Management of Malignancies in Maxillo-ethmoid Complex

Adharsh Anand, Deepak Balasubramanian

● INTRODUCTION

Sinonasal tumors are uncommon and represent a heterogeneous group of head and neck lesions. Malignancies of this area comprise approximately 3% of all head and neck tumors. Approximately, 50% of paranasal neoplasms are benign, principally inverting and other squamous papillomas although fibro-osseous neoplasms are more commonly identified in children. Most paranasal sinus malignancies arise in the maxillary sinus (70–80%), followed by ethmoid sinus (10–20%), and rarely in the sphenoid and frontal sinus.

● PATTERNS OF SPREAD

Direct Spread

Maxillary Sinus

The pattern of spread depends on the site of origin within the sinus. Lesions of the antero-inferior infrastructure tend to invade the lateral inferior wall and present in the oral cavity where the tumor erodes the maxillary gingiva or the gingivolabial sulcus. Tumor is at first submucosal causing elevation of the mucosa, loosening of the teeth or improper fitting of a denture. Ulceration may lead to oro-antral fistula. Lesions arising from the medial infrastructure extend into the nasal cavity.

Lesions of the posterior infrastructure erode the posterolateral wall to enter the infratemporal fossa, or invade directly posterior to the pterygopalatine fossa and pterygoid plates. Cancer in the ptertygopalatine fossa has access to the middle cranial fossa through the foramen rotundum; the foramen lacerum through the pterygoid canal, the nasopharynx through the sphenopalatine foramen; the infratemporal fossa through the pterygomaxillary fissure; and the orbital apex through the inferior orbital fissure.

Extension to the orbit may occur through the roof of the maxillary sinus, the ethmoid sinus, or the pterygopalatine fossa, and inferior orbital fissure. Tumors of the suprastructure may grow laterally and invade the malar process of the maxilla and zygomatic bone, producing a mass below the lateral floor of the orbit. Anterior spread can cause invasion of the soft tissue of the cheek and later causing involvement and ulceration of the skin. Suprastructure cancers can also invade medially into the nasal cavity, ethmoid sinus, frontal sinus, lacrimal apparatus, and medial inferior orbit.

Tumors invading the roof of the antrum may extend perineurally along the infraorbital nerve, through the inferior orbital fissure, across the pterygopalatine fossa, and then into the middle cranial fossa through the foramen rotundum.

Ethmoid Sinus

From the ethmoid sinus, the tumor can extend into the nasal cavity, maxillary sinus, orbit, sphenoid sinus, nasopharynx, and contralateral ethmoid sinus. Tumor can also spread superiorly through the ethmoidal roof, cribriform plate to invade dura, and spread intracranially.

Lymphatic Spread

The lymphatic drainage of the paranasal sinuses goes primarily into the retropharyngeal nodes, lateral pharyngeal nodes along the base of the skull, and then to the upper jugular nodes. Cancer that erodes the maxilla into the soft tissues of the face can spread to the submandibular and upper jugular nodes. Regional disease is evident on initial presentation in approximately 10% of the patients and an additional 15% develop lymph node metastasis at some point after treatment.

Distant Spread

For squamous cell carcinoma of the maxillary sinus, the distant metastasis is approximately 10%.

● PRESENTING SIGNS AND SYMPTOMS

- Early lesions may be asymptomatic.
- *Nasal symptoms:* Epistaxis, blood-stained nasal discharge, nasal block, and nasal mass.
- *Eye symptoms:* Diplopia, proptosis, epiphora, and diminution of vision (late).
- *Oral symptoms:* Mass/ulceration palate, upper GB sulcus, loosening of teeth, ill-fitting dentures.
- *Trismus:* Due to posterior extension, due to the involvement of the pterygoids.
- Soft tissue swelling/ulceration of the face.
- Extension of skull base can lead to involvement of cranial nerves, anosmia, blurred vision, and hypoesthesia along the branches of the trigeminal nerve.

- Neck masses due to metastatic nodal involvement (rare).

● OHNGREN'S CLASSIFICATION

This classification divides the antrum by an imaginary line drawn from the angle of the mandible to the medial canthus of the eye. Patients with tumor located above the Ohngren's line (suprastructure) had a significantly worse prognosis than those with tumors located below (infrastructure).

● TNM STAGING, AJCC 8TH EDITION

The T staging remains the same. However, the N staging is revised and is similar to other nonviral sites. Overall staging is also similar **(Tables 1 to 3)**. Table 4 shows modified Kadish staging for esthesioneuroblastoma.

● EVALUATION

Imaging

Radiographic studies provide information related to the location, size, extent, and anatomic structures involved. In addition, imaging may guide appropriate biopsy, surgical approaches, staging, and treatment. Computed tomography (CT) has essentially rendered plain films obsolete in the evaluation of sinonasal masses, providing higher accuracy in assessing bony framework and anatomic detail.

Magnetic resonance imaging (MRI) may differentiate tumor from inflammatory soft tissue and is useful in defining intracranial, intraorbital extension, and perineural spread.

Angiographic studies, including magnetic resonance angiography (MRA), may assist in the evaluation of vascular tumors and carotid artery involvement.

Nasal Endoscopy and Biopsy

Most tumors can be adequately assessed with nasal endoscopes and may be biopsied with

Table 1: T staging.

Maxillary sinus	
T stage	**T criteria**
TX	Primary tumor cannot be assessed
Tis	Carcinoma *in situ*
T1	Tumor limited to maxillary sinus mucosa with no erosion or destruction of bone
T2	Tumor causing bone erosion or destruction including extension into the hard palate and/or middle nasal meatus, except extension to posterior wall of maxillary sinus and pterygoid plates
T3	Tumor invades any of the following—bone of the posterior wall of maxillary sinus, subcutaneous tissues, floor or medial wall of orbit, pterygoid fossa, ethmoid sinuses
T4	Moderately advanced or very advanced local disease
T4a	Moderately advanced local disease Tumor invades anterior orbital contents, skin of cheek, pterygoid plates, infratemporal fossa, cribriform plate, sphenoid, or frontal sinuses
T4b	Very advanced local disease Tumor invades any of the following—orbital apex, dura, brain, middle cranial fossa, cranial nerves other than maxillary division of trigeminal nerve (V2), nasopharynx, or clivus
Nasal cavity and ethmoid sinus	
TX	Primary tumor cannot be assessed
Tis	Carcinoma *in situ*
T1	Tumor restricted to any one subsite, with or without bony invasion
T2	Tumor invading two subsites in a single region or extending to involve an adjacent region within the nasoethmoidal complex, with or without bony invasion
T3	Tumor extends to invade the medial wall or floor of the orbit, maxillary sinus, palate, or cribriform plate
T4	Moderately advanced or very advanced local disease
T4a	Moderately advanced local disease Tumor invades any of the following—anterior orbital contents, skin of nose or cheek, minimal extension to anterior cranial fossa, pterygoid plates, sphenoid, or frontal sinuses
T4b	Very advanced local disease Tumor invades any of the following—orbital apex, dura, brain, middle cranial fossa, cranial nerves other than (V2), nasopharynx, or clivus

topical anesthesia, using the instruments used in endoscopic sinus surgery. It is recommended that adequate imaging be completed before the biopsy to assure the absence of a mass that contains cerebrospinal fluid or a vascular neoplasm. Immunohistochemistry may have to be done to confirm the diagnosis.

● TREATMENT GUIDELINES (FLOWCHART 1)

The primary treatment modality for tumors in the maxillary and ethmoidal sinus is surgery.

Early lesions can be managed by single modality surgery (or radiation in selected cases) whereas advanced lesions would require a combined modality approach.

Squamous cell and adenocarcinoma are managed according to stage. In cases of early maxillary sinus tumors (T1 and T2) surgery is the preferred modality of treatment. The presence of adverse features namely margin positivity and perineural invasion warrants adjuvant treatment. In cases of advanced tumors (T3 and T4a), combined modality

Table 2: N staging and M staging.

Clinical N (cN)	
NX	Regional lymph nodes cannot be assessed
N0	No regional lymph node metastasis
N1	Metastasis in a single ipsilateral lymph node, 3 cm or smaller in greatest dimension and ENE (–)
N2	Metastasis in a single ipsilateral node larger than 3 cm but not larger than 6 cm in greatest dimension and ENE (–) ;or metastases in multiple ipsilateral lymph nodes, none larger than 6 cm in greatest dimension and ENE (–); or in bilateral or contralateral lymph nodes, none larger than 6 cm in greatest dimension and ENE (–)
N2a	Metastasis in a single ipsilateral node larger than 3 cm but not larger than 6 cm in greatest dimension and ENE (–)
N2b	Metastasis in multiple ipsilateral nodes, none larger than 6 cm in greatest dimension and ENE (–)
N2c	Metastasis in bilateral or contralateral lymph nodes, none larger than 6 cm in greatest dimension and ENE (–)
N3	Metastasis in a lymph node larger than 6 cm in greatest dimension and ENE (–); or metastasis in any node (s) with clinically overt ENE (+)
N3a	Metastasis in a lymph node larger than 6 cm in greatest dimension and ENE (–)
N3b	Metastasis in any node (s) with clinically overt ENE (+)
Pathological N (pN)	
NX	Regional lymph nodes cannot be assessed
N0	No regional lymph node metastasis
N1	Metastasis in a single ipsilateral lymph node, 3 cm or smaller in greatest dimension and ENE (–)
N2	Metastasis in a single ipsilateral node, 3 cm or smaller in greatest dimension and ENE (+); or metastasis in a single ipsilateral node larger than 3 cm but not larger than 6 cm in greatest dimension and ENE (–); or metastases in multiple ipsilateral lymph nodes, none larger than 6 cm in greatest dimension and ENE (–); or in bilateral or contralateral lymph nodes, none larger than 6 cm in greatest dimension and ENE (–)
N2a	Metastasis in a single ipsilateral node, 3 cm or smaller in greatest dimension and ENE (+); or metastasis in a single ipsilateral node larger than 3 cm but not larger than 6 cm in greatest dimension and ENE (–)
N2b	Metastasis in multiple ipsilateral nodes, none larger than 6 cm in greatest dimension and ENE (–)
N2c	Metastasis in bilateral or contralateral lymph nodes, none larger than 6 cm in greatest dimension and ENE (–)
N3	Metastasis in a lymph node larger than 6 cm in greatest dimension and ENE (–); or in a single ipsilateral node larger than 3 cm in greatest dimension and ENE (+); or multiple ipsilateral, contralateral, or bilateral nodes any with ENE (+)
N3a	Metastasis in a lymph node larger than 6 cm in greatest dimension and EN E (–)
N3b	Metastasis in a single ipsilateral node larger than 3 cm in greatest dimension and ENE (+); or multiple ipsilateral, contralateral, or bilateral nodes any with ENE (+)

Note: A designation of "U" or "L" may be used for any N category to indicate metastasis above the lower border of the cricoid (U) or below the lower border of the cricoid (L).
Similarly, clinical and pathological ENE should be recorded as ENE (–) or ENE (+).

Distant metastasis M	
M0	No distant metastasis
M1	Distant metastasis

Table 3: AJCC prognostic stage groups.

When T is...	And N is...	And M is...	Then the stage group is...
Tis	N0	M0	0
T1	N0	M0	I
T2	N0	M0	II
T3	N0	M0	III
T0, T1, T2,T3	N1	M0	III
T4a	N0,N1	M0	IVA
T0, T1, T2,T3,T4a	N2	M0	IVA
Any T	N3	M0	IVB
T4b	Any N	M0	IVB
Any T	Any N	M1	IVC

Table 4: Kadish staging for esthesioneuroblastoma.

Stage	Location
A	Tumor confined to nasal cavity
B	Tumor extending to the paranasal sinuses
C	Tumor extending beyod the sinonasal cavity locally
D	Tumor with regional or distant spread

Flowchart 1: Algorithm for the management of patients with sinonasal malignancy.

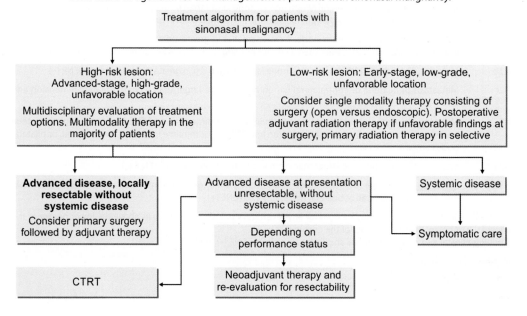

treatment is preferred. Surgery followed by adjuvant radiation is recommended. In case of margin positivity or extracapsular nodal spread, chemoradiation is preferred.

Adenoid cystic carcinomas irrespective of the stage require combined modality treatment due to their propensity for perineural spread and recurrence.

Very advanced tumors (T4b) can be treated with definitive radiation or chemoradiation as they are surgically unresectable tumors. Upfront chemotherapy for unresectable tumors and then surgery (if possible) followed by adjuvant treatment is also an option.

● MANAGEMENT OF NECK

The management of the neck has been controversial. The N+ neck has to be addressed surgically in the form of a neck dissection. However, considering the first echelon lymph nodes are the retropharyngeal nodes, the adjuvant radiotherapy for the primary site can be used to address the neck in the N0 neck.

● MANAGEMENT OF THE ORBIT

The orbit requires special mention. The involvement of the globe, the extraocular muscles, and orbital apex require orbital exenteration. However, in cases of early orbital invasion, there can be an attempt to preserve the orbit. When the tumor has breached the orbital periosteum, frozen section control can be used to resect the orbital fat until a negative margin is obtained, thus preserving the globe. If there is gross involvement of the fat and inability to obtain negative frozen margins, then an orbital exenteration is to be performed. Involvement of the intraconal fat, extraocular muscles, orbital apex, and globe are indications of orbital exenteration **(Flowchart 2)**.

● RECONSTRUCTION AND REHABILITATION

The goals of reconstruction are oronasal separation (surgical, interim, and permanent obturators), cranionasal separation (fascia grafts and vascularized galea-pericranial flap), eye and cheek support (implants, pedicled muscle flaps,

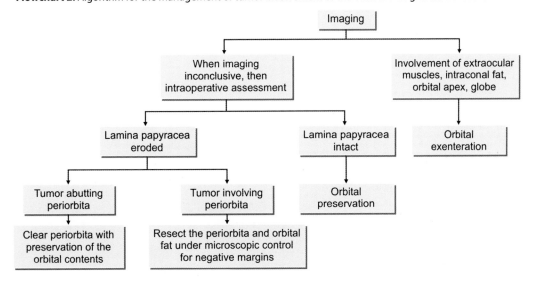

Flowchart 2: Algorithm for the management of tumor involvement of the orbit in malignant sinonasal tumors.

and microvascular free flaps), dental restoration (dentures and osteointegrated implants), and restoration of facial defects (local skin flaps, regional flaps, microvascular free flaps, and prostheses).

● OUTCOME

The 5-year survival rates of sinonasal malignancies vary depending on tumor stage (91% in T1 and 49% in T4), site of origin (77% in nasal cavity, 62% in maxillary sinus, and 48% in ethmoid sinus), histology (squamous cell carcinoma 60% and undifferentiated carcinoma 40%), and treatment modality (surgery only: 79%, RT only: 57%, combined surgery and RT: 66%). The main pattern of failure is local recurrence, and efforts to improve survival should be directed towards improved local control.

● FURTHER READING

1. Day TA, Beas RA, Schlosser RJ, et al. Management of paranasal sinus malignancy. Curr Treat Options Oncol. 2005;6(1):3-18.
2. Iyer S, Thankappan K. Maxillary reconstruction: Current concepts and controversies. Indian J Plast Surg. 2014;47(1):8-19.
3. Resto VA, Deschler DG. Sinonasal malignancies. Otolaryngol Clin North Am. 2004;37(2):473-87.
4. Suárez C, Ferlito A, Lund VJ, et al. Management of the orbit in malignant sinonasal tumors. Head Neck. 2008;30(2):242-50.

CHAPTER 24

Principles of Surgery in the Management of Tumors of Maxillo-ethmoid Complex

Adharsh Anand, Deepak Balasubramanian

● INTRODUCTION

The nasal and paranasal sinus malignant tumors pose a challenge to the clinicians due to their rarity, diversity in histological profile, delay of presentation, and considerable adjacent site involvement at the time of presentation.

● SURGICAL ANATOMY

The nose and paranasal sinuses are in close proximity to the skull base, cranial cavity, and the orbit. These areas are potential sites of involvement. A brief review of the relevant anatomy is essential to understand the pathways of spread and surgical management.

The maxillary sinus is a pyramidal shaped sinus within the walls of the maxilla. The maxillary sinus is related to the adjacent structures, namely the orbit, nasal cavity, skull base, and the oral cavity. The maxillary sinus opens into the nasal cavity via the ostium in the lateral nasal wall. The floor of the maxillary sinus is formed by the alveolar process and the palate. The posterior wall of the maxilla is in relation to the infratemporal fossa. The floor of the orbit forms the roof of the maxillary sinus. All of these structures are potential sites of involvement in maxillary sinus tumors.

The ethmoid sinuses form a bony labyrinth of multiple air cells in the roof of the nasal cavity. The roof of the ethmoid sinus is the fovea ethmoidalis which separates it from the anterior cranial fossa. The sinus is related laterally to the orbit being separated by a thin bone called the lamina papyracea. The anterior and posterior ethmoidal arteries traverse the roof of the sinus. Tumors arising or involving the ethmoidal sinus have a propensity to superior spread into the anterior cranial fossa and laterally to the orbit.

The orbit is of critical importance in the management of paranasal sinus tumors. The bony orbit is formed by contributions from the maxilla, frontal, sphenoid, lacrimal, zygomatic, and ethmoidal bones. The orbit communicates to the infratemporal fossa via the inferior orbital fissure and to the cavernous sinus via the superior orbital fissure, and these are pathways of spread from the orbit.

The lymphatic drainage of the nasal vestibule and columella are to the submandibular lymph nodes. Lymph node metastasis from primary sinus tumors is rare, and the retropharyngeal lymph node is a potential site of involvement.

● SURGICAL TREATMENT

There are various surgical procedures described for the management of paranasal sinus tumors. The extent of surgical resection depends upon the extent of involvement. The surgical options include:

- Maxillectomy and its subtypes
- External ethmoidectomy
- Craniofacial resection
- Endoscopic approaches.

Maxillectomy

It is the surgical removal of the walls of the maxilla and its contents. There are various terminologies associated with maxillectomy and this is based on the extent of the walls removed.

Indications

Malignant tumors of the maxilla involving the inferior, superior, anterior or posterior walls. Extension through the orbital periosteum superiorly will necessitate orbital clearance. Preoperatively the patient should consult a prosthetic orthodontist to take an impression of the upper alveolus for future reconstruction.

Contraindications

Extension superiorly to the skull base will require an additional craniofacial approach.

Surgical Approaches to the Maxilla

There are two principle approaches to the maxilla namely the open approach and the endoscopic approach. The open approach is usually performed via a mid-facial degloving or a Weber Fergusson incision.

- *Midfacial Degloving*: It allows access to the midface without an external skin incision. The incision is usually a sublabial incision combined with an intercartilaginous and transfixation incision in the nose and the elevation of the skin and soft tissues of the nose and maxilla.
  Indications: Tumors involving the nasal cavity and maxilla **(Fig. 1)**.
- *Weber Fergusson and lateral rhinotomy*: Traditional approaches to the maxillary sinus involve the use of a facial incision and raising of a cheek flap to expose the maxilla. The incision commonly used is the Weber Fergusson incision. The incision usually incorporates an upper median or paramedial lip split, skin incision along the ala, and upper extension along the nasofacial crease. Most commonly this incision is extended along the infraorbital area as a subciliary incision. This approach gives excellent exposure for a total maxillectomy. For more limited procedures, a Moure incision is used which is limited to the nasofacial area **(Fig. 2)**.
- *Mandibulotomy approach*: Tumors extending posteriorly, with involvement of the pterygoid plates and muscles may require a mandibulotomy approach for infratemporal fossa clearance.

Types

- *Medial maxillectomy*: It is currently used for inverted papillomas and other tumors confined to the lateral nasal wall. The surgical approach is usually through a lateral rhinotomy using a Moure's or a Weber Fergusson approach. Recently the endoscopic medial maxillectomy has become popular for inverted papillomas of the lateral nasal wall **(Fig. 3)**.
- *Inferior (infrastructure maxillectomy)*: This involves resection of the inferior maxillary sinus below the level of the infraorbital nerve. This is the most commonly used for the neoplasms of the alveolar process of the maxilla with minimal extension to the maxillary antrum. This procedure can be accomplished by a sublabial approach **(Fig. 4)**.
- *Total maxillectomy*: It is removal of all of the walls of the maxilla along with the contents. It is usually performed for tumors of the maxillary sinus. The total maxillectomy can be combined with removal of the orbital contents (orbital exenteration). It is commonly performed through a Weber Fergusson incision. The incision can be extended depending upon the extent of the tumor **(Fig. 5)**.

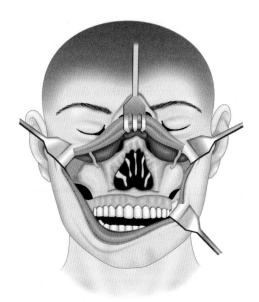

Fig. 1: Midfacial degloving approach.

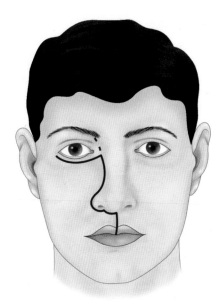

Fig. 2: Lateral rhinotomy and Weber Fergusson.

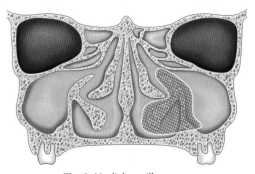

Fig. 3: Medial maxillectomy.

Steps of Total Maxillectomy

A Weber Fergusson incision is used for the cheek skin. The upper lip is split using a median or paramedian incision. Another incision is made in the sublabial mucosa from anterior to the maxillary tuberosity posteriorly. The incision is then continued between the hard and soft palate and then across the midline palate.

The cheek flap is elevated exposing the maxilla, pyriform aperture, lateral zygomaticomaxillary buttress, and frontal process of maxilla.

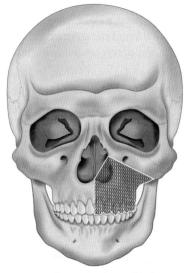

Fig. 4: Infrastructure maxillectomy.

The nasolacrimal duct is sectioned and the orbital floor is exposed by raising the orbital contents subperiostally exposing the inferior orbital fissure.

The maxilla is mobilized by performing osteotomies which are through the pyriform

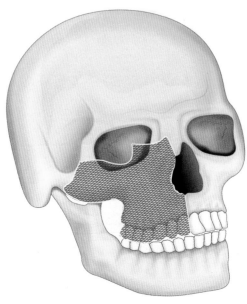

Fig. 5: Total maxillectomy.

aperture, the hard palate, frontal process of maxilla, orbital floor, lateral zygomaticomaxillary area, and finally pterygopalatine disjunction.

Note: In cases of extension of the maxillary tumor posteriorly and involvement of the pterygoid plates, pterygomaxillary disjunction is to be avoided as it is blind, and there is no en bloc tumor removal. In such cases, the posterior maxilla and the ITF are exposed through a mandibulotomy approach and the pterygoid plates are separated from the skull bases and included in the resected specimen.

Note: Anterior spread of tumor to the facial skin may necessitate sacrifice and repair with a local pedicled flap or a microvascular free flap. Posterior extension often involves the pterygoid plates obscuring oncological resection margins and adversely affects prognosis. Limited areas of the pterygoid muscle can be removed. Pterygopalatine and infratemporal fossa clearance can be undertaken keeping in mind their close relation with ICA.

External Ethmoidectomy

This is rarely performed nowadays. The ethmoid sinuses can be exposed through a lynch incision. Due to the advanced presentation of ethmoidal tumors and its proximity to the skull base, most of the patients would require a craniofacial resection.

Craniofacial Resection

Craniofacial resection forms the gold standard in the surgical treatment of paranasal sinus tumors that cross the fovea ethmoidalis and the cribriform plate involving the anterior cranial fossa. The concept was first reported by Smith in 1954 and popularized by Ketcham a decade later. The en bloc resection of the tumor includes removal of the upper septum, cribriform plate, and floor of the anterior cranial fossa. The procedure is usually done through a combined transcranial (bifrontal craniotomy) and transfacial approach. Transfacial approaches can be either lateral rhinotomy or Weber Fergusson or mid facial degloving. Neurosurgery assistance is essential for the transcranial approach **(Figs. 6A to C)**.

Certain tumors, however, are considered unresectable and they include patients with extensive frontal lobe involvement, optic chiasma involvement, bilateral orbital apex involvement, and extensive cavernous sinus involvement.

Endoscopic Resection

Endoscopic resection of malignant tumors of the skull base can be pure endoscopic approaches or combined (with craniotomy) endoscopic approaches. The endoscopic resection of tumors should be limited to tumors confined to the nasal cavity with minimal invasion of the skull base. The oncological principles should not be violated and an attempt to remove the tumor with adequate margins should always be made. Also surgical expertize is paramount and one should be proficient in repairing the dural

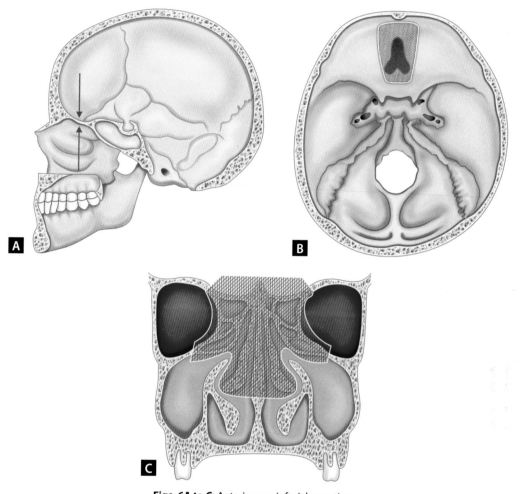

Figs. 6A to C: Anterior craniofacial resection.

defect endoscopically. Tumors with extensive skull base, orbital, and intracranial involvement are not amenable to endoscopic excision.

● **FURTHER READING**

1. Bhattacharyya N. Cancer of the nasal cavity: Survival and factors influencing prognosis. Arch Otolaryngol Head Neck Surg. 2002;128(9):1079-83.

2. Bradley P, Jones NS, Robertson I. Diagnosis and management of esthesioneuroblastoma. Curr Opin Otolaryngol Head Neck Surg. 2003;11(2):112-8.

3. Carrau RL, Segas J, Nuss DW, et al. Squamous cell carcinoma of the sinonasal tract invading the orbit. Laryngoscope. 1999;109(2 Pt 1):230-5.

4. Devaiah A, Larsen C, Tawfik O, et al. Esthesio-neuroblastoma: Endoscopic nasal and anterior craniotomy resection. Laryngoscope. 2003;113(12):2086-90.

Section 5

Oral Cavity and Oropharynx

Chapters

CHAPTER 25

Imaging in Oral and Oropharyngeal Tumors

Sandya CJ, Akshay Kudpaje, Shreya Bhattacharya

● ORAL CAVITY

Squamous cell carcinoma (SCC) accounts for more than 90% of the malignant neoplasms of the oral cavity. Risk factors include long-term use of alcohol and tobacco chewing. The various subsites in the oral cavity are lips, floor of mouth, oral tongue, cheek, gingival, hard palate, and retromolar trigone (RMT). Tongue and buccal mucosa are the most commonly affected sites.

Staging

Squamous cell carcinoma of oral cavity and oropharynx are staged by TNM classification. Differentiation between early stage (I, II) and late stage (III, IV) tumors is important because early stage tumors may be treated by single modality therapy alone and late stage tumors require multimodality therapy which includes combination of surgery, radiation, and chemotherapy.

Lips

Lip is composed of orbicularis oris muscle which is derived from multiple facial muscles like levator labii superioris, levator angularis oris, zygomaticus major, platysma, risorius, and buccinator. It is lined externally by keratinizing stratified squamous epithelium and internally by nonkeratinizing stratified squamous epithelium. Lymphatic drainage

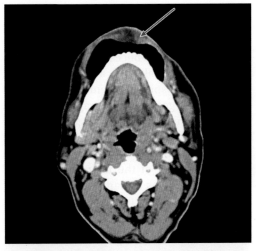

Fig. 1: Axial CT image showing normal lip.

is into submental and submandibular lymph nodes **(Fig. 1)**.

Squamous cell carcinoma of the lip spreads laterally to involve the skin and deep to involve the orbicularis oris muscle. Lesion later may spread deep to involve the gingiva of maxilla and mandible. Early stage disease is difficult to assess by imaging and better assessed by direct clinical examination. Advanced stage disease is assessed by computed tomography (CT) scan for both primary extent and nodal involvement. Key features to be looked for in advanced disease are osseous involvement and perineural invasion along the alveolar nerves.

Buccal Mucosa and Gingiva

Vestibule of the mouth is a cleft lined by buccal mucosa which separates lips and cheeks from the teeth and gums. The junction between the gingiva and buccal mucosa is termed gingivo-buccal sulcus and is a common site for SCC.

On imaging, patient should be instructed to puff the cheek to separate the mucosal surfaces. Deep to buccal mucosa is the buccal space. This includes masseter, buccinator muscle, buccal pad of fat, angular branch of facial artery, facial vein, buccal artery and nerve, terminal part of parotid duct, and facial nodes **(Fig. 2)**. Superficial spread can be assessed clinically while deeper involvement requires imaging techniques.

Evaluation of the buccal and gingival mucosal lesions must take into account the extent of submucosal spread, extent of involvement of RMT, pterygomandibular raphe, bone and cervical lymph node. Pterygomandibular raphe is a thick fascial band extending from the hamulus of medial pterygoid plate to the posterior border of the mylohyoid ridge of mandible. It forms the anterior boundary of the prestyloid compartment of parapharyngeal space. Lymphatics drain to levels I, II and III nodes.

Very early, superficial lesions detected as ulcers on the cheek usually do not require imaging for assessing the primary lesion. Ultrasound evaluation of the neck using high-frequency linear probe (8–12 MHz) is done to exclude cervical nodes. Deep-seated lesions need cross-sectional imaging to determine the exact extent including bone erosions. CT scan is the preferred imaging modality **(Figs. 3 to 5)**.

● RETROMOLAR TRIGONE

Retromolar trigone is a triangular shaped area posterior to the last molar tooth. It extends behind the last molar tooth along the ascending ramus of mandible up to the last maxillary molar tooth. Pterygomandibular raphe lies posterior to this mucosa. RMT can be seen in entire extent in an oblique plane reformatted CT scan **(Fig. 6)**. Imaging is required to assess the lesion for involvement of masticator space, osseous involvement, perineural spread, and infratemporal spread **(Figs. 7 and 8)**.

Retromolar trigone provides easy access to many routes of spread. Based on the outcomes,

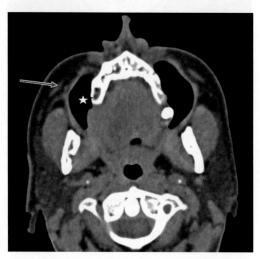

Fig. 2: Axial CT image (puffed cheek view), illustrating normal cheek.

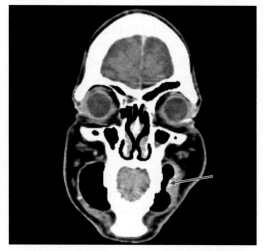

Fig. 3: Coronal CT image (puffed cheek) showing mass in the left cheek.

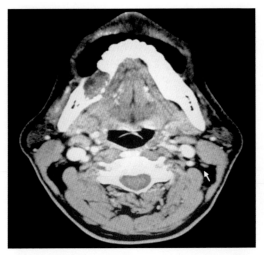

Fig. 4: Axial CT scan showing erosion of the mandible in a case of alveolar carcinoma.

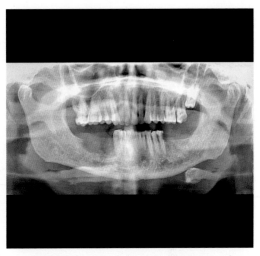

Fig. 5: OPG erosion of the alveolar margin of mandible.

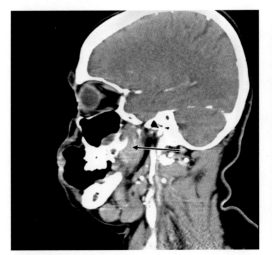

Fig. 6: Sagittal CT image showing mass in the retromolar trigone with extension into the infratemporal fossa.

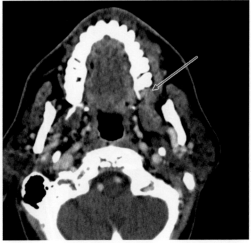

Fig. 7: Axial CT image showing asymmetry in the retromolar trigone with a mass on the left side.

such lesions have been subdivided into supra- and infranotch using mandibular notch between the coronoid and condyloid process as line of demarcation. Supranotch carries a poor prognosis and this space includes lateral pterygoid and upper two-thirds of pterygoid plate. Infranotch includes medial pterygoid and masseter muscles and carries a better prognosis **(Fig. 9)**. Involvement of skull base with perineural spread through foramen ovale and involvement of ICA makes it very advanced disease which may be unresectable **(Fig. 10)**.

Computed tomography scan provides highest specificity for bone involvement.

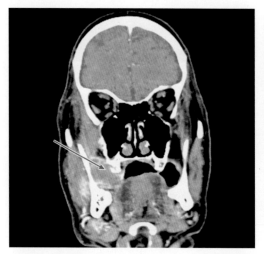

Fig. 8: Coronal CT image showing mass in the right retromolar trigone.

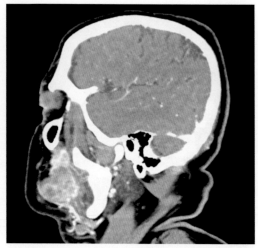

Fig. 9: Infranotch retromolar trigone lesion involving the medial pterygoid (CT image).

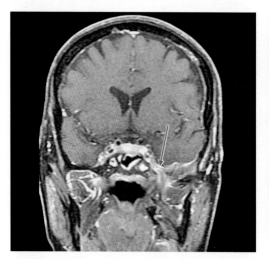

Fig. 10: Coronal MRI image showing enhancement along the left foramen ovale suggesting perineural extension.

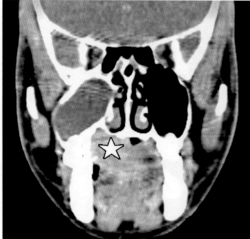

Fig. 11: Coronal CT image showing mass lesion on the hard palate on the right side eroding the bone.

Perineural spread is best evaluated by an MRI scan which shows enhancement along the foramina and loss of normal fat plane. CT depicts the perineural spread as foramina widening and excessive enhancement within the foramen. T1W, T2W, postcontrast T1 with fatsat axial and coronal MR images are ideal to demonstrate the lesion and its spread **(Fig. 11)**.

Hard Palate

Primary tumor is rare; usually it is an extension from gingival lesion. Imaging is needed to assess the osseous erosion, extension into the floor of nasal cavity, maxillary sinus, and soft palate. Lesions are best demonstrated using sagittal or coronal CT **(Fig. 12)**. Perineural spread can occur along the greater and lesser palatine nerves. Perineural spread is best evaluated by MRI.

Floor of the Mouth

Floor of mouth extends from the inferior aspect of tongue to the mylohyoid sling. It is divided in half by the lingual frenulum. Mylohyoid muscle

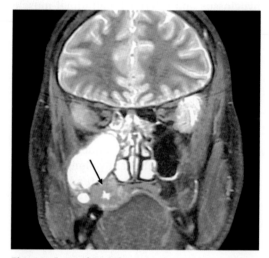

Fig. 12: Coronal T2 MR image depicts lesion in the hard palate (bright lesion in the right maxillary sinus is pooled secretions).

serves as the anatomical landmark in separating sublingual space from the submandibular space even though there is continuity of spaces along the posterior aspect. Submandibular salivary gland lies inferior to the mylohyoid muscle and the deep lobe goes above the muscle. Paired geniohyoid muscle runs above the mylohyoid, lies in paramedian position, and inserts itself to hyoid. Sublingual space is superomedial to mylohyoid and lateral to genioglossus. It contains lingual artery, lingual nerve, sublingual gland, and deep part of submandibular salivary gland. Floor of mouth is best demonstrated in CT or MR in coronal sections **(Figs. 13A and B)**. Imaging is required to define the extent of disease and depth of involvement, neurovascular invasion, osseous erosion, and cervical lymph node involvement.

Oral Tongue

Oral tongue consists of anterior two-thirds of the tongue. Posterior third of tongue is considered part of the oropharynx. Tongue is composed of four intrinsic muscles—superior and inferior longitudinal, transverse and vertical, which form the bulk of the tongue **(Figs. 13A and B)**. They interdigitate with each

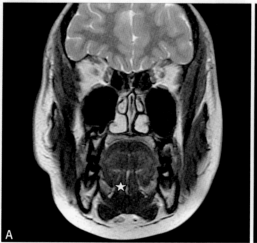
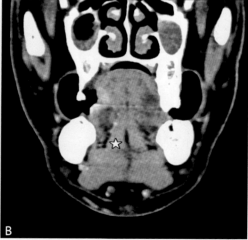

Figs. 13A and B: Normal anatomy of tongue and mouth (MR and CT).

other, which is well delineated on MR imaging. Intrinsic muscles originate and insert within the tongue and have no bony attachments. In contrast, extrinsic muscles have one bony attachment and the other end inserts to the tongue. Extrinsic muscles include genioglossus, styloglossus, hyoglossus and palatoglossus and are demarcated on T2-weighted MR images in various planes. These muscles anchor tongue to hyoid bone, mandible, and styloid process.

Genioglossus is the largest muscle of the tongue and takes origin from the superior genial tubercle, located on the inner aspect of the mandible and fans out superiorly to terminate in the connective tissue of the lingual dorsum. Inferiorly, it is attached to hyoid bone also (best appreciated in sag images). They can be divided into three main components—vertical, oblique, and horizontal. Genioglossus is absent in the tip of the tongue where it is composed of only intrinsic muscles. Two genioglossus muscles are separated by fibrofatty median raphe. Lateral to genioglossus is paramedian septum separating genioglossus from the hyoglossus, styloglossus and inferior longitudinal muscle. Septum contains lingual artery, vein and hypoglossal nerve, and lingual nodes.

Hyoglossus is seen lateral to genioglossus, takes origin from greater cornu of hyoid and inserted to the sides of the tongue, best seen in axial or coronal images. Hyoglossus is bordered by genioglossus and inferior longitudinal muscle medially and styloglossus laterally. Lateral side of paramedian septum lies between hyoglossus and inferior longitudinal muscle and contains hypoglossal, lingual nerves, and sublingual gland. Styloglossus arises from anteromedial surface of styloid process and stylomandibular ligament and interdigitate with hyoglossus. Palatoglossus is the smallest muscle of all; it arises from oral surface of soft plate and passes anterior to the tonsil and blend with hyoglossus.

Squamous cell carcinoma of the oral tongue occurs predominantly along its lateral and ventral surface. Lesions tend to spread along the submucosa, involve the floor of mouth and mandibular gingiva **(Figs. 14 to 17)**. Involvement of gingiva leads to osseous involvement and perineural spread.

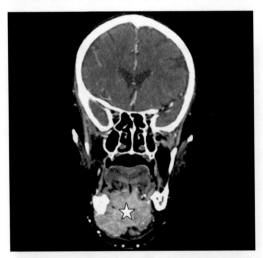

Fig. 14: Coronal CT image carcinoma tongue with floor of mouth invasion.

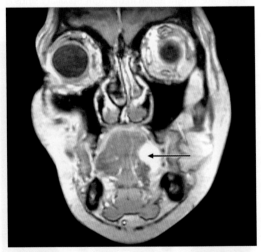

Fig. 15: Coronal postcontrast MR image showing enhancing lesion in the left lateral border of oral tongue in a case of carcinoma.

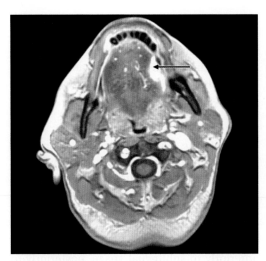

Fig. 16: Axial postcontrast MR image showing enhancing lesion in the left lateral border of oral tongue in a case of carcinoma.

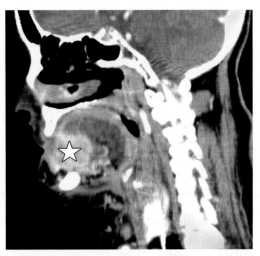

Fig. 17: Sagittal CT image showing infiltration of floor of mouth in a case of carcinoma tongue.

Surgery is considered the mainstay in the management of oral tongue and floor of mouth tumors. MRI is the optimal imaging modality for evaluating the tongue, floor of mouth, and neurovascular bundle complemented by CT for osseous involvement.

Early SCC is seen as shallow ulcer, may not be detected on primary imaging. Intraoral USG is helpful in such cases to assess the tumor depth but is used less frequently. Ultrasound with a high frequency transducer is the imaging modality of choice for evaluation of the nodal deposits in the neck. Tumor thickness of more than 4 mm is associated with increased incidence of occult cervical nodal deposits. MRI is a useful tool to study the depth of involvement by the tumor.

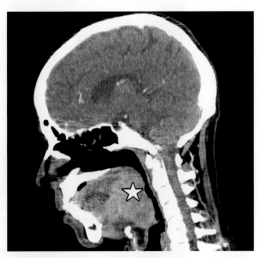

Fig. 18: Sagittal CT image showing lesion in the oropharynx.

Oropharynx

Oropharynx includes posterior third of tongue behind the circumvallate papilla, palatine tonsils, soft palate, and posterior pharyngeal wall. Majority of tumors are SCC followed by lymphoma, minor salivary gland tumors, and rare mesenchymal tumors **(Fig. 18)**.

Palatine Tonsil

It includes anterior and posterior tonsillar pillars and tonsils. Anterior tonsillar pillar is a mucosal fold over the palatoglossus muscle. The lesion arising from this fold spreads superiorly to soft palate. From the palate the lesion can spread to skull base via pterygoid muscles and tensor and levator veli palatini. Extensive lesion can spread to involve the ipsilateral nasopharynx and masticator space. Lymphatic drainage is to level I, II and III nodes.

Posterior tonsillar fold is formed by mucosal fold over palatopharyngeus muscles. Superiorly lesion extends to palate, inferiorly to pharyngoepiglottic fold, middle pharyngeal constrictors and posteriorly lesion spreads to retropharyngeal space. Primary lymphatic drainage is to the level II and retropharyngeal nodes.

The evaluation of tonsillar SCC includes extent of lesion, involvement of pterygoid muscles, extension along pterygomandibular raphe, osseous involvement, and cervical nodes. CT imaging in coronal and axial planes is usually the modality of choice. Positron emission tomography-CT may be useful for assessing the response to therapy and for distant metastasis **(Fig. 19)**.

Base of Tongue

Base of the tongue extends from the circumvallate papilla anteriorly to the vallecula inferiorly. Thorough clinical evaluation is a must. T2 and contrast enhanced T1-weighted MR imaging in sagittal plane is helpful to visualize the full extent of the lesion. These tumors can spread to tonsils, pharyngeal wall, anteriorly to sublingual space, posteriorly to vallecula, and supraglottic larynx.

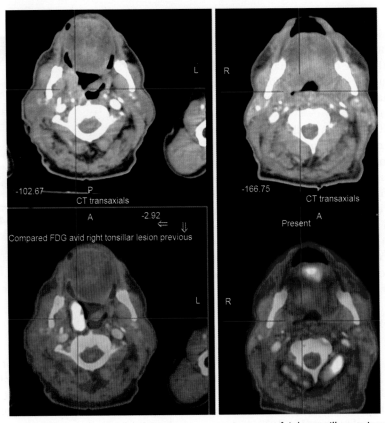

Fig. 19: PET–CT images showing treatment response in a case of right tonsillar carcinoma.

Tongue base has rich lymphatic network and there is high incidence of lymph node metastasis. Lymphatic drainage is to levels II and III nodes. 30% of patients already have cervical nodal metastasis at initial presentation. For MRI images are acquired in T2W, T2 with fatsat, T1W and postcontrast T1W with fatsat in all planes. Sagittal and coronal planes are ideal to demonstrate the intrinsic anatomy of tongue and relation of the lesion to the floor of the mouth and mandible. MR imaging findings that are indicative of osseous involvement include loss of low signal intensity cortex, replacement of high signal intensity marrow on T1W low signal tumor, and contrast enhancement within the bone. False-positive results may occur in cases of recent tooth extraction, radiation-induced inflammation, and osteoradionecrosis. These features influence the choice of therapy (single or multimodality) and extent of surgical resection that can vary from wide excision to partial glossectomy to total glossectomy.

• LYMPHATIC EVALUATION

Imaging assessment includes determination of nodal size, morphology, and margination.

The crucial factors are large nodal size (15 mm for jugulodigastric node and 10 mm for other nodes in short axis) and central necrosis and extracapsular spread. Ultrasound-guided fine needle aspiration cytology is the most reliable technique to assess nodal metastases. Involvement of node with carotid of more than 270° and invasion of prevertebral soft tissue by tumor is a contraindication for surgery (**Figs. 20 and 21**).

• METASTASES

Distant metastases adversely affect the survival and may significantly alter treatment planning. The patients with advanced nodal disease have a high incidence of distant metastases. Pulmonary metastasis is the most frequently encountered. Other sites are bone, liver, skin, and mediastinum. Preoperative chest CT is a must in excluding the lung parenchymal deposits. Annual chest X-ray or chest CT is advised on follow-up.

• CONCLUSION

Imaging plays a significant role in the treatment of oral cancers. It provides information about

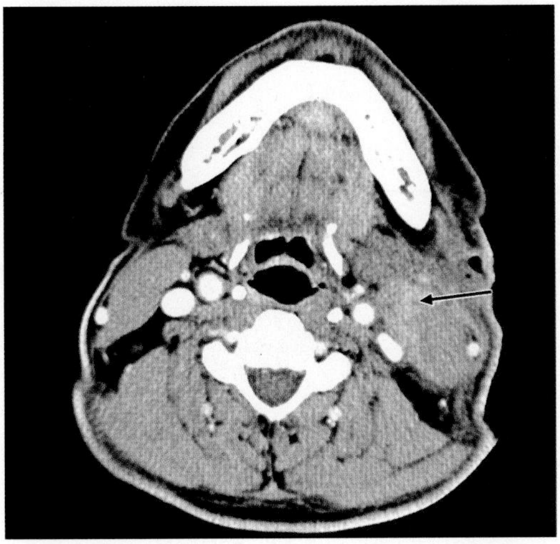

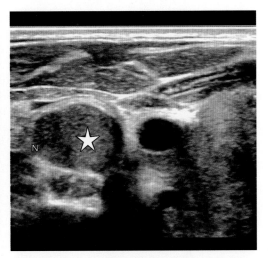

Fig. 20: Axial CT image showing a large nodal mass with perinodal infiltration.

Fig. 21: Ultrasound image of a large node with absent fatty hilum.

the extent of tumor, resectability, reconstruction option, and the prognosis and treatment outcomes.

• FURTHER READING

1. Arya S, Chaukar D, Pai P. Imaging in oral cancers. Indian J Radiol Imaging. 2012;22(3):195-208.
2. Mukherji SK. The pharynx. In: Som PA, Curtine HD (Eds). Head and Neck Imaging, 4th edition. London: Mosby Publishers; 2003. pp. 1465-520.
3. Okura M, Iida S, Aikawa T, et al. Tumor thickness and paralingual distance of coronal MR imaging predicts cervical node metastases in oral tongue carcinoma. AJNR Am J Neuroradiol. 2008;29(1):45-50.
4. Ong CK, Chong VF. Imaging of tongue carcinoma. Cancer Imaging. 2006;6:186-93.
5. Piazza C, Montalto N, Paderno A, et al. Is it time to incorporate 'depth of infiltration' in the T staging of oral tongue and floor of mouth cancer? Curr Opin Otolaryngol Head Neck Surg. 2014;22(2):81-9.
6. Preda L, Chiesa F, Calabrese L, et al. Relationship between histologic thickness of tongue carcinoma and thickness estimated from preoperative MRI. Eur Radiol. 2006;16(10):2242-8.
7. Sigal R, Zagdanski AM, Schwaab G, et al. CT and MR imaging of squamous cell carcinoma of the tongue and floor of the mouth. Radiographics. 1996;16(4):787-810.
8. Trotta BM, Pease CS, Rasamny JJ, et al. Oral cavity and oropharyngeal squamous cell cancer: Key imaging findings for staging and treatment planning. Radiographics. 2011;31(2):339-54.
9. Yousem DM, Chalian AA. Oral cavity and pharynx. Radiol Clin North Am. 1998;36(5):967-81, vii.

CHAPTER 26

Guidelines in the Management of Oral Cavity Cancers

Sivakumar Vidhyadharan, Anoop R, Krishnakumar Thankappan

● INTRODUCTION

The oral cavity comprises the seven subsites: lips, buccal mucosa, retromolar trigone, floor of the mouth, hard palate, oral tongue, and upper and lower alveolar ridge. The area has a rich lymphatic supply. The tumor and the consequences of its treatment can profoundly affect one or more of the several important functions of the oral cavity. Changes of the functions such as mastication, speech, taste, swallowing, oral sensation, and continence can have a devastating impact on the patient's quality of life.

● EPIDEMIOLOGY

Over 57% of the world's head and neck cancers occur in Asia. Oral cancer is the third most common cancer in Southeast Asia. Head and neck cancers account for about 30% of all cancers in India. Head and neck malignancies within the Indian population are very unique with regard to its demographic profile, risk factors, diet, and personal and family history. Oral cavity cancers constitute about 11.5% of the head and neck cancers. Over 90% of tumors of the oral cavity are squamous cell carcinomas.

TNM staging (AJCC, 8th Edition): The major changes are:

- *Definition of primary tumor (T):* Clinical and pathological depth of invasion (DOI) are now used to increase the T category. Extrinsic tongue muscle invasion is no longer used in T4 because this is a feature of DOI.
- Definition of regional lymph node (N).

The new TNM staging and the prognostic stage groups are given in **Tables 1 and 2**.

● CLINICAL PRESENTATION

Even though the oral cavity is a clearly available site for examination by both the patient and the clinician, a remarkably huge number of oral cancers present at an advanced stage due to the painless and indefinable nature of the symptoms.

Alveolar ridge carcinomas, usually present with pain during mastication, but patients may also complain of occasional bleeding and loose teeth. Edentulous patients may give a history of ill-fitting dentures. At a locally advanced stage, trismus, paresthesia or anesthesia of the lower teeth and lip can be present (because of the involvement of the mandibular canal and the inferior alveolar nerve). This is an important sign of locally advanced disease.

Floor of mouth lesions are painful due to their infiltrative nature. They could extend to invade bone anteriorly, muscles of the floor of mouth inferiorly, or the ventral tongue posteriorly. The most common complaint for these patients is the food getting trapped

Table 1: TNM staging lip and oral cavity (AJCC, 8th edition).

T stage	
TX	Primary tumor cannot be assessed
T0	No evidence of primary tumor
Tis	Carcinoma *in situ*
T1	Tumor less than or equal to 2 cm, less than or equal to 5 mm DOI. DOI is depth of invasion and not thickness
T2	Tumor less than or equal to 2 cm, DOI >5 mm and less than or equal to 10 mm OR tumor >2 cm but less than or equal to 4 cm, and DOI less than or equal to 10 mm
T3	Tumor >4 m OR any tumor DOI >10 mm and less than or equal to 20 mm
T4	Moderately advanced or very advanced disease
T4a	Moderately advanced local disease (Lip) Tumor invades through cortical bone or involves the inferior alveolar nerve, floor of mouth, or skin of face (i.e. chin or nose). (Oral cavity) Tumor invades adjacent structures only (through the cortical bone of the mandible or the maxilla, or involves the maxillary sinus or skin of the face) or extensive tumor with bilateral tongue involvement and/or DOI more than 20 mm. *Note:* Superficial erosion of the bone/tooth socket (alone) by a gingival primary is not sufficient to classify a tumor as T4
T4b	Very advanced disease Tumor invades masticator space, pterygoid plates, or skull base and/or encases carotid artery
Clinical N (cN)	
NX	Regional lymph nodes cannot be assessed
N0	No regional lymph node metastasis
N1	Metastasis in a single ipsilateral lymph node, 3 cm or smaller in greatest dimension and ENE (–)
N2	Metastasis in a single ipsilateral node larger than 3 cm but not larger than 6 cm in greatest dimension and ENE (–); or metastases in multiple ipsilateral lymph nodes, none larger than 6 cm in greatest dimension and ENE (–); or in bilateral or contralateral lymph nodes, none larger than 6 cm in greatest dimension and ENE (–)
N2a	Metastasis in a single ipsilateral node larger than 3 cm but not larger than 6 cm in greatest dimension and ENE (–)
N2b	Metastasis in multiple ipsilateral nodes, none larger than 6 cm in greatest dimension and ENE (–)
N2c	Metastasis in bilateral or contralateral lymph nodes, none larger than 6 cm in greatest dimension and ENE (–)
N3	Metastasis in a lymph node larger than 6 cm in greatest dimension and ENE (–); or metastasis in any node(s) with clinically overt ENE (+)
N3a	Metastasis in a lymph node larger than 6 cm in greatest dimension and ENE (–)
N3b	Metastasis in any node (s) with clinically overt ENE (+)
Pathological N (pN)	
NX	Regional lymph nodes cannot be assessed
N0	No regional lymph node metastasis
N1	Metastasis in a single ipsilateral lymph node, 3 cm or smaller in greatest dimension and ENE (–)
N2	Metastasis in a single ipsilateral node, 3 cm or smaller in greatest dimension and ENE (+); or metastasis in a single ipsilateral node larger than 3 cm but not larger than 6 cm in greatest dimension and ENE (–) or metastases in multiple ipsilateral lymph nodes, none larger than 6 cm in greatest dimension and ENE (–); or in bilateral or contralateral lymph nodes, none larger than 6 cm in greatest dimension and ENE (–)

Contd...

Contd...

Pathological N (pN)	
N2a	Metastasis in a single ipsilateral node, 3 cm or smaller in greatest dimension and ENE (+); or metastasis in a single ipsilateral node larger than 3 cm but not larger than 6 cm in greatest dimension and ENE (−)
N2b	Metastasis in multiple ipsilateral nodes, none larger than 6 cm in greatest dimension and ENE (−)
N2c	Metastasis in bilateral or contralateral lymph nodes, none larger than 6 cm in greatest dimension and ENE (−)
N3	Metastasis in a lymph node larger than 6 cm in greatest dimension and ENE (−); or in a single ipsilateral node larger than 3 cm in greatest dimension and ENE (+); or multiple ipsilateral, contralateral, or bilateral nodes any with ENE (+)
N3a	Metastasis in a lymph node larger than 6 cm in greatest dimension and ENE (−)
N3b	Metastasis in a single ipsilateral node larger than 3 cm in greatest dimension and ENE (+); or multiple ipsilateral, contralateral, or bilateral nodes any with ENE (+)

Note: A designation of "U" or "L" may be used for any N category to indicate metastasis above the lower border of the cricoid (U) or below the lower border of the cricoid (L). Similarly, clinical and pathological ENE should be recorded as ENE (−) or ENE (+).

Distant metastasis M	
M0	No distant metastasis
M1	Distant metastasis

Table 2: AJCC prognostic stage groups.

When T is ...	And N is ...	And M is ...	Then the stage group is ...
Tis	N0	M0	0
T1	N0	M0	I
T2	N0	M0	II
T3	N0	M0	III
T0, T1, T2, T3	N1	M0	III
T4a	N0, N1	M0	IVA
T0, T1, T2, T3, T4a	N2	M0	IVA
Any T	N3	M0	IVB
T4b	Any N	M0	IVB
Any T	Any N	M1	IVC

under the tongue. Spread to the alveolus and periosteum of the mandible is a common and initial finding. Fixation of the tumor to the mandible indicates periosteal involvement, and direct bone invasion is not uncommon.

Most tumors of the oral tongue **(Fig. 1)** begin as a small ulcer that progressively infiltrates the musculature of the tongue until its motility is limited. Early lesions appear as small granular outgrowth, which may be suspicious either because of a subtle difference from adjacent normal mucosa or because the patient is anxious about the nature of the lesion. Advanced tumors present either as exophytic or ulcerative lesions **(Fig. 2)**. Endophytic infiltrative or submucosal lesions may be more difficult to identify, and

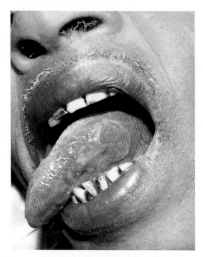

Fig. 1: Infiltrative carcinoma of lateral tongue.

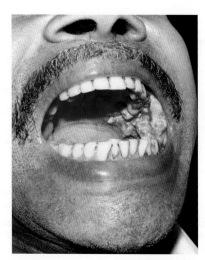

Fig. 2: Proliferative carcinoma of buccal mucosa extending to the gingivobuccal sulcus and alveolus.

their extent may not be apparent until an adequate evaluation under a general anesthetic is performed. Patients may complain of difficulty swallowing or speaking, which becomes even more obvious if the tumor spreads to the floor of the mouth. Cancer of the tongue is usually painful even in its early stage. However, painless lesions may contribute to a significant delay in diagnosis. Any painful ulcer in the oral cavity that fails to heal within a week after a supposed irritant has been removed must be investigated by a biopsy. Cervical lymph node metastases occur early in the course of the disease; patient may also present with a lump in the neck.

Buccal mucosal cancer is more common in developing countries as a consequence of chewing tobacco abuse. Lesions may be proliferative or erosive and are often located near the dental occlusal line. Leukoplakia of the surrounding mucosa may be a prominent feature. Buccal cancers are more commonly exophytic than other oral cancers, but they rarely present as T1 tumors as pain is not an obvious symptom. The presence of trismus indicates possible extension into pterygoid musculature and signifies locally advanced disease.

There should be a thorough examination of the lesion and the rest of the upper aerodigestive tract. A TNM-staged documentation during initial examination is essential and helps with information from further staging investigations.

Imaging

Ultrasonogram of the neck for clinically N0 neck; USG with FNAC increases the specificity.

The investigations for bony involvement can be orthopantomogram (OPG), computed tomographic (CT) scan, or magnetic resonance imaging (MRI). OPG is not preferred because a minimum of 30% bone erosion is required to be detected **(Fig. 3)**. Moreover, it may not be the best for assessing the midline lesions of the mandible due to the overlap by the spine.

CT scan is most commonly used to detect mandibular invasion **(Fig. 4)**. It is preferred over the OPG as it gives information about soft tissue extent along with bony invasion. It is used to assess early bone involvement, in midline lesions and in sites as buccal mucosa, upper and lower alveolus, RMT and hard palate.

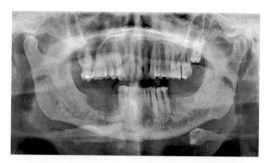

Fig. 3: Orthopantomogram showing mandibular erosion.

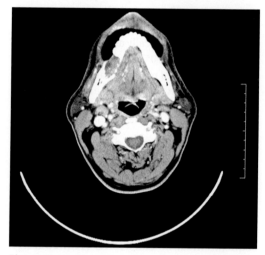

Fig. 4: Contrast-enhanced computed tomography image showing carcinoma eroding the mandibular cortex.

It can also give the extent of infratemporal fossa involvement and the nodal involvement.

MRI is preferred for tongue and floor of mouth lesions and for extension in oropharynx or parapharyngeal space. MRI may be better in assessing the bone marrow infiltration.

Positron emission tomography-CT scan (PET-CT) is helpful for evaluation of post-treatment residual or recurrent disease.

Biopsy

Accessible oral cavity lesions may be biopsied in the outpatient clinic after complete assessment of the DOI, and palpation of neck nodes. Biopsy may be achieved with a knife, punch biopsy forceps. Trucut needle and/or fine needle aspiration may be used for nodes.

● TREATMENT: GENERAL PRINCIPLES

Generally, squamous carcinoma of the oral cavity is managed either by surgery or by radiation alone or in combination. Currently, chemotherapy and targeted immunotherapy protocols are for patients with incurable disease or for those patients in whom conventional treatment has failed. The choice of the best initial therapy for each patient must take into account a variety of interrelated factors (tumor, patient, and clinician) and discussed in a multidisciplinary tumor board and must be tailored individually.

The chronological age by itself should not be a deterrent to aggressive treatment. Rather, the risk of treatment should be assessed based on comorbidity conditions, cardiopulmonary status, and other factors. The patient's motivation and acceptance of a particular plan of management should be considered. Treatment decisions may also be influenced by the patient's lifestyle (i.e. unwillingness to give up smoking and alcohol) and by their occupation and socioeconomic status.

Multidisciplinary team involvement is particularly important for this site, because critical physiologic functions may be affected such as mastication, deglutition, and articulation of speech. The team approach to treatment planning by combined clinic with physicians, surgeons, radiotherapists, medical oncologists, medical social worker, dieticians, swallowing, and rehabilitation specialists is of great importance. It is important to counsel the patient of the potential for failure of treatment and that management of complications of treatment may require staged procedures over a long period of time, and informed consent can be obtained. Cessation of smoking in the period leading up to treatment, especially major surgery or radiation therapy, is important in minimizing complications.

Margins

The tumor has to be resected with clear margins. The general consensus for clear margins is a measured distance of 5 mm from the tumor to the edge of the specimen. For a three-dimensional structure like oral tongue, this may be appropriate and possible. Generally, at least tumor free 1 cm free mucosal and deep soft tissue margin is taken intraoperatively to achieve this 5 mm microscopic clearance. However, this may not be universally applicable in all subsites of oral cavity. An anatomical method is most practicable; if the tumor involves a particular tissue plane, it is wise to take the adjacent next anatomical tissue plane as a margin to get an adequate surgical clearance. For floor of mouth carcinomas, minimal margins of 1 cm, including deep margin should be planned, the deep margin of resection might also include one or both submandibular ducts or the sublingual glands. For buccal mucosal lesion, 1 cm mucosal clearance is possible, but the three-dimensional depth clearance may be possible only by an anatomical approach. A marginal or segmental mandibulectomy may also be required as appropriate. When there is infratemporal fossa invasion, a large compartmental excision along with pterygoid muscles and the pterygoid plates is usually performed.

Assessment of Resectability

The criteria for resectability of a tumor may vary according to the surgical expertise and reconstructive backup. However, in general, tumor involvement of the following structures is considered technically unresectable in a squamous cell carcinoma of the oral cavity.

- Erosion of skull base, sphenoid bone, widening of foramen ovale
- Encasement of internal carotid artery, defined radiologically as tumor surrounding the carotids >270°
- Involvement of mediastinal structures
- Involvement of prevertebral fascia or cervical vertebrae

Early Stage (Stages I and II)

For early lesions (T1–2), a single modality treatment, using either radiation or surgery offers comparable control rates, but factors including functional results, compliance of the patient, cost of treatment, and long-term sequelae must be considered **(Flowchart 1)**. Surgical treatment involves wide resection of the primary lesion with adequate margins and neck dissection. For a node-negative neck, elective selective neck dissection levels I to III

Flowchart 1: Management algorithm for early-stage oral cancers.

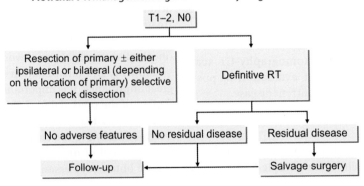

is the recommendation. Removal of level IV is recommended by few authors, considering the potential skip metastasis. However, it is controversial. In a node-positive neck, the recommendation is a comprehensive neck dissection, usually a modified radical neck dissection.

Advanced Lesions (Stages III and IV)

A combined modality approach, primary surgery followed by adjuvant radiation therapy/chemoradiotherapy is generally accepted as standard treatment. The specific treatment for oral cavity subsites is dictated by the TN stage and, if N0 at diagnosis, by the risk of nodal involvement. Surgical management is mostly recommended as primary mode of therapy, since functional outcome is good with the advances in reconstruction using microvascular techniques. Therefore, organ preservation using chemotherapy has less recommendation for the initial management of patients with oral cavity cancers **(Flowchart 2)**.

Postsurgical adjuvant treatment options depend on whether adverse features are present on pathology.

Indications of Adjuvant Radiotherapy

- Advanced T stage (T3/T4)
- Presence of lymphovascular invasion
- Presence of perineural invasion
- Positive surgical margins
- Multiple lymph node involvement
- Extracapsular nodal extension.

Flowchart 2: Management algorithm for advanced-stage oral cancers.

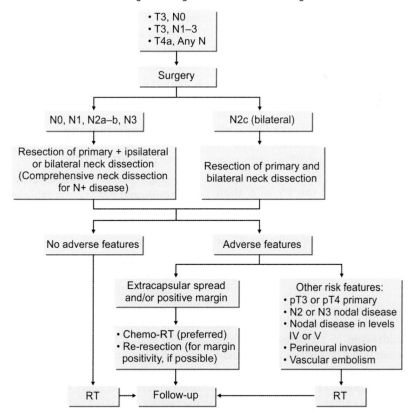

Indications of Adjuvant Chemoradiotherapy

- Positive tumor margins
- Extracapsular nodal extension.

For patients with positive surgical margins, management options include reresection or chemoradiotherapy.

In adjuvant setting, postoperative adjuvant external beam radiation therapy (EBRT) is given in conventional fractionation, with a dose of 60 Gy in 30 fractions to the surgical bed and first echelon nodal stations, while the low-risk nodal stations are treated with 50–54 Gy in conventional fractionation. In case of high-risk features like perinodal spread or positive/close margins, patients are treated with concurrent chemoradiation and the high-risk regions are treated to a total dose of 66 Gy.

Very Advanced-stage Tumors (Stage IVB)

For very advanced stage IVB disease (either T4b with any N stage or any T stage with N3 neck), the patient has the options of either participating in a clinical trial or undergoes standard therapy depending on his performance status (PS) as described by Eastern Cooperative Oncology Group (ECOG). If PS is between 0 and 1, concurrent systemic therapy/RT or induction chemotherapy followed by RT/chemoradiation therapy may be tried. If the PS is 2, then definitive RT+/– concurrent systemic therapy is recommended. With a PS of 3, the patient is suggested to undergo either palliative RT or single agent chemotherapy or best supportive care.

Neck

For clinically node-negative necks, the neck has to be addressed in all cases where the chance of occult nodal metastasis is more than 20%. This will include all tumors of oral cavity except T1T2 hard plate, T1T2 lip lesions, and T1 buccal mucosa cancers. The neck can be managed expectantly in patients with early-stage carcinoma of oral tongue with a thickness of <4 mm. The problem with this approach is that there is no reliable and cost-effective method to determine the thickness of the lesion preoperatively. If the primary is treated with radical radiotherapy, this can be elective neck irradiation; and if the primary is treated with surgery, this is usually elective selective neck dissection levels I to III (supraomohyoid neck dissection).

Byers et al. reported "skip metastases" in patients with tongue carcinoma. He discussed that level IV may be the only involved level, or level III may be involved with no disease present in level I or II. Hence, a selective dissection of levels I–IV may be performed for oral tongue lesions. Bilateral staging neck dissection must be performed, if the primary oral tongue carcinoma is either close to or involving the midline as the patient will have an increased risk of bilateral regional lymph node metastasis.

For clinically and radiologically positive necks, a comprehensive neck dissection, usually a modified radical neck dissection clearing all five levels of neck nodes is appropriate.

Radical Radiotherapy

Primary Radiotherapy

Early-stage cancers of the oral cavity (lip, floor of the mouth, and RMT) are curable by surgery or radiation therapy. Radical radiotherapy is used in treating T1 or T2 tumors with a proliferative component, where the functional or cosmetic result is likely to be better, with similar chances of local control and survival.

Radiation therapy can be administered by EBRT or interstitial implantation alone. Small superficial tumors away from bone may be treated with interstitial brachytherapy alone, while for tumors more than 2 cm, usually both the modalities are combined. The addition of brachytherapy to EBRT has shown to improve the results compared with EBRT alone, but the time interval between them has to be as short as possible. Increasing the overall treatment time has shown to affect the treatment outcome adversely.

When treating with brachytherapy alone, the recommended dose is 66–70 Gy with LDR brachytherapy and 45–60 Gy with 3–6 Gy per fraction with HDR brachytherapy.

The dose when EBRT is used alone is 66–70 Gy in conventional fractionation over 6–7 weeks, or hypofractionated RT 5250 cGy in 15 fractions over 3 weeks.

● FURTHER READING

1. Byers RM, El-Naggar AK, Lee YY, et al. Can we detect or predict the presence of occult nodal metastases in patients with squamous carcinoma of the oral tongue? Head and Neck. 1998;20(2):138-44.

2. Diaz EM Jr, Holsinger FC, Zuniga ER, et al. Squamous cell carcinoma of the buccal mucosa: One institution's experience with 119 previously untreated patients. Head and Neck. 2003;25(4):267-73.

3. Inoue T, Inoue T, Teshima T, et al. Phase III trial of high and low dose rate interstitial radiotherapy for early oral tongue cancer. Int J Radiat Oncol Biol Phys. 1996;36(5):1201-4.

4. Looser KG, Shah JP, Strong EW. The significance of "positive" margins in surgically resected epidermoid carcinomas. Head Neck Surg. 1978;1(2):107-11.

5. Mohit-Tabatabai MA, Sobel HJ, Rush BF, et al. Relation of thickness of floor of mouth stage I and II cancers to regional metastasis. A J Surg. 1986;152(4):351-3.

6. Nair MK, Sankaranarayanan R, Padmanabhan TK. Evaluation of the role of radiotherapy in the management of carcinoma of the buccal mucosa. Cancer. 1988;61(7):1326-31.

7. O'Brien CJ, Lauer CS, Fredricks S, et al. Tumor thickness influences prognosis of T1 and T2 oral cavity cancer—but what thickness? Head Neck. 2003;25(11):937-45.

8. Pernot M, Malissard L, Hoffstetter S, et al. The study of tumoral, radiobiological, and general health factors that influence results and complications in a series of 448 oral tongue carcinomas treated exclusively by irradiation. Int J Radiat Oncol Biol Phys. 1994;29(4):673-9.

9. Schwartz GJ, Mehta RH, Wenig BL, et al. Salvage treatment for recurrent squamous cell carcinoma of the oral cavity. Head Neck. 2000;22(1):34-41.

10. Shah JP, Cendon RA, Farr HW, et al. Carcinoma of the oral cavity. Factors affecting treatment failure at the primary site and neck. Am J Surg. 1976;132(4):504-7.

11. Thomas G, Hashibe M, Jacob BJ, et al. Risk factors for multiple oral premalignant lesions. Int J Cancer. 2003;107(2):285-91.

12. Urist MM, O'Brien CJ, Soong SJ, et al. Squamous cell carcinoma of the buccal mucosa: Analysis of prognostic factors. Am J Surg. 1987;154(4):411-4.

13. Woolgar JA. Histopathological prognosticators in oral and oropharyngeal squamous cell carcinoma. Oral Oncol. 2006;42(3):229-39.

14. Woolgar JA. T2 carcinoma of the tongue: The histopathologist's perspective. Br J Oral Maxillofac Surg. 1999;37(3):187-93.

CHAPTER 27

Guidelines in the Management of Oropharyngeal Cancers

Prameela CG

● INTRODUCTION

Oropharynx is the part of pharynx, between the nasopharynx superiorly and the laryngopharynx inferiorly. Pharynx extends from skull base superiorly to the level of inferior border of cricoid cartilage, where it continues as the esophagus, and lies posterior to nasal and oral cavities, and is also posterior to larynx. This position arbitrarily divides pharynx into the three subdivisions. Malignancies of the oropharynx affect normal swallowing and speech by obstructing the cavity, by causing pain or by infiltration of the surrounding structures and musculature. Radiotherapy is the preferred mode of treatment and may require concurrent chemotherapy to enhance results. High tumoricidal doses can be delivered with less impairment of the functional aspects. Still, curative intent treatment to some extent can hamper structural and functional outcomes.

● EPIDEMIOLOGY

Approximately 10% of head and neck tumors, world over, annually have their origin in oropharynx. Geographic variations in the prevalence have been noted. Increase in the incidence of oropharyngeal cancers has been observed as opposed to malignancies of other sites of head and neck, especially in the nonsmokers and nonconsumers of alcohol. This has been attributed to the oncogenic human papilloma virus. A 28% increase in the incidence has been noted during the period of 1998–2004 with a 225% increase in HPV-associated oropharyngeal cancers, while HPV-unassociated oropharyngeal cancers have come down by 50%. There is a higher prevalence of the disease in males with a ratio of 4:1, probably because the major factor leading to the tumor is tobacco smoking and/or excessive consumption of alcohol-containing beverages. Common presentation is in the 5th to 6th decades.

● ETIOLOGY

About 95% of oropharyngeal malignances are squamous cell carcinomas. Most important factor associated with its carcinogenesis is chronic exposure to tobacco and alcohol, as in the entire mucosa of the aerodigestive tract. Clinically recognized premalignant lesions are leukoplakia, and erythroplakia. An erythroplakic lesion transforms more frequently to a malignant lesion. Multiple independent premalignant and malignant foci can also be present. Annual incidence of a second squamous cell carcinoma in the head and neck region is estimated to be about 4–7%. Apart from tobacco and alcohol, other factors attributed are diet low in fruits and vegetables, drinking mate, a stimulant drink common in South America, chewing betel quid, a common practice in India and other parts of Asia, and human papilloma virus infection.

Association between HPV-16 and other oncogenic HPV viruses and oropharyngeal carcinomas have been documented. This is especially true for tonsillar carcinoma. HPV associated carcinomas are found to be more in younger patients, who are most often nonsmokers and are not abusers of alcohol, and hence have a better risk profile, and also respond better to treatment. HPV-positive tumors have less incidence of recurrence, and the patients are less likely to die of disease.

Discontinuing smoking and chewing tobacco and alcohol consumption are known to reduce the risk of a second primary in the head and neck area. Patients who continue to smoke even after the diagnosis and treatment for an index cancer is known to have twice the risk of developing a second primary malignancy. Those who consume more than 14 alcoholic drinks a week after treatment for an index cancer is known to have a 50% risk of developing a second primary cancer.

● ANATOMY

Oropharynx extends from uvula and soft palate superiorly to the level of hyoid bone and superior border of epiglottis inferiorly. Anteriorly it communicates with oral cavity through oropharyngeal isthmus. The oropharyngeal isthmus superiorly has the soft palate, laterally the palatoglossal arches and inferiorly the tongue. Mucous membrane of epiglottis reflects over the base of tongue and on to the lateral wall of pharynx, forming the median glossoepiglottic fold and epiglottic vallecula on either side. Anterior wall of oropharynx is formed by base of tongue, and epiglottic valleculae. Lateral wall of oropharynx has palatoglossal and palatopharyngeal arches. Triangular recess between the two arches is occupied by the tonsil. Roof of oropharynx is bound by the uvula and the soft palate. Opening of the nasopharynx to the oropharynx is the pharyngeal isthmus, bound by free edge of soft palate, the palatopharyngeal folds, and the posterior pharyngeal wall.

● SUBSITES OF OROPHARYNX

The anatomical subsites of oropharynx are the base of tongue, the tonsillar regions, the soft palate and the pharyngeal walls. All these structures play important roles in swallowing and speech. Lymphatic spread of malignancies of oropharynx differs based on the subsite of origin.

● PATHOLOGY

Almost 95% of oropharyngeal tumors are squamous cell carcinomas. The other histology that can occur though rare, are minor salivary gland tumors. Abundance of lymphoid tissue and the Waldeyer's ring makes both Hodgkin and non-Hodgkin lymphoma a probability in this region.

● CLINICAL FEATURES

Oropharyngeal tumors are usually asymptomatic in the initial stages. As the disease progress they can manifest with localized pain. Deep-seated pain in the ear mediated by irritation of glossopharyngeal nerve (9th cranial nerve) through the petrosal ganglion to the tympanic nerve of Jacobson is another presenting complaint. Often they present with mobile, firm and nontender lymph nodal mass in the neck. Later on they can become fixed masses indicating extranodal extension and infiltration of adjacent tissues. Increase in size and extent of the lesion can lead to dysphagia, and/or odynophagia, when there is invasion of the pharyngeal musculature, or obstruction due to mass lesions, and hoarseness when tumor infiltrates larynx. Necrosis of tumor can result in bad odor. Infiltration of oral tongue makes articulation difficult producing dysarthria. Impairment of tongue protrusion and its movement in the anterior or lateral direction suggests involvement of the root of tongue. Lesions of soft palate and tonsillar regions are easily visualized and can be picked up at earlier stages. Extensive lesions of soft palate or lesions infiltrating soft palate can impair normal elevation of soft palate during deglutition leading to nasal regurgitation. Due to difficulty in visualizing the tumors of base tongue, they are usually detected at a late stage. Trismus manifests with involvement of the pterygoid fossa and pterygoid muscles.

Lymphatic Spread

Rouvier in 1938 described the lymphatic spread of the oropharynx. Ipsilatral level II nodes are the most common nodal groups involved in an oropharyngeal lesion. The lymphatic spread is usually systematic in a nonviolated neck, with progression from upper jugular chain nodes (level I/II) the first echelon, to mid cervical (level III), and then to the lower cervical nodes (level IV) inferiorly. Isolated skip metastasis are rare in oropharyngeal cancers. Involvement of level I or level V nodes are usually associated with involvement of other levels. Probability of nodal metastasis depends on size and extent of primary tumor.

● DISTANT METASTASIS

Only about 15% of patients with oropharyngeal cancers in the normal course of their disease develop distant metastasis. The common site of distant metastasis is lung parenchyma, followed by bone and hepatic metastasis. Locoregionally advanced disease with N2 or N3 nodal status and recurrent tumors are the ones usually having distant metastasis. Other factors associated with distant metastases are—perinodal spread, lymphadenopathy in lower cervical levels, and lymphovascular emboli.

● EVALUATION

Physical Examination

Thorough clinical evaluation requires assessment of primary tumor, in terms of extent and involvement of adjacent sites, and presence and nature of lymph nodal involvement. The size of the primary tumor and nodal disease forms the basis of the American Joint Committee

on Cancer (AJCC) staging system. Most oropharyngeal tumors present as ulcerated masses with surrounding erythema and neovascularization. Tenderness, evidence of any recent bleeding, obstruction to airway, skin invasion, alteration of gagreflex, and extent of trismus (measured from upper to lower incisors or alveolar ridges in edentulous patients) carry importance. Bulging of parapharyngeal space can indicate retropharyngeal lymphadenopathy. Lymph nodal size and character need also to be noted. Confirmatory biopsy of the primary site should be performed.

Direct visualization should be followed by fiberoptic examination whenever possible, as it facilitates optimal inspection of base of tongue, posterior-inferior tonsil, valecula, as well as spread to laryngeal and pharyngeal subsites. Tumor extensions into larynx, pyriform sinus, and superiorly to nasopharynx need to be assessed and documented.

Imaging: Computed Tomography (CT)

Imaging of head and neck with intravenous contrast should be performed for all newly diagnosed oropharyngeal cancer patients to assess extent of primary tumors and to determine presence or absence of cervical lymph node metastases. Scan slice thickness 3 mm is desirable to optimize the detection of smaller sized lesions and to provide best anatomic delineation of both primary and nodal disease. Primary tumors appear as contrast-enhancing masses, distorting normal anatomic relationships. Primary tumor measurements are to be assessed in both longitudinal and transverse planes **(Fig. 1)**.

Important findings to be assessed in the CT images–

▪ Tumor size
▪ Tumor extent
▪ Involvement of medial pterygoid, larynx, hard palate, mandible
▪ Lateral pterygoids, pterygoid plates, skull base or carotid artery.

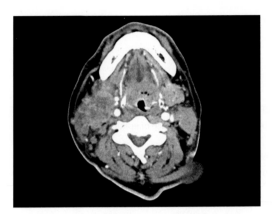

Fig. 1: CT scan of oropharynx showing primary disease and lymph nodal extension.

Thoracic CT scan should be performed to look for pulmonary spread of oropharyngeal cancer, in patients with N2 or greater nodal disease, as well as those with advanced primary tumors, given the risks of pulmonary metastases.

Positron Emission Tomography and Computed Tomography (PET–CT) Scan

PET-based imaging can assess locoregional burden of disease and also distant metastases. For oropharyngeal cancer patients, specifically the ability to detect occult pathologic cervical lymphadenopathy renders PET a powerful tool, as ipsilateral radiotherapy volumes are used in specific circumstances like early stage ipsilateral tonsillar lesion. PET-CT for oropharyngeal cancer patients demonstrates high sensitivity of 99%, and a specificity of 60% for pathologically proven tumor. Recent biopsies and infections can show elevated metabolic activity in PET.

Magnetic Resonance Imaging

Squamous cell carcinoma appears as low signal in T1 MRI and corresponding high signal in T2 sequences. MRI can differentiate tumor from soft tissues, which is particularly useful in base tongue lesions to delineate extension to oral tongue, if brachytherapy is being planned. MRI is useful in patients with compromised renal function who are not candidates for iodine-based CT contrast agents.

Biopsy

Confirmatory tissue diagnosis is mandatory before proceeding to the management of the lesion as in any other suspicious lesion. Most of the oropharyngeal tumors are accessible through an intraoral approach. A posterior oropharyngeal tumor would require a biopsy under general anesthesia, which can be combined with endoscopic evaluation.

TNM Staging (AJCC 8th Edition, 2010)

The Eighth Edition has introduced a separate TNM staging system for HPV mediated (p16+) oropharyngeal cancer **(Tables 1 to 4)**.

- *Definition of T staging:* There is no *Tis* included, there is no separation of T4 into T4a and T4b.
- *Definition of Clinical N(CN):* There are no divisions for N2 or N3. Extranodal extension has no relevance.
- *Pathological N(PN):* This staging is different from CN. There is no PN3 stage
- For p16- oropharyngeal cancers, T staging has no T0 and *Tis*, N staging is similar to other non-HPV related cancers.

● MANAGEMENT

Primary goal in the treatment of any malignancy is to achieve maximum tumor control, while conserving functional aspects of the organ and minimizing cosmetic deformities.

The oropharyngeal tumors are classified as:
- *Early disease*—disease confined locally— stage I and II tumors
- *Locoregionally advanced disease*—stage III and IV—non-metastatic disease
- Metastatic disease.

Table 1: TNM staging p16+ oropharyngeal cancer (AJCC 8th Edition).

T Stage	
TX	Primary tumor cannot be assessed.
T0	No primary identified.
T1	Tumor 2 cm or smaller in greatest dimension.
T2	Tumor larger than 2 cm but not larger than 4 cm in greatest dimension.
T3	Tumor larger than 4 cm in greatest dimension or extension to lingual surface of epiglottis.
T4	Moderately advanced local disease. Tumor invades the larynx, extrinsic muscle of tongue, medial pterygoid, hard palate, or mandible or beyond*. *Note:* *Mucosal extension to lingual surface of epiglottis from primary tumors of the base of the tongue and vallecula does not constitute invasion of the larynx.

Clinical N (cN)	
NX	Regional lymph nodes cannot be assessed.
N0	No regional lymph node metastasis.
N1	One or more ipsilateral lymph nodes, none larger than 6 cm.
N2	Contralateral or bilateral lymph nodes. none larger than 6 cm.
N3	Lymph node(s) larger than 6 cm.

Pathological N (PN)	
NX	Regional lymph nodes cannot be assessed.
N0	No regional lymph node metastasis.
N1	Metastasis in 4 or fewer lymph nodes.
N2	Metastasis in more than 4 lymph nodes.

Distant metastasis M	
M0	No distant metastasis
M1	Distant metastasis

Table 2: AJCC prognostic stage groups (p16+ oropharyngeal cancer).

Clinical CTNM				
When p16 status is	**When T is ...**	**And N is ...**	**And M is ...**	**Then the stage group is ...**
Positive	T0, T1, T2	N0 or N1	M0	I
Positive	T0, T1, T2	N2	M0	II
Positive	T3	N0, N1 or N2	M0	II
Positive	T0, T1, T2,T3,T4	N3	M0	III
Positive	T4	N0, N1, N2, N3	M0	III
Positive	Any T	Any N	M1	IV
Pathological pTNM				
When p16 status is	**When T is...**	**And N is...**	**And M is...**	**Then the stage group is...**
Positive	T0, T1, T2	N0 or N1	M0	I
Positive	T0, T1, T2	N2	M0	II
Positive	T3 or T4	N0, N1	M0	II
Positive	T3 or T4	N2	M0	III
Positive	Any T	Any N	M1	IV

Table 3: TNM staging p16– oropharyngeal cancer (AJCC 8th Edition).

T Stage

TX	Primary tumor cannot be assessed.
Tis	Carcinoma *in situ*.
T1	Tumor 2 cm or smaller in greatest dimension.
T2	Tumor larger than 2 cm but not larger than 4 cm in greatest dimension.
T3	Tumor larger than 4 cm in greatest dimension or extension to lingual surface of epiglottis.
T4	Moderately advanced or very advanced disease.
T4a	Moderately advanced local disease. Tumor invades the larynx, extrinsic muscle of tongue, medial pterygoid, hard palate, or mandible or beyond*.
T4b	Very advanced local disease. Tumor invades lateral pterygoid muscle, pterygoid plates, lateral nasopharynx, or skull base or encases carotid artery.
	Note: *Mucosal extension to lingual surface of epiglottis from primary tumors of the base of the tongue and vallecula does not constitute invasion of the larynx.

Clinical N (cN)

NX	Regional lymph nodes cannot be assessed.
N0	No regional lymph node metastasis.
N1	Metastasis in a single ipsilateral lymph node, 3 cm or smaller in greatest dimension and ENE (–).
N2	Metastasis in a single ipsilateral node larger than 3 cm but not larger than 6 cm in greatest dimension and ENE (–); or metastases in multiple ipsilateral lymph nodes, none larger than 6 cm in greatest dimension and ENE (–); or in bilateral or contralateral lymph nodes, none larger than 6 cm in greatest dimension and ENE (–).
N2a	Metastasis in a single ipsilateral node larger than 3 cm but not larger than 6 cm in greatest dimension and ENE (–).
N2b	Metastasis in multiple ipsilateral nodes, none larger than 6 cm in greatest dimension and ENE (–).
N2c	Metastasis in bilateral or contralateral lymph nodes, none larger than 6 cm in greatest dimension and ENE (–).
N3	Metastasis in a lymph node larger than 6 cm in greatest dimension and ENE (–); or metastasis in any node(s) with clinically overt ENE (+).
N3a	Metastasis in a lymph node larger than 6 cm in greatest dimension and ENE (–).
N3b	Metastasis in any node(s) with clinically overt ENE (+).

Pathological N (pN)

NX	Regional lymph nodes cannot be assessed.
N0	No regional lymph node metastasis.
N1	Metastasis in a single ipsilateral lymph node, 3 cm or smaller in greatest dimension and ENE (–).
N2	Metastasis in a single ipsilateral node, 3 cm or smaller in greatest dimension and ENE (+); or metastasis in a single ipsilateral node larger than 3 cm but not larger than 6 cm in greatest dimension and ENE (–) or metastases in multiple ipsilateral lymph nodes, none larger than 6 cm in greatest dimension and ENE (–); or in bilateral or contralateral lymph nodes, none larger than 6 cm in greatest dimension and ENE (–).
N2a	Metastasis in a single ipsilateral node, 3 cm or smaller in greatest dimension and ENE (+); or metastasis in a single ipsilateral node larger than 3 cm but not larger than 6 cm in greatest dimension and ENE (–).
N2b	Metastasis in multiple ipsilateral nodes, none larger than 6 cm in greatest dimension and ENE (–).
N2c	Metastasis in bilateral or contralateral lymph nodes, none larger than 6 cm in greatest dimension and ENE (–).

Contd...

Contd...

Pathological N (pN)	
N3	Metastasis in a lymph node larger than 6 cm in greatest dimension and ENE (–); or in a single ipsilateral node larger than 3 cm in greatest dimension and ENE (+); or multiple ipsilateral, contralateral, or bilateral nodes any with ENE (+).
N3a	Metastasis in a lymph node larger than 6 cm in greatest dimension and EN E (–).
N3b	Metastasis in a single ipsilateral node larger than 3 cm in greatest dimension and ENE (+); or multiple ipsilateral, contralateral, or bilateral nodes any with ENE (+).

Note: A designation of "U" or "L" may be used for any N category to indicate metastasis above the lower border of the cricoid (U) or below the lower border of the cricoid (L). Similarly, clinical and pathological ENE should be recorded as ENE (–) or ENE (+)

Distant metastasis M	
M0	No distant metastasis
M1	Distant metastasis

Table 4: AJCC Prognostic stage groups (p16– oropharyngeal cancer).

When T is ...	And N is ...	And M is ...	Then the stage group is ...
Tis	N0	M0	0
T1	N0	M0	I
T2	N0	M0	II
T3	N0	M0	III
T0, T1, T2, T3	N1	M0	III
T4a	N0, N1	M0	IVA
T0, T1, T2, T3,T4a	N2	M0	IVA
Any T	N3	M0	IVB
T4b	Any N	M0	IVB
Any T	Any N	M1	IVC

Early stage tumors of all subsites of oropharynx are usually well controlled with single local modality treatment, either in the form of surgery or radiotherapy. Treatment modality is decided based on primary site, size and extent of disease. Locally advanced diseases require the use of combined approaches using radiotherapy, chemotherapy, and surgery.

● SUBSITE-WISE TREATMENT APPROACHES

Base of Tongue

Definitive radiotherapy or surgery gives equivalent results in terms of overall survival and locoregional control for early stage lesions of base of tongue. Radiotherapy is most of the time the treatment opted in view of better functional and quality-of-life outcomes compared to surgery.

Surgical Options

Surgery has very limited role in base of tongue malignancy. This is because a large or a midline lesion necessitates near-total or total glossectomy. A well lateralized lesion of base of tongue, with no cervical lymphadenopathy can be addressed with a surgical procedure. Being close to the laryngeal apparatus, lesions of vallecula may require a supraglottic or a total laryngectomy for achieving adequate negative margins. In view of the high propensity for nodal involvement, any surgical procedure would need to be combined with bilateral lymph nodal dissection. Most often a surgical procedure would require adjuvant external beam radiotherapy, in case of inadequate or close margins and microscopic positive nodes.

For an early primary lesion of base of tongue, primary radiation or surgery often with adjuvant postoperative radiation therapy can give similar local and regional control rates. Possibility of maximal functional outcome with radiotherapy makes it the choice of treatment. Surgery is often reserved for patients who cannot receive radiation, or for locally advanced lesion which would not be adequately controlled with radiation alone.

If primary tumor is treated with radiation alone, patients with nodal lesions will require surgical dissection, which is usually done at the completion of RT. If an upfront surgery of the nodal volume is being planned, this can be combined with placement of catheters for interstitial implant, and treatment delivered at a later date.

The traditional surgical approaches for a base of tongue lesion have been a transoral approach or through a mandibulotomy, and transhyoid pharyngotomy, or a lateral mandibulotomy, or floor drop procedures. Transoral approach is used for small, superficial, well-delineated lesions. Evidence of bone invasion or adherence to bone needs a mandibulectomy. Flap or plate reconstructions are combined with resection depending on amount of tissue resected, age of the patient, and the anticipated functional impairment.

Radiation Therapy Options

Preferred definitive treatment in base of tongue tumors is radical radiation therapy. A T1, T2, and an exophytic T3 tumor can be treated using primary radiotherapy as the sole modality. Infiltrative T3 and all T4 lesions require combined approach using concurrent chemoradiation, which also is a functionally viable option in view of the organ preservation achieved. Another option in advanced tumors of base of tongue is primary surgery followed by postoperative radiotherapy (PORT).

Target volume includes primary tumor with the base of tongue, and adequate margin to include a part of the oral tongue, vallecula, the pharyngeal walls, the suprahyoid epiglottis and the superior aspect of the preepiglottic space. Probability of nodal metastasis is high in base of tongue tumors. Incidence of pathological lymph nodes in ipsilateral clinical N0 neck is around 22–33%. Contralateral nodal metastasis at presentation is seen in 37% of patients. Hence, the volume should electively include bilateral level II–IV cervical nodes and retropharyngeal group of lymph nodes, even in patients with clinically negative neck electively.

Intensity modulated radiation therapy (IMRT) is the preferred mode of EBRT in base of tongue, though three-dimensional conformal radiation therapy (3DCRT) can also be used. Interstitial brachytherapy using iridium-192 as a primary mode in early tumors or to boost EBRT dose to augment dose received by primary tumor can be considered. EBRT dose of 50–54 Gy in 1.8–2.0 Gy fractions is followed by brachytherapy boost of 20–30 Gy, performed approximately 3 weeks after treatment. Iridium-192 after-loading catheters are used for implant through submental approach. Temporary tracheostomy and nasogastric tube feeding is required prior to implant. If neck dissection is planned upfront, placement of interstitial catheter can be combined with the procedure, and treatment delivered at a later date. Palate has to be protected during brachytherapy using customized shields. Intraoral cone is another option of treatment.

Neck is managed with EBRT alone in node negative and N1 nodal status. For more advanced disease of neck, chemotherapy is given concurrently with radiation to improve results. Surgical approach is warranted in patients with early stage disease, treated with radiotherapy, when there is residual nodal mass six weeks after completion of treatment.

Outcomes

Primary EBRT alone or in combination with planned neck dissection following RT has high local control rate of 80–90% in T1 and T2 tumors, and 70–85% for T3 tumors of base of tongue. Surgical results are also equivalent being 75–85%. Overall survival is similar in both treatment modes though RT has lower incidence of complications. Combination of EBRT with brachytherapy in early T1 and T2 tumors has local control rates of 80–100%. Five-year local control rates of 93% for T1 and 72% for T2 tumors and 5-year disease-free survival of 76% and 62%, respectively have been reported, with EBRT, brachytherapy combination.

Tonsillar Cancers

Early lesions of tonsillar region are preferably treated with radiotherapy as the results and functional outcomes are excellent, though both surgery and radiotherapy can be used.

Surgical Options

Surgery can be considered as an option for treating small, (<1 cm) superficial, early stage lesions of tonsil confined to anterior tonsillar pillar, or tonsillar fossa. Wide local excision most of the time achieves a tumor-free margin. For lesions of palatine tonsils, radical tonsillectomy is usually required. Preferred approach is transoral, with primary closure. Larger lesions extending to tongue, mandible, and other surrounding structures, need to be addressed by a composite resection with resection of tonsil, tonsillar fossa, tonsillar pillars, part of soft palate, tongue and mandible. Tumor, not adherent or adjacent to mandible can have

midline mandibulotomy approach, while for those adherent to mandible, or superficial periosteal extension would need a partial mandibulectomy. Closure is done with myocutaneous flaps. Postsurgery complications depend on extent of resection. A clinically negative neck is addressed by a modified supraomohyoid neck dissection, as a staging procedure. Positive nodes need the addition of postoperative radiotherapy. Swallowing can be compromised when there is a substantial resection of tongue and soft palate.

Radiation Therapy Options

Definitive radiotherapy is the treatment of choice in T1, T2, and T3 (exophytic) tumors. Well-lateralized, early stage, N0 or N1 tumor of tonsil can be considered for ipsilateral curative intent radical external beam radiation, sparing contralateral side. Target volume in ipsilateral treatment should include primary tumor with a margin of 2 cm, ipsilateral jugular vein, and lateral retropharyngeal nodes. Contralateral sparing reduces treatment related morbidity substantially. Incidence of xerostomia is reduced in these patients and the outcomes are excellent in well selected group of patients. 3DCRT or IMRT can be used for treatment. Most of the T1 and T2 tumors either with no nodal disease or a single ipsilateral nodal status are treated with ipsilateral plans.

Extensive lesions, crossing the midline, involving surrounding structures with multiple cervical nodal diseases would require treatment of ipsilateral and contralateral neck. Extension to base of tongue needs to be addressed with additional dose, and interstitial implants and brachytherapy is a preferred option. Adjacent normal structure tolerances are to be respected while planning radical dose to target volume.

In case of infiltrative endophytic, T3 lesions and in T4 lesions concurrent chemotherapy with external beam radiation therapy is opted. In selected cases surgery followed by PORT can be the choice of treatment, with concurrent chemotherapy depending on pathological status.

Outcomes

Surgery as the sole treatment of early tonsillar tumors is rare. However, local control rates of 80–90% have been reported with surgery alone. Extension to lateral pharyngeal wall or to base of tongue, leads to poor local control with recurrence rates of 33–47%, respectively. Local control rates depend on extension of tumor beyond tonsillar fossa.

There are no randomized controlled trials comparing surgery and EBRT. For most early stage disease EBRT is the treatment of choice. Conventional fractionated radiotherapy using 1.8–2 Gy fractions per day to a total dose of 66–70 Gy spanning over 6.5–7 weeks gives excellent results in early stage tumors. Local control rates of 100% for T1, 89% for T2, 68% for T3, and 24% for T4 lesions have been reported, with EBRT alone. Cervical control rates were around 95%. Planned neck dissection improved neck control rates to 100%. Distant metastasis was 10% and primary treatment option was not found to influence this. Tumors arising from glossopalatine sulcus which can involve the tongue were found to have inferior local control rates, when compared to tumors arising from other subsites of tonsil. Lower doses of radiation resulted in poor locoregional control.

Soft Palate Cancers

Small early stage lesions of soft palate can be treated with either surgery or radiotherapy, and have equivalent results. Radiotherapy is usually preferred as the results are excellent and functional results are superior. Usually the lesions are in the midline or cross the midline and radiotherapy addresses both primary and bilateral neck nodal regions better. Morbidity of surgery can be aggravated if a postoperative radiation therapy is required.

Surgical Options

Tumors of soft palate are rarely considered for surgical management. This is because resections can lead to nasal regurgitation during swallowing even with the use of customized palatine prosthesis. Tumors of palate usually are midline and have rich bilateral lymphatic drainage, and hence require elective bilateral nodal dissection. When surgery is opted, a transoral approach is preferred and a full thickness wide local dissection is done, when the tumor is confined to soft palate. For lesions involving surrounding structures, extensive composite resection is usually done. Velopharyngeal competence, which can be lost with surgery, can be preserved with use of customized prosthesis, or with proper flap reconstruction. Nasal twang of speech is another postsurgery consequence.

Radiation Therapy Options

Majority of T1 or T2 tumors of soft palate are treated using radiotherapy. Early, well lateralized lesions, less than 1 cm in size, can be addressed with radiotherapy only to the primary site, without addressing the neck, to a dose of 66–70 Gy in conventional fractionation. T1 and T2 lesions require treatment of primary along with ipsilateral neck. Larger T1–T3 lesions though can be treated with surgery, associated functional morbidity makes radiotherapy a better option. EBRT to a dose of 70–75 Gy to the primary or a combination of EBRT (40–50 Gy) with brachytherapy boost to the primary site gives good results. Advanced diseases need concurrent chemotherapy along with radical radiotherapy.

Brachytherapy implant using iridium-192 has been in use for soft palate tumors either as a single modality approach or as a boost to primary EBRT. Fractionated high dose rate brachytherapy using twice a day fractions of 3.0–5.4 Gy to a dose of 15–20 Gy delivered after 1–2 weeks of completion of EBRT has been tried, with the EBRT dose being 46–50 Gy. Pulsed dose rate brachytherapy has also been tried in these situations with brachytherapy dose of 20–28 Gy.

Outcomes

Five-year locoregional control rates of 90%, 92%, 84%, and 64% for stage I–IV have been documented with EBRT followed by salvage surgery. Local failure rates of 25% for EBRT alone, 0% for brachytherapy alone, and 18% for combination treatment have been quoted. Radiotherapy is effective for early stage disease but is certainly suboptimal for advanced diseases of soft palate.

The surgical procedures used for oropharyngeal malignancies are–

- Transoral surgical approaches
- Transoral laser surgery
- Transoral robotic surgery.

● TRANSORAL SURGICAL APPROACHES

Transoral surgical approaches are preferred alternative procedures to open surgical options. This is used for early stage, limited tonsillar lesions, and other oropharyngeal tumors. As opposed to an open procedure, transoral approaches are less morbid and postsurgery recovery is faster. Prospective trials comparing advantages of transoral approaches are still in the early stages and further robust evidence is required in this area.

Transoral Laser Surgery

Transoral laser microsurgery with or without elective neck dissection is a newer area and favorable results have been documented from small series. This requires adjuvant radiation or chemoradiation based on pathological data. Resected margin clearance depends on primary tumor site and extent of lesion. Results quoted for stage I and II tumors are 87–100%, while for stage III and IV tumors, high local recurrence rates of 20–30% have been reported. Swallowing complications are less and normal diet tolerance is found to be good in these patients.

Transoral Robotic Surgery (TORS)

Use of a computer-aided interaction between the surgeon and the patient is commonly referred to as robotic surgery. The da Vinci Surgical System is the most common robotic surgical system used. Movements of the surgeons are translated to micromovements of the instrument. The advantage is the motion scaling which leads to better precision and reduced hand tremor and fatigue. Enhancement in visualization over transoral approach has been highlighted. Better local control with TORS debulking, which can lead to minimal acute complications have been suggested by advocates of this. Further studies are required for convincing evidence in the use of TORS in oropharyngeal cancers.

● ADJUVANT TREATMENT

It is decided based on pathological findings after a definitive surgery. Indications for adjuvant treatment are:

- Advanced primary stage—T3 or T4
- Lymphovascular space invasion
- Perineural invasion
- Positive resected margins
- Multiple pathologically involved cervical lymph nodes
- Extranodal extension of the tumor.

All these features have shown to increase the risk locoregional recurrence. Postoperative radiotherapy (PORT) either with or without concurrent chemotherapy has been shown to improve local control rates in oropharyngeal tumors. RTOG 73-03 had shown superior locoregional control of 70% with PORT versus preoperative radiotherapy (58%), though there was no survival advantage.

Adjuvant Radiotherapy

Conventional fractionation using 2 Gy daily fractions to a cumulative dose of 60–66 Gy to the high-risk areas, like the primary tumor bed with positive margin, and the extranodal spread, has been used in most of the randomized studies using concurrent chemotherapy with PORT. A dose of 50–54 Gy to areas at risk of microscopic disease is given. A significant benefit for patients with positive margins and extranodal spread has been documented, and this is the recommended conventional dose in a postoperative setting, with concurrent chemotherapy.

Volumes in Postoperative Setting

Treatment volumes in PORT would include the primary tumor site and bilateral neck nodal stations. A well-lateralized lesion, whose pattern of spread can be considered to involve only the ipsilateral neck, can be treated with ipsilateral PORT. Opinions are differed as to the inclusion of the neck in a patient with negative nodes after adequate neck dissection, when there is only primary tumor-site margin positivity, and suggest treating only the primary site with PORT. Similarly with a radical primary surgery with wide negative margins and positive neck nodes, the need for primary site radiation is questioned, and only neck irradiation is advised by few authors.

• DEFINITIVE RADIOTHERAPY

Early stage oropharyngeal cancers can be treated with curative intent single modality external beam radiotherapy. The outcomes are good with the advantage of functional preservation.

Pretreatment Dental Evaluation and Prophylaxis

A radical EBRT for oropharyngeal tumors can lead to transient and permanent changes in oral cavity and oropharynx. These include mucositis, xerostomia, and infections. Reduced salivary flow and change in oral saliva pH enhances bacterial growth and proliferation and this in turn can cause or aggravate and already existent dental caries. Detailed dental evaluation and

prophylactic treatment of dental caries and any other coexistent pathology hence is mandatory before taking up for EBRT. Prophylactic fluoride gel applications are advised to prevent dental caries during treatment, which need to be continued for an extended period after completion of treatment.

Simulation and Planning

Pretreatment CT simulation with optimal immobilization is mandatory for treatment planning. Patients are treated in the supine position with neck extended using a neck roll and also a bite-block, when indicated. A thermoplastic mask is custom made for patient immobilization (**Fig. 2**). CT images are taken in 3 mm cuts, from the vertex to the carina. If better delineation is needed 2 mm cuts can be chosen. A contrast enhanced CT simulation can also be performed. Fiducials are placed for anatomical reproducibility and daily set-up matching.

Once simulation is done, images acquired are transferred to contouring stations and gross tumor volumes, clinical target volume, and planning volumes are contoured, as per RTOG guidelines. Normal structures and organs at risk are also contoured. Planning is done on the treatment planning systems and the generated

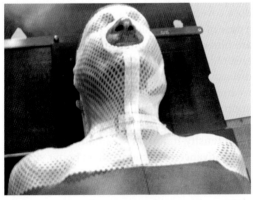

Fig. 2: Immobilization for RT planning in a head and neck malignancy.

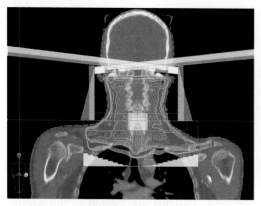

Fig. 3: Field arrangement in 3DCRT in a base of tongue lesion.

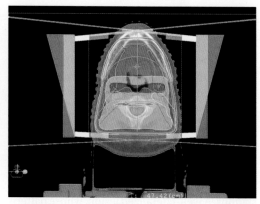

Fig. 4: Dose distribution in a base of tongue lesion.

plans are evaluated for adequate target volume coverage and at risk organ sparing, before plan execution.

The treatment portals for oropharyngeal tumors should encompass the primary tumor and the locoregional extensions. Neck portals should extend superiorly up to the level of c1 for a node negative patient and up to the base of skull (retrostyloid space) for a node positive one.

In a conventional 3-dimensional plan, lateral parallel opposed portals are used for upper neck. Lower neck is usually treated using a single anteroposterior field, with a compensatory posterior portal, for adequate dose coverage. Initial treatment is continued to a dose of 44–45 Gy following which spinal cords are blocked. Gross tumor dose of 66–70 Gy is ensured, and a dose of 50–60 Gy for microscopic disease. Usually 6 MV photons are used for treatment. Once the spinal cord is blocked appropriate energy electrons are used for the treatment of the posterior neck **(Figs. 3 to 5)**.

Intensity-modulated radiation therapy, a more advanced technique offers better sparing of organs at risk while not compromising dose to target. Parotid sparing is best possible with IMRT, and hence the consequent xerostomia is lesser with this.

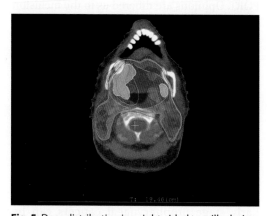

Fig. 5: Dose distribution in a right-sided tonsillar lesion.

● ALTERED FRACTIONATION SCHEDULES

The common fractionation schedules tried in head and neck malignancies are:

- *Conventional fractionation:* 2 Gy daily fractions, 5 days a week to 70 Gy in 7 weeks.
- *Split course accelerated fractionation:* Dose of 1.6 Gy BID, to a total dose of 67.2 Gy in 6 weeks, with an intentional 2-week break after 38.4 Gy, and an interfraction interval of 6 hours.
- *Delayed concomitant boost:* Daily morning treatments of 1.8 Gy, and a 1.5 Gy afternoon

concomitant boost during the last 12 days of treatment with an interfraction interval of 6 hours, and a total dose of 72 Gy in 6 weeks.

- *Pure hyperfractionation:* 1.2 Gy twice daily fractions with an interfraction interval of 6 hours to a total dose of 81.6 Gy over 7 weeks.

Hyperfractionated Radiotherapy

Oropharyngeal cancers show definite advantage with hyperfractionated radiotherapy, as was proven by the EORTC 22791 trial. A dose of 1.5 Gy twice daily, to a total dose of 80.5 Gy has been used. Significant improved locoregional control rates have been observed with this. Improved overall survival was also observed especially in advanced stages.

Accelerated Radiotherapy

Accelerated radiotherapy is another altered fractionation schedule which has shown a benefit in oropharyngeal cancers. Instead of 5 days in the conventional fractionation, 6 days treatments are delivered in this. Total dose of

66–70 Gy has shown a trend towards improved overall survival and a significant locoregional control also. More intense accelerated regimens of twice a day fractions of 1.8 Gy each, to a total dose of 59.4 Gy in stage III and IV oropharyngeal cancers have failed to show an added advantage.

Simultaneous Integrated Boost Radiotherapy

Intensity modulated radiotherapy has shown advantages in the treatment of head and neck tumors. With the use of IMRT techniques, it has become possible to treat different volumes with differential doses, thereby achieving higher tumoricidal doses to the targets at the same time lower doses to the microscopic diseases **(Flowcharts 1 and 2)**.

Doses of 2.2 Gy to the gross tumor, 2.0 Gy to the intermediate risk areas, and 1.8 Gy to the low risk planning target volumes have been studied in T1–T2, N0–N2 tumors by the RTOG 00–22 trial. Two-year overall survival rates of 95% and disease-free survival rates of 82% have

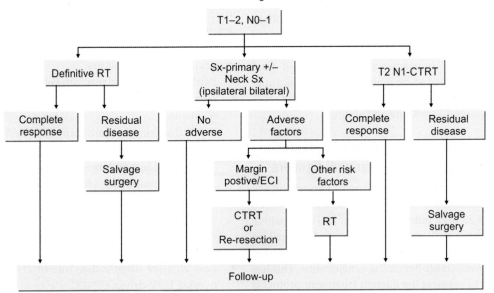

Flowchart 1: Treatment algorithm T1–2, N0–1.

Flowchart 2: Treatment algorithm T3,4 N0,1.

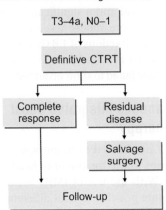

Flowchart 3: Treatment algorithm any T, N2–3.

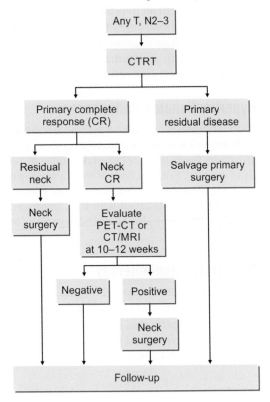

been reported. Simultaneous integrated boost is now the preferred treatment option in most of the IMRT plans in oropharyngeal tumors **(Flowchart 3)**.

● TREATMENT SEQUELAE

Complications of radiotherapy can be classified as acute and late. These depend on the dose per fraction, fractionation schedules, total volume irradiated, total dose delivered, previous surgery or concurrent or adjuvant chemotherapy. Acute toxicities observed while patient is on treatment are mucositis, skin changes, sore throat, loss of taste, and xerostomia. Infections of the mucosa with *Candida* species are also observed. Oral hygiene need to be maintained for continuing treatment without interruptions and this requires diligent care and support.

Treatment De-escalation Strategies in HPV-related Oropharyngeal Cancers

HPV-driven oropharyngeal cancers have significantly better survival rates than tobacco and alcohol induced cancers. As HPV-positive patients are younger, healthier, and more likely to survive their disease, long-term treatment side effects are becoming a major issue. This has led to reassess the current treatment protocols

in order to develop less toxic strategies while maintaining good oncological outcomes.

Various strategies that are currently undergoing clinical trials are:

- Replacement of cisplatin with cetuximab
- *Less "aggressive" radiation/chemoradiation regimens:*
  - Induction chemotherapy followed by decreased radiation doses or volumes in good responders
  - Chemoradiation with decreased dose of radiation and chemotherapy
  - Removal of chemotherapy
  - Alternative to the "conventional" photon beam therapy
- *Less invasive surgery:* The role of TORS in treating HPV-driven OPSCC.

CHAPTER 28

Principles of Surgery in Oral Cavity Cancers

Sivakumar Vidhyadharan, Subramania Iyer, Krishnakumar Thankappan

● SURGICAL ANATOMY

The oral cavity extends from the muco-cutaneous junction of the vermillion border of the lips to the oropharyngeal inlet posteriorly. The junction between the oral cavity and oropharynx is bounded, superiorly by the demarcation between hard and soft palate, laterally by the anterior pillar of tonsil on either side, and inferiorly by the circumvallate papillae of tongue. The oral cavity is lined by nonkeratinized stratified squamous epithelial mucous membrane. The submucosa is rich with minor salivary glands, concentrated more within the hard and soft palates.

The oral cavity is divided into numerous anatomical subsites **(Fig. 1)**.

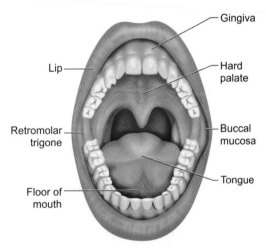

Fig. 1: Subsites of oral cavity.

Buccal Mucosa

The site includes all the surface epithelium of the inner surface of the cheeks and lips, extending from the oral commissure anteriorly to the retromolar gingiva posteriorly. Both superiorly and inferiorly, the mucosa terminates at the gingiva-buccal sulcus of both the maxillary and mandibular gingiva. The papule of Stenson's duct is situated opposite to the second maxillary molar. The buccinator muscle lies just deep to the thin mucosa with the buccal fat pad just beyond.

The buccal mucosa gets its blood supply from branches of the transverse facial artery that runs along the parotid duct from its origin from the superficial temporal branch of the external carotid artery. The buccal branch of the mandibular nerve (branch of the trigeminal nerve) supplies most of the buccal mucosa. Lymph drains into the parotid, submental, and submandibular lymph nodes, and ultimately into the upper deep cervical nodes or to the facial node on the margin of the mandible and then to the submandibular lymph nodes.

Floor of Mouth

The floor of the mouth (FOM) is a horseshoe-shaped space above the mylohyoid and hyoglossus muscles, extending from the inner surface of the lower alveolar ridge to the ventral surface of the tongue. The posterior boundary is the base of the anterior pillar of the tonsil, and is divided into right and left sides by the frenulum of the tongue. A muscular sling composed of the mylohyoid, the geniohyoid, and the genioglossus muscles supports the FOM. The sling also supports the submucosal sublingual glands, the Wharton's ducts, and the minor salivary glands. Surgery or radiotherapy to the anterior FOM may interfere with free salivary flow and can result in salivary gland obstruction. Lymphatic channels from the FOM drain to the submental and submandibular lymph nodes.

Anterior (Oral) Tongue

The mobile part of the tongue extends anteriorly from the line of the circumvallate papillae to the undersurface of the tongue at the junction of the FOM. It is composed of four regions: the tip, lateral borders, dorsum, and the ventral surface. The surface epithelium is interspersed with fungiform, filiform, and circumvallate papillae. The dorsum of the tongue bears no mucus or serous glands.

The intrinsic muscles of the tongue (superior and inferior longitudinal, transverse, and vertical) are not attached to bone and are responsible for agility of the tongue, important in fine motions of articulation and bolus preparation. The extrinsic muscles are attached to bone—genioglossus (mandible and hyoid), hyoglossus (hyoid), styloglossus (styloid process), and palatoglossus (hard palate). The genioglossus is the largest and makes up the bulk of the tongue. The extrinsic muscles elevate, depress, protrude, and retract the tongue.

The lingual artery supplies the tongue, coursing deep in the extrinsic musculature below the digastric tendon and the posterior border of the hyoglossus muscle. The midline of the tongue is an avascular plane due to the tough fibrous septum that prevents anastomosis of blood vessels of the two muscular halves.

The lingual vein accompanies the lingual artery and usually joins the internal jugular vein near the greater cornu of the hyoid. The tip of the tongue is drained by the deep lingual vein seen on ventral tongue on either side of the midline. It traverses posteriorly and superficially on the hyoglossus and is united at its anterior limit by the sublingual vein to form the vena comitans of the hypoglossal nerve, draining eventually into the internal jugular vein.

The hypoglossal nerve supplies all the muscles of the tongue except the palatoglossus, which is supplied by the pharyngeal plexus. The lingual nerve (V3) supplies the sensory distribution to the anterior two-thirds of the tongue and adjacent FOM. Taste fibers course with the lingual nerve after originating in the geniculate ganglion and traversing in the chorda tympani, then joining the lingual nerve.

With regard to the lymphatic drainage of the tongue, the tip drains to the submental nodes while the rest of the anterior tongue drains to the submandibular nodes. A distinctive feature of these lymphatics is that lymph from one side may reach nodes of both sides of the neck, particularly when ipsilateral lymphatic channels are obstructed. Therefore, patients may require bilateral neck management to optimize loco-regional control. In some instances, lymphatics from the tip of the tongue as from the anterior FOM may go directly from the submental nodes to the jugulo-omohyoid node at the junction of levels III and IV, thus missing out the submandibular and upper cervical nodes, thereby leading to skip metastasis.

Hard Palate

The hard palate is a semilunar area bounded by the inner surface of superior alveolar ridge anteriorly and laterally and the soft palate junction posteriorly. The submucosa here is tough and thick; it is strongly united with the underlying periosteum, which in turn is secured to the bone by Sharpey's fibers. The mucosa also contains numerous minor salivary glands from which minor salivary gland tumors may arise.

The hard palate is supplied by branches of the greater palatine artery, which emerges from the greater palatine foramen of the palatine bone near the second molar tooth and passes laterally around the palate to enter the nose through the incisive foramen. The maxillary nerve (V2) innervates the larger part of the palate up to the incisive foramen by its greater palatine branch via the pterygopalatine ganglion. The premaxillary region between the incisor teeth and incisive foramen is supplied by nasopalatine nerve. Lymphatic channels drain first to the retropharyngeal and then to the deep cervical nodes.

Alveolar Ridges

The alveolar ridges include only the alveolar processes of the mandible and the maxilla, and their covering mucosa. These are bony structures supporting the teeth and periodontal tissues arise from the FOM and descend from the hard palate. As the mucosa is thin and tightly adherent to the periosteum, tumors of both alveolar ridges may invade the alveolar bone of the jaws quite early in their natural history.

The lower alveolus receives its sensory innervation from the branches of the mandibular nerve (inferior alveolar, buccal, and lingual nerves); whereas the upper alveolus is innervated by branches of the maxillary nerve (superior alveolar, greater palatine, and nasopalatine nerves). The primary echelons of lymphatic drainage are the nodes in the submental and submandibular triangle. Tumors of the mandible are more likely to metastasize to the neck than those of the maxilla.

● RETROMOLAR TRIGONE

The retromolar trigone (RMT) area is bounded posteromedially by the anterior tonsillar pillar, laterally by the buccal mucosa, and superiorly by the maxillary tubercle. Submucosa here is very thin with bone near the surface, since the retromolar mucosa is not exposed to masticatory loads. Sensory innervation to the area is by the buccal branch of the mandibular division of the trigeminal nerve. Lymphatic drainage is to the ipsilateral submandibular and deep cervical nodes.

● SURGICAL MANAGEMENT AND TECHNIQUES

The location and behavior of oral cavity cancers make surgery the treatment of choice in the majority of cases. Oral squamous cell carcinoma, minor salivary gland tumors, and sarcomas are associated with a more limited response to nonsurgical treatment. Treatment goals for carcinoma of the oral cavity are as follows:

- Achieving cure of the cancer
- Preserving or restoring physical form and function
- Minimizing consequences of treatment
- Preventing second primary cancers.

Surgical Access to Tumors within Oral Cavity

Surgical approach depends on the size, site, and location of the tumor; proximity of the tumor to the mandible or maxilla and the necessity for either neck dissection, reconstruction or both. The different approaches are described below:

- Transoral/peroral approach
- combined transoral/transcervical approaches to the oral cavity
- Lingual release
  - Visor flap for mandibulectomy
  - Cheek flap
  - Mandibular swing approach.

Marginal mandibulectomy and mandibulotomy are types of mandible sparing approaches.

Transoral/Peroral Approach

Most early (T1 or T2) tumors are easily excised via a transoral approach, without external incisions, or extensive dissection to achieve adequate exposure. Transoral exposure may be augmented by use of circumferential cheek retractors, dental bite blocks, self-retaining mouth gags, or handheld retractors for the tongue and the buccal mucosa.

When limited transoral resection is combined with surgical management of the neck, care should be taken to avoid communication of the oral and the neck wounds when possible to minimize the risk of fistula formation. However, such concerns must always be secondary to oncologic considerations and achieving the exposure necessary for appropriate tumor extirpation.

When oral cavity tumors extend into the oropharynx, assisted technology can afford improved visualization with transoral robotic surgery using three-dimensional visualization and robotic instruments. Transoral laser surgery has also been suggested for tumors of the oral cavity and the oropharynx. When the transoral approach is employed, a separate neck incision and neck dissection is performed, avoiding entry into the oral cavity when possible.

Combined Transoral/Transcervical Approaches to the Oral Cavity

For large (T3 or T4) or large invasive tumors of the oral cavity, attaining adequate exposure may not be possible via a transoral approach. In combination with surgical management of the neck, variations of either the mandibular lingual release or the visor approach allow excellent access to the oral cavity through exposure via the neck. A level I neck dissection is performed prior to the combined approach to allow exposure of the external carotid branches, the lingual and the hypoglossal nerves, and the suprahyoid muscles.

A long horizontal incision in a cervical skin crease is primarily done. A subplatysmal flap elevated up to the inferior border of the mandible can be utilized in a unilateral fashion for the mandible or tongue with anterior FOM lesions or bilaterally when large defects and bilateral tumors are treated. Unilateral approach is usually intended for lateral mandibular body, RMT, lateral FOM, or lateral tongue defects.

Lingual release: Lingual release refers to the separation of the lingual aspect of the mucosal surfaces from the inner aspect of the mandible 270° from the glossotonsillar sulcus on one side, anteriorly around the mandible to the contralateral glossotonsillar sulcus.

Indications:
- Large anterior, lateral, or posterior tumors of the oral cavity
- Tumors of the oral cavity extending to the lateral or posterior oropharynx
- Tumors of the anterior tongue extending to the base of tongue
- Alternative to lip-split approach providing esthetic benefit, also prevents interruption of the buccal or labial periosteum and the inferior alveolar vessels of the mandible, thereby preserving the blood supply to the lower jaw especially in patients needing adjuvant radiation.

Contraindications:
- Tumor extending and involving the skin of chin
- Patient has already undergone a lip-split procedure
- If an osteocutaneous flap reconstruction has been planned, difficulties during insetting of the flap will be encountered.

The steps of lingual release are as follows:
1. Horizontal neck crease incision is made from a point below the ipsilateral mastoid tip and across neck at hyoid level going across midline and extending to an equivalent

point on the contralateral side for more posterior lesion.

2. A level I neck dissection is performed prior to allow exposure of the external carotid branches, the lingual and the hypoglossal nerves, and the suprahyoid muscles. Marginal mandibular branch is preserved.

3. Mandibular periosteum is incised along inferior border of mandible. If a segmental mandibulectomy has been planned, the periosteum is not elevated in the area of involved mandible and parts bone cuts are planned. The part of mandible to be resected has to remain attached to the FOM and be released with the tongue and FOM for en bloc resection of the tumor.

4. The digastric, genioglossus, and hyoglossus muscle attachments to mandible are released.

5. Periosteum of inner cortex of mandible from below up to FOM is elevated.

6. After freeing the soft tissue and muscular attachments to the mandible, intraoral releasing incision is made and extended from ipsilateral RMT to contralateral RMT.

7. For edentulous patients, intraoral incision is placed on superior gingival crest, thereby dividing the keratinaceous tissue along the alveolar crest. In a dentate patient, incision is made along the gingival margin of dentomucosal interface, thereby preserving interdental papillae needed during closure.

8. The posterior releasing incision on the contralateral side may be "back cut" along the lateral FOM to prevent tearing and increase exposure. This back cut should be through mucosa only to avoid injury to the contralateral lingual nerve.

9. If mandibulectomy is planned, the releasing incision should join the mucosal incisions over bone cuts. Remaining periosteum from the inner cortex is released.

10. The entire tongue and the FOM is "released", brought down into the neck and dissected via the neck incision.

11. If mandibular resection is not planned, mandibular lingual release may be performed without dissection of the soft-tissue envelope overlying the mandible. The anterior attachments of the digastric, the mylohyoid, the geniohyoid and the genioglossus muscles are released and subperiosteal dissection is performed along the inner cortex of the mandible. The intraoral mucosa is released at the dental mucosal junction. Following mucosal release, the tongue and the FOM are delivered into the neck.

12. During closure, the interdental papillae have to be replaced back to their normal anatomic position. Adequate restoration of the oral diaphragm is important. The suprahyoid muscles must be reattached to the anterior mandibular arch using vicryl sutures through drill holes in the mandible.

Visor flap for mandibulectomy: Visor flap is a bilateral neck and cheek flap elevated cephalad beyond the mandible to expose the body of the mandible bilaterally **(Fig. 2)**. In most cases, a level I dissection is performed prior to the combined approach to allow exposure of the

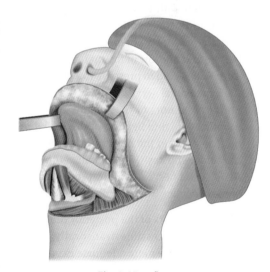

Fig. 2: Visor flap.

external carotid branches, the lingual and the hypoglossal nerves, and the suprahyoid muscles. The steps of a visor flap are as follows:

- For mandibular resection, a visor flap is made by subplatysmal dissection stretched superiorly over the lateral surface of the mandible necessitating division of mental nerves on either side. Patients must be counseled preoperatively regarding the resulting sensory deficit.
- If the mandible does not require resection on one side, the mental nerve can be preserved.
- The mandibular release requires a releasing incision along the gingivolabial and gingivobuccal sulcus.
- Preplating with the transosseous plate prior to osteotomy is performed. This may preserve occlusion and cosmesis of the mandibular contour and height. Otherwise, intermaxillary fixation (IMF) may be necessary to maintain mandibular position for reconstruction.
- Once appropriate releasing incisions are completed, the mandible, the tongue, and the FOM are delivered into the neck. Tumor is resected with osteotomies on the bone where indicated, and margins are taken peripherally, deep, and in the neurovascular bundle and marrow of the mandible.
- Attention is paid to preserve the lingual and the hypoglossal nerves.
- For large tumors of the tongue, exposure, mobilization, and ligation of the ipsilateral lingual artery in the neck prior to resection may aid hemostasis, and mobilization of the hypoglossal nerve can allow preservation of some branches when oncologically safe.

Cheek flaps: Tumors of the posterior oral cavity are not easily accessible transorally, and a cheek flap may give more adequate exposure in appropriate cases.

The steps are as follows:

- An upper cheek flap **(Fig. 3)** is raised using a median upper lip-split and incision is extended around the nose with the corresponding mucosal incision in the upper gingivobuccal sulcus.
- The lower cheek flap **(Fig. 4)** uses a midline lip-split that continues down to the neck. The flap is raised subplatysmally, but care should be taken not to strip the periosteum off the mandible. Cervical incision along the papillae of teeth is most suited.
- A midfacial degloving flap through bilateral gingivobuccal incisions is preferable in appropriate cases as this avoids midfacial scars.

Mandibular swing (Lip-split + mandibulotomy): The mandibular swing approach signifies a parasymphyseal or midline osteotomy with a lip-split, allowing the mandible and lip/cheek complex to "swing" laterally, leaving a wide open access to the oral cavity, the RMT, the deep tongue, the oropharynx, and the parapharyngeal space without limitation by position of the lips and the cheek **(Fig. 5)**. A variety of incisions dividing the lower lip and the chin have been described, including straight line, zigzag, and chin button among others. A visible facial scar is unavoidable; hence patient has to be appropriately counseled. Paramedian mandibulotomy is most commonly performed due to its advantages of giving wide exposure, preserving the hyomandibular complex, avoids denervation and devascularization of skin, easy fixation with plates, and away from the radiation field.

Indications:

- The approach may also provide access to the upper oropharynx for oral tumors extending into the soft palate, the tonsillar fossa, the glossopharyngeal sulcus, or the base of tongue or the mandible.
- With a neck extension, this approach may also be used to gain access to the

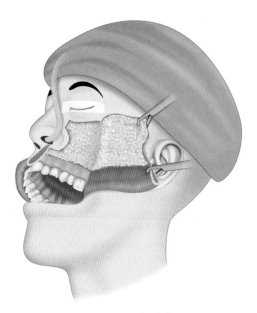

Fig. 3: Upper cheek flap.

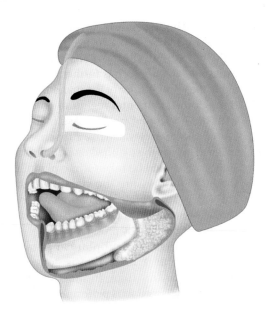

Fig. 4: Lower cheek flap.

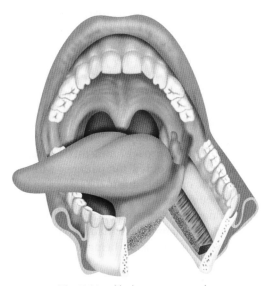

Fig. 5: Mandibulotomy approach.

parapharyngeal space for excision of tumors in this area.

- Access to the cervical spine can be obtained by a midline mandibulotomy and median glossotomy.

Contraindications:

- Due to esthetic reasons, patients who are not keen for a lip-split incision should be considered for a lingual releasing approach.
- Relative contraindications to this technique are patients with small atrophic mandible. Better tissue healing can be obtained with a lingual release.
- In cases where questionable presence of tumor invasion of the more distal part of mandible, extent of mandibular resection required for tumor excision is to be determined prior to a midline mandibulotomy.

The steps are as follows:

- Planned dental extractions should be performed prior to mandibulotomy or mandibulectomy.
- The lip-split incision is made utilizing modified zigzag stepped technique. In other words, a midline-Z incorporating the mental crease is used. The skin incision over the lip is deepened towards the mucosal surface, cutting the orbicularis muscle sharply along

the way. The incision is deepened down to the muscular fascia in a longitudinal direction cutting the mentalis muscle to expose the mandible. It is further extended along the lower border of the mandible and through the submental region to connect with the horizontal neck crease incision. The cheek flap is elevated in a subperiosteal plane to expose the planned mandibultomy side. Care should be taken while planning the incision to assure the viability of the cheek flap. The marginal mandibular nerve should be identified and elevated along with the cheek flap, thereby preserving it.

- After raising the subplatysmal and cheek flaps, neck dissection is generally performed at this time. In most cases, a level I neck dissection is performed prior to the combined approach to allow exposure of the external carotid branches, the lingual and the hypoglossal nerves, and the suprahyoid muscles.

- Subperiosteal dissection is performed around both the inner and outer cortices at the planned mandibulotomy site and along the inferior and anterior surfaces to fix 2.5 mm miniplates (preplating). In the dentate patient, preplating prior to mandibulotomy is done to optimize dental occlusion. No such preparation is required in the edentulous patient.

- The mental nerve should be identified and preserved. Dissection along the inner surface of the symphysis should be avoided when possible in order to minimize disruption of dense muscular attachments at the genial tubercle. Due to the preservation of the muscular floor comprising the oral diaphragm, this approach may offer better speech and swallowing outcomes than lingual release techniques.

- The site for mandibulotomy is marked on the mandible. The vertical mandibulotomy is usually performed between the lateral incisors and canine roots. Multiple anterior mandibulotomy techniques have been described, including straight-line symphyseal or parasymphyseal cuts and angled cuts. If only wire fixation is planned, incorporation of a step-off or angle into the mandibulotomy may improve precise reapproximation of bone. With the use of miniplates presently, vertical mandibultomy is routinely performed.

- A more commonly performed technique is a straight vertical cut in the parasymphyseal region, which is later fixed with titanium plates. This minimizes disruption of ipsilateral genioglossus and the geniohyoid muscles from the genial tubercle, thereby preventing disruption of the oral diaphragm. A powered sagittal, or reciprocating saw may be helpful.

- Following mandibulotomy, the FOM mucosa is released at the dental mucosal junction, and the mandible is laterally retracted. A mucosal incision is extended from the alveolus to the margin of planned tumor resection, and the resection is performed. If the lingual and hypoglossal nerves have been exposed in the neck, they may be further dissected into the FOM and free of the tumor, if possible.

- The risk of postoperative fistula and oral incompetence may be higher with a mandibulotomy approach compared with a delivery approach, and this approach should be avoided for patients with an atrophic mandible due to the increased risk of nonunion or fracture.

- During closure, osteotomies must be draped with gingival mucosa or flap reconstruction to avoid the suture line being directly in line with the osteotomy.

● MANAGEMENT OF THE MANDIBLE

Mechanism of Invasion of the Mandible

Tumors of the FOM, the ventral tongue, and the gingivobuccal sulcus may extend along the mucosa to the adjacent gingiva. The periosteum plays the role of a barrier to mandibular invasion. Involvement of the mandible increases the tumor staging, risk of inferior alveolar nerve invasion within the mandibular canal leading to perineural spread of the tumor toward the skull base.

In the dentate mandible **(Fig. 6)** tumor spreads up from the gingiva, through the dental socket into the cancellous bone. On the contrary, the resistance offered by an edentulous mandible **(Fig. 7)** is much less and tumor invasion of cancellous bone occurs through the dental pores of the alveolar process. Invasive cancer enters into the marrow space and mental nerve canal when there is a lack of cortex in an empty tooth socket. The tumor may then spread laterally and medially to the extent of the marrow space in the absence of obvious external signs.

Recent studies report that tumor enters at the point of abutment; most often at the junction of attached and free mucosa in both dentulous and edentulous mandible in the nonirradiated mandible spread along the medullary cavity is associated with fibrosis in the place of hemopoetic tissue. The presence of hemopoetic marrow at the lateral most resection margin

indicates that margins have adequate clearance. Tumor extension in the marrow cavity beyond the superficial mucosal and soft-tissue extent of the disease is insignificant.

● ASSESSMENT OF BONY INVASION

Early cortical invasion of the mandible is extremely difficult to image radiographically even with modern technology. A number of imaging investigations are available: plain radiography, cephalometric orthognathic films, orthopantomogram (OPG), dental occlusal films, radionuclide bone scans, CT scans, MRI, and positron emission tomography (PET) scans. The accuracy of conventional radiography in detecting early invasion is limited by the fact that 30–50% mineral loss must occur before the changes are radiologically apparent.

The OPG is a first-line investigation, but early invasion of the lingual cortex, especially in the region of the mental symphysis, may not be evident **(Fig. 8)**. The OPG evaluation is similar to X-rays except it reduces overlap of bone images in the ramus and the body. Since OPG can detect bony erosion only after 30% mineral loss, high false-negative results are obtained.

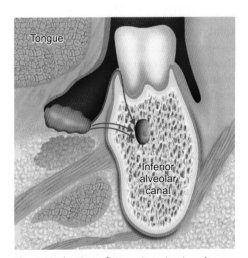

Fig. 6: Mechanism of tumor invasion in a dentate mandible.

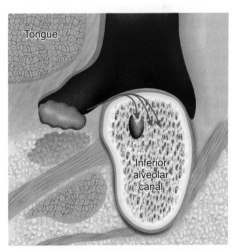

Fig. 7: Mechanism of tumor invasion in an edentulous mandible.

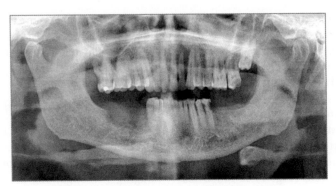

Fig. 8: Orthopantomogram showing tumor invasion.

The symphysis is sometimes difficult to image accurately due to overlap of the spine.

It has been reported that computed tomography (CT) scans are accurate in demonstrating bone invasion in edentulous patients. The accuracy of a CT scan during evaluation of bone invasion is limited by artifact produced by an irregular dental socket and by patient motion. CT scan is a standard imaging technique for the mandible.

Computerized tomography multiplanar reformation (CT/MPR or Dentascan) is a computer software technique that uses information from CT scan slices to generate true cross-sectional images and panoramic views of the mandible and maxilla. The oblique sagittal view on Dentascan reportedly allows accurate evaluation of buccal and lingual cortical bone margins as well as clear visualization of the incisive and inferior alveolar canals. As a formatted high-resolution tool of the mandible, it has sensitivity of 95% and specificity of 79%.

The MRI scan gives the additional advantage of soft-tissue imaging. According to some studies, the MRI has high sensitivity but low specificity and overestimates the tumor invasion. Some studies also claim that clinical examination and direct visualization with periosteal stripping had the greatest accuracy and should be done whenever in doubt. The role of MRI has also been investigated, and reports indicate that though a negative study virtually excludes periosteal or cortical involvement, the overall usefulness of this investigation is hampered by the high rate of false-positive results in dental infections, previously irradiated mandibles, and in osteoradionecrosis.

In summary, the most sensitive investigations for assessing mandibular invasion are the SPECT (97%) and bone scan (93%). The most specific are CT (88%) and MRI (86%) scans. When there is clinically evident bony involvement, it can be confirmed with an OPG.

● MANDIBULECTOMY

Careful preoperative clinical and radiographic assessment of the mandible is critical during evaluation of oral cavity cancer. Lesions abutting periostium of mandible or those exhibiting only superficial cortical invasion may be treated with marginal or rim mandibulectomy in select cases. Edentulous patients with significant loss of vertical mandibular height are poor candidates for marginal mandibulectomy due to the great risk for pathologic fracture, especially in the postirradiation period. Such situations warrant a segmental resection. Segmental mandibulectomy is indicated when there is widespread cortical or cancellous invasion, primary or metastatic bone tumor, or invasion of the marrow, inferior alveolar nerve or canal.

Adequate exposure is most important, regardless of whether a marginal or segmental resection is planned, an exclusively transoral approach with marginal mandibulectomy may be successful for the occasional early-stage lesion, which abuts the periosteum, but does not grossly invade the cortex. In cases requiring mandibular resection, more extensive access must be achieved either via a lip-splitting incision or transcervical approach.

Segmental Mandibulectomy

A very select low-grade group of lesions limited to the mandible may be amenable to resection via a relatively small transoral or cervical incision. Segmental resection via a small cervical incision may be also permissible for larger lesions limited to the mandible. However, the degree and duration of superior retraction of the soft-tissue envelope required by a small incision puts the marginal mandibular nerve at risk of traction injury, hence must be performed with caution. A lip-split or visor flap minimizes such risk. Once adequate exposure is achieved, proximal, and distal mandibulectomy sites are marked and any necessary dental extractions are performed.

In the dentate patient, precontouring and preplating with an appropriate reconstruction plate for planned defect is performed, with at least three holes predrilled on each side of the defect. For situations where tumor significantly deforms the outer contour of the mandible and prevents accurate molding of hardware, there are commercially available three-dimensional models based upon preoperative imaging, which may be customized and altered to assist with reconstruction planning.

Indications for Segmental Mandibulectomy

- Invasion of the mandibular canal and inferior alveolar nerve
- Gross invasion of the mandible

- Significant paramandibular tumor involvement
- Primary mandibular osseous tumor
- Metastatic carcinoma.

For lesions posterior to the mental foramen, requiring resection of the posterior mandibular body or RMT, it may be necessary to extend a vertical cut from the mandibular angle to the sigmoid notch. This allows removal of the anterior ramus and coronoid process, while preserving the condyle and a length of posterior ramus sufficient to fix reconstruction plates **(Fig. 9)**.

Although it is useful to delineate the intraoral mucosal margins, performing bone cuts for segmental mandibulectomy early in the resection will greatly improve exposure and facilitate the remainder of the soft-tissue dissection. For lesions that are limited to the medial or superior aspect of the bone, dissection in a subperiosteal plane over the lateral surface of the mandible is usually sufficient. However, if tumor extends onto the buccal surface of the mandible or into the gingivobuccal surface, the margin of resection must include a cuff of overlying normal appearing soft tissue.

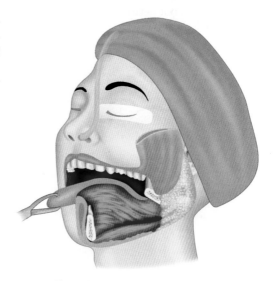

Fig. 9: Segmental mandibulectomy.

Marginal/Rim Resection of the Mandible

The cortical part of the bone containing the mandibular canal lies inferior to the dental roots, remains relatively uninvolved in early-stage disease, and can be safely spared during marginal resection of bone. There are three types of marginal mandibulectomy—vertical, horizontal and oblique **(Fig. 10)**.

Indications for Marginal Mandibulectomy

- Primary tumor abutting against the mandible
- Minimal involvement of the alveolar process
- Minimal cortical erosion.

Contraindication for Marginal Mandibulectomy

- Gross bony involvement
- Deep soft-tissue involvement (significant paramandibular involvement); resect mandible for third dimension clearance
- Post-radiotherapy
- Edentulous mandibles where the overall height does not permit a residual segment of 1 cm.

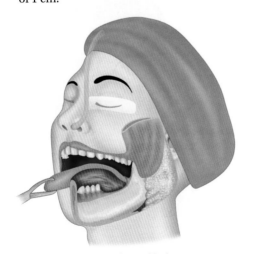

Fig. 10: Marginal mandibulectomy.

The practical feasibility to perform a marginal mandibulectomy depends upon the vertical height of the body of the mandible. In elderly patients, resorption of the mandible with age results in recession of the alveolar process, and the mandibular canal with the inferior alveolar nerve is at increased risk of involvement. In edentulous patients, marginal resection is unsafe, as the residual bone is very liable to iatrogenic or spontaneous fracture. The risk of mandibular fracture after a marginal mandibulectomy can be minimized with smooth, rounded bone cuts; since sharp angles tend to concentrate the forces of stress, thereby increase the chances of fracture. Acceptable tumor clearance in edentulous patients may necessitate a segmental mandibulectomy.

Marginal mandibular resection is also best avoided in previously irradiated patients because of the more variable routes of tumor entry and multiple foci of tumor invasion coupled with the high risk of osteoradionecrosis. Resection of the normal uninvolved mandible to accomplish an en bloc resection can no longer be justified in view of the realization that there are no lymphatic channels passing through the mandible.

● FURTHER READING

1. Brown JS, Lowe D, Kalavrezos N, et al. Patterns of invasion and routes of tumor entry into the mandible by oral squamous cell carcinoma. Head Neck. 2002;24(4):370-83.
2. Christopoulos E, Carrau R, Segas J, et al. Transmandibular approaches to the oral cavity and oropharynx. A functional assessment. Arch Otolaryngol Head Neck Surg. 1992;118(11):1164-7.
3. Dubner S, Spiro RH. Median mandibulotomy: A critical assessment. Head Neck. 1991;13(5):389-93.
4. Genden EM, Rinaldo A, Jacobson A, et al. Management of mandibular invasion: When is a marginal mandibulectomy appropriate? Oral Oncol. 2005;41(8):776-82.
5. Marchetta FC, Sako K, Murphy JB. The periosteum of the mandible and intraoral carcinoma. Am J Surg. 1971;122(6):711-3.
6. McGregor AD, MacDonald DG. Routes of entry of squamous cell carcinoma to the mandible. Head Neck Surg. 1988;10(5):294-301.

7. Spiro RH, Gerold FP, Strong EW. Mandibular "swing" approach for oral and oropharyngeal tumors. Head Neck Surg. 1981;3(5):371-8.

8. Stanley RB. Mandibular lingual releasing approach to oral and oropharyngeal carcinomas. Laryngoscope. 1984;94(5 Pt 1):596-600.

9. Stringer SP, Jordan JR, Mendenhall WM, et al. Mandibular lingual releasing approach. Otolaryngol Head Neck Surg. 1992;107(3):395-8.

10. van der Brekel MW, Runne RW, Smeele LE, et al. Assessment of tumor invasion into mandible: The value of different imaging techniques. Eur Radiol. 1998;8(9):1552-7.

11. Wolff D, Hassfeld S, Hofele C. Influence of marginal and segmental mandibular resection on the survival rate in patients with squamous cell carcinoma of the inferior parts of the oral cavity. J Craniomaxillofac Surg. 2004;32(5):318-23.

Section 6

Larynx, Hypopharynx and Nasopharynx

Chapters

CHAPTER 29

Imaging in Laryngeal and Hypopharyngeal Tumors

Sandya CJ, Akshay Kudpaje

● INTRODUCTION

Although laryngoscopy is crucial in the evaluation and diagnosis, cross-sectional imaging helps to further study the tumor extent, extralaryngeal spread, nodal status, and metastasis. Laryngeal and hypopharyngeal tumors harbor a high-risk of developing synchronous malignancies in the lung and upper esophagus and have to be further evaluated by imaging studies.

● ANATOMY OF LARYNX

Larynx is anatomically divided into three sites—supraglottis, glottis, and subglottis (**Figs. 1A to C**).

Supraglottis extends from epiglottis to laryngeal ventricle and includes epiglottis, aryepiglottic folds, arytenoids, ventricles, and false cords. The supraglottis is further divided into infra- and suprahyoid region by the hyoepiglottic ligament. The supraglottis and glottis is divided by an imaginary line passing through the ventricle. The glottis lies at the level of vocal cord and comprises of the true vocal cord, anterior, and posterior commissure. Subglottis starts 5 mm below the free edge of the vocal cord to inferior border of cricoid cartilage.

Laryngeal framework consists of the hyoid bone, thyroid cartilage, and cricoid cartilage externally. The interior includes the epiglottis, arytenoids, corniculate, and cuneiform cartilages. Cricoid cartilage is the only complete ring in the aerodigestive tract, shaped like a signet ring with wider end facing posteriorly. On the upper surface of cricoid lies the arytenoid which is about 5–8 mm lateral to the midline. Corniculate and cuneiform cartilages are superior to arytenoids, almost buried in aryepiglottic fold.

Epiglottis is an elastic fibrocartilage which seldom calcifies and is attached inferiorly to the thyroid cartilage by thyroepiglottic ligament just above the anterior commissure. The tip of epiglottis is free. Hyoepiglottic ligament attaches to the epiglottis of the hyoid bone. Pre-epiglottic space lies just below the hyoepiglottic ligament.

The quadrangular membrane is formed by paired membranes from the lateral edge of the epiglottis extending posteriorly to the arytenoids. The aryepiglottic folds form the free superior border. The quadrangular membrane is wider superiorly and narrows down inferiorly to form the false cords (**Fig. 2**).

Conus elasticus is a thin continuous membrane that has the vocal ligament as the superior border. This vocal ligament extends from the vocal process of the arytenoids cartilage to the angle of the thyroid cartilage, and forms the true vocal cord. Thyroarytenoid muscle forms the main mass of vocal cord which lies below the vocal ligament.

Pre-epiglottic and paraglottic spaces lie between the external framework of the thyroid

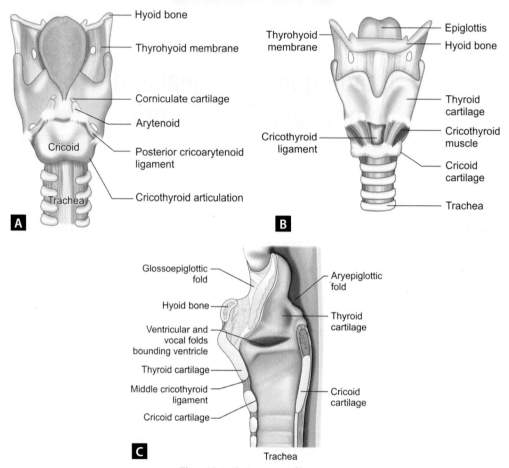

Figs. 1A to C: Anatomy of larynx.

cartilage and hyoid bone and inner framework of the epiglottis and intrinsic muscles, and ligaments. These spaces contain fat, blood vessels, and lymphatics.

● IMAGING TECHNIQUES

CT Scan

Contrast-enhanced multidetector computed tomography (MDCT) scan provides excellent images of neck where scanning starts from base of skull to the level of aortic arch. Patient lies in supine position and breathes quietly and should refrain from swallowing, and coughing when volume acquisition of the area is done. Multiplanar reconstruction can be performed in coronal and sagittal planes with the thin slices obtained. All the images should be reviewed, both in bone and soft tissue windows.

The appearance of vocal cords differs with the phase of respiration. While quiet respiration, the vocal cords are slightly abducted. But when the breath is forcefully held, the cords adduct and clear visualization of paraglottic fat can be achieved. Anterior commissure normally should exhibit air closely lining the cartilage.

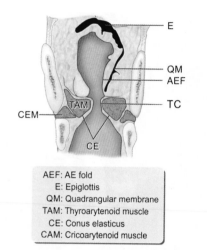

AEF: AE fold
E: Epiglottis
QM: Quadrangular membrane
TAM: Thyroarytenoid muscle
CE: Conus elasticus
CAM: Cricoarytenoid muscle

Fig. 2: Anatomy of larynx showing conus elasticus and quadrangular membrane.

If this appearance is seen, one can be certain that no lesion is present. At subglottic level, the configuration changes to an oval form.

Dual Energy CT

It is difficult to differentiate materials of different chemical composition such as iodine, bone, and cartilage by conventional CT scanner as they have the same CT density. Dual energy CT, in which two different X-ray tubes working at different tube voltages, i.e. 100 and 140 KV, helps to differentiate among these materials. Dual energy CT has exact potential to define the distribution of iodine in the tissue and the area can be color coded. The areas of tumor extension into the cartilage can be better revealed with this modality.

MRI Imaging

A 1.5 tesla MRI scanner with dedicated neck coil is employed. Neck is placed in a relaxed position and patient is instructed to breathe quietly. T1 WI, T2 WI, T2 with fat sat and T1 postcontrast with fat sat is attained. Section thickness of 4 mm with a gap of 1 mm is favored. Patient

should abstain from coughing or swallowing during the procedure. Flow compensation technique is performed to avoid flow artifacts from carotids. Images are acquired in axial, sagittal, and coronal planes depending on the area of interest.

Sagittal images demonstrate the epiglottis, vallecula, and base of tongue. Pre-epiglottic fat is seen clearly in this plane. Postcricoid area is also well-visualized. Coronal imaging demonstrates the laryngeal ventricle, upper margin of cord, and paraglottic fat.

MRI is a useful tool in cases with suspicious cartilage involvement. T2 and contrast enhanced T1 signal intensity of the tumor can be compared with that of the cartilage. If the cartilage shows similar signal intensity as tumor, possibility of cartilage invasion is to be considered. However, specificity of MR for tumor invasion is only 56% since peritumoral inflammation, fibrosis, and edema can also cause abnormal signal in the cartilage.

● SUPRAGLOTTIC CANCERS

Supraglottic tumors usually present with locally advanced disease. Due to rich lymphatic drainage in this region nodal disease is a frequent finding. Supraglottic carcinoma can arise from supra- or infrahyoid compartment, line of separation is formed by hyoepiglottic ligament.

Suprahyoid—Anteromedial Compartment

Epiglottis

Tumors from epiglottis can spread to pre-epiglottic space (PES) and base of tongue through vallecula. Through PES, it can reach the glottis or subglottis via anterior commissure. Axial imaging can demonstrate the glossoepiglottic folds and vallecula. Sagittal images are better suited to evaluate epiglottis, pre-epiglottic space, and base of tongue **(Figs. 3 and 4)**.

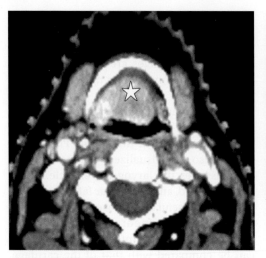

Fig. 3: Axial CT scan section showing lesion involving epiglottis and pre-epiglottic fat.

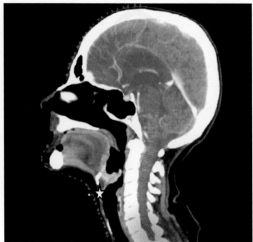

Fig. 4: Computed tomography sagittal image showing involvement of epiglottis with pre-epiglottic fat being clear.

Suprahyoid—Posterolateral Compartment

Aryepiglottic Fold and False Cord

Infrahyoid supraglottic larynx is bounded by aryepiglottic (AE) folds. Lesion on the anterior aspect of AE fold can spread through epiglottis to pre-epiglottic space. Lesion on the posterior margin can spread to pharyngeal wall. Laterally the lesion can extend into the pyriform sinus. On imaging, involvement of PES is demonstrated as replacement of fat density by soft tissue. Resection line for a supraglottic laryngectomy is through the ventricle. Coronal sections are needed to localize the ventricle and to determine the relationship of lower edge of tumor to ventricle.

Invasive supraglottic tumors can extend through the quadrangular membrane into the paraglottic space and around the lateral margin of ventricle along the mucosa to the outer border of the cord. Tumor and muscle have same density in CT and difficult to differentiate. On MRI, tumor has relatively higher signal intensity than normal muscle on T2-weighted images. Sometimes, squamous cell carcinoma can incite inflammatory response exhibiting a higher signal on T2-weighted images beyond the actual limit of the tumor. Contrast enhanced images is proved useful in such situations **(Fig. 5)**.

False Cord

These tumors have a strong preference for submucous spread to pre-epiglottic space. More extensive tumor can further destroy the thyroid cartilage and spread transglottically into glottis and subglottis. Axial and coronal images, both are helpful in such scenarios **(Fig. 6)**.

Glottis

Glottis ranges from laryngeal ventricle to a plane 1 cm below this level. It includes true cord, anterior, and posterior commissures. Due to sparse lymphatic drainage, lymph node metastases are rare **(Fig. 7)**.

Key areas in the assessment of glottic tumors are:

- Inferior extension
- Anterior commissure

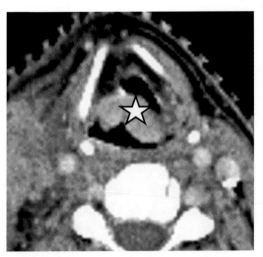

Fig. 5: Axial CT image showing mass from the right aryepiglottic fold.

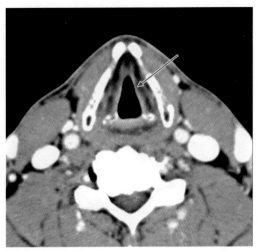

Fig. 6: Axial CT scan showing normal false cord.

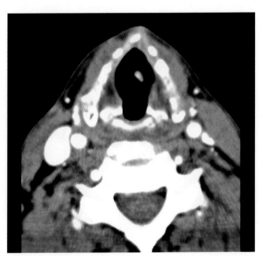

Fig. 7: Axial CT scan showing normal true cord in "EE" phonation.

- Arytenoid
- Thyroid cartilage
- Paraglottic space.

Conus elasticus play a significant role in regulating inferior growth of the glottic tumor. This membrane forms the lower border of paraglottic space and extends from vocal cord to upper border of cricoid. Tumor invading mucosa and growing caudally is separated from the deeper tissues by conus. Caudal to the conus, tumor invading the mucosa can immediately invade the cricoid cartilage. If tumor is extending deep into the true cord, conus elasticus prevents its inferior growth and directs it laterally where it may grow between the cricoid and thyroid cartilages to extralaryngeal tissues. These situations may be evident on axial or coronal scans.

Anterior commissure disease is demonstrated as a soft tissue thickness of 1–2 mm and easily involves the thyroid cartilage, opposite cord, and cricothyroid membrane **(Fig. 8)**. Posteriorly the tumor extends to posterior commissure, arytenoids, cricoarytenoid joint, and cricoid cartilage. Cartilage invasion is evident as sclerosis, erosion, lysis, and presence of extralaryngeal tumor on CT scan. MRI has a high sensitivity but lower specificity as compared to CT for detection of cartilage **(Fig. 9)**. T1WI, T2WI, and gadolinium-enhanced T1WI may be used to assess cartilage erosion and differentiation of peritumoral inflammation from tumor.

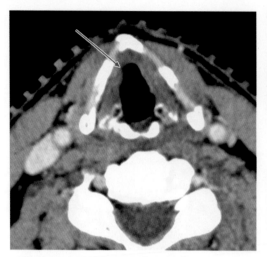

Fig. 8: Axial CT scan showing carcinoma vocal cord extending to the anterior commissure.

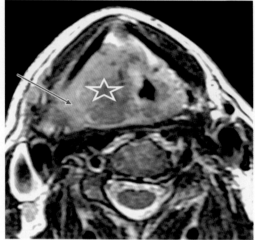

Fig. 9: Axial T2 MRI image showing mass lesion in right paraglottic fat with thyroid cartilage erosion.

Subglottis

It comprises about 5% of all laryngeal cancers. Lymph node metastasis may be seen. Imaging shows a soft tissue thickening in the cricoid **(Fig. 10)**.

Transglottis

Tumors encroaching on both glottis and supraglottis with or without subglottic component is labeled as transglottic tumors. Coronal images are useful in assessing the transglottic extension of tumor **(Fig. 11)**.

Laryngeal Ventricle

These lesions encompass the undersurface of false cord and upper surface of true cord and classified as either supraglottic or glottic **(Fig. 12)**.

● TNM STAGING

Only imaging can carefully assess the clinical and endoscopic blind spots like laryngeal submucosal spaces, spread across commissures,

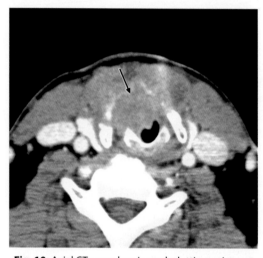

Fig. 10: Axial CT scan showing subglottic carcinoma.

cartilage invasion, transglottic, deep subglottic, and extralaryngeal extension. Diseases in the PES and paraglottic space are more likely to have nodal spread, which can be better assessed with imaging. Pretreatment tumor volume has been shown to have an impact in the prognosis and response to treatment.

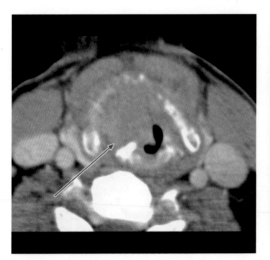

Fig. 11: Axial CT scan showing transglottic carcinoma eroding the thyroid cartilage.

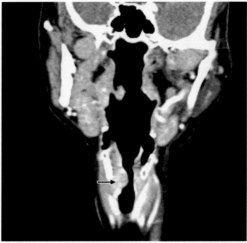

Fig. 12: Coronal CT scan image of larynx showing mass involving right true and false cord.

Nodes

Nodal involvement increases the risk of recurrence and affects long-term survival. Short axis diameter of more than 10 mm, necrotic nodes, and nodes with indistinct margins are the established criteria to diagnose malignant nodes at CT or MRI. Ultrasound-guided fine needle aspiration cytology (FNAC) may be used for the accurate diagnosis of nodal metastases.

Metastasis

Lung and bone are the frequent sites of metastases. Chest CT is sufficient to assess lung nodules. Whole body positron emission tomography (PET)-CT is recommended for patients with advanced laryngeal SCC.

Recurrence

Radiation can cause significant edema, blurring of fat planes, swelling of epiglottis, AE fold, and arytenoids **(Figs. 13 and 14)**. PET-CT provides a superior diagnostic accuracy in detecting tumor recurrence than conventional CT, since it lights up the areas of tumor recurrence **(Fig. 15)**.

Post-treatment neck is also better evaluated with PET-CT. Guided biopsy is also essential for confirmation.

Baseline scan is to be done within 4–6 weeks after surgery or radiotherapy. Most tumor recurrences occur within 2 years after initial treatment. Hence, most patients should receive routine surveillance scans at 6 monthly intervals for the first year and yearly scans thereafter.

Other Cancers

Lymphoma, paraganglioma, and tumors form laryngeal cartilages like chondroid malignancy. Imaging findings are nonspecific. Role of imaging is only to define extent of the lesion and to guide the clinician for appropriate sites for biopsy.

Hypopharynx

This includes pyriform sinus, posterior pharyngeal wall **(Fig. 16)**, and postcricoid region **(Fig. 17)**. Hypopharynx extends from the hyoid superiorly to the lower border of cricoid inferiorly, at C5/C6 level where pharynx meets

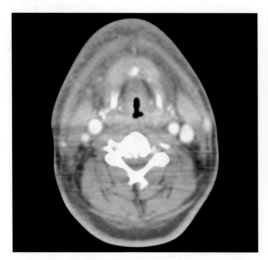

Fig. 13: Axial CT image showing larynx postradiotherapy changes.

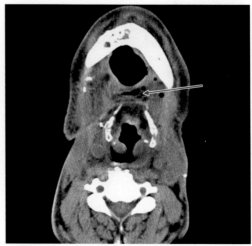

Fig. 14: Axial CT image in a case that had undergone surgery followed by radiotherapy showing anatomical distortion.

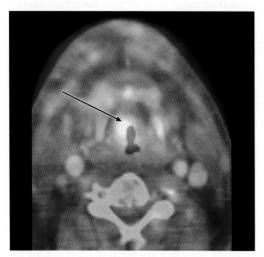

Fig. 15: Positron emission tomography-CT scan image showing uptake in right cord and anterior commissure area, in a postradiotherapy case suggesting recurrence.

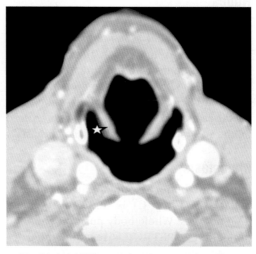

Fig. 16: Axial CT image showing normal pyriform sinus and posterior pharyngeal wall.

the esophagus. Pyriform sinus lies between the aryepiglottic folds medially and thyroid cartilage and thyrohyoid membrane laterally. Paraglottic space lies anterior to it. Apex of pyriform sinus reaches up to the cricoid cartilage. Posterior

wall of oropharynx communicates down to the posterior pharyngeal wall of hypopharynx.

Postcricoid pharynx lies behind the cricoid where it becomes continuous with the esophagus at C6 level. It extends from the

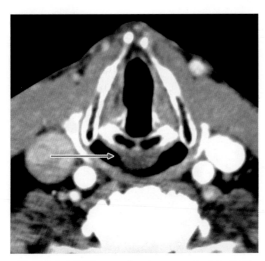

Fig. 17: Axial CT image showing normal postcricoid pharynx.

cricoarytenoid joint to the lower border of cricoid cartilage.

Lymphatic drainage goes to the level II and III nodes. Occasionally from the lower end of hypopharynx it drains to high lateral retropharyngeal nodes behind the skull base. Postcricoid region drains to level III and level IV and VI nodes. Primary tumors from the false cord and ventricle can extend through aryepiglottic fold to the hypopharynx.

Hypopharyngeal SCC is more aggressive than laryngeal SCC and has a rich lymphatic drainage with a high incidence of metastasis. Up to 75% of patients with hypopharynx have metastasis to cervical lymph nodes at the time of diagnosis. Up to 15% of SCC will present with synchronous (25%) or metachronous (40%) second primary tumor.

Carcinoma is most commonly originated in pyriform sinus (60%) followed by postcricoid (25%) and posterior pharyngeal wall (15%). Tumors from the pyriform sinus can spread to involve the paraglottic and pre-epiglottic spaces and base of tongue anteriorly, medially to AE fold, false cord, and arytenoid cartilage. Tumors

from the lateral wall can invade the thyroid cartilage.

Tumors of postcricoid area spread anteriorly to larynx and inferiorly it can involve the cervical esophagus and it has the worst prognosis. Tumors of posterior pharyngeal wall invade retropharyngeal space and prevertebral muscles. Prevertebral muscle invasion is better seen on MRI where prevertebral muscles show abnormal bright signal like tumor on T2-weighted images.

Imaging Technique

CT Scan

CT is the preferred imaging technique for evaluating the larynx and hypopharynx. Patient lies supine in quite respiration with neck slightly extended and symmetrically positioned. The patient should be imaged with "EE" phonation or Valsalva technique to open up the pyriform sinus. A 100 mL of iodinated contrast 300 mg iodine/mL is injected intravenously at the rate of mL/second and scanning started 45 seconds later. Scan range is from base of skull to carina. Coronal and sagittal images are reconstructed later at 2 mm thickness **(Figs. 18 to 20)**.

MR Imaging

It is performed with patient lying supine in quiet breathing. T1- and T2-weighted images are acquired in axial planes with scan plane parallel to vocal cords. Slice thickness is 3 mm with 1 mm interslice gap. The axial T1-weighted image with fat saturation is done after the administration of intravenous gadolinium. 3D T1- and T2-weighted images are acquired from 1 cm above the hyoid down to the inferior border of cricoid to evaluate cartilage invasion. Images in sagittal plane are acquired to evaluate the pre-epiglottic space and coronal plane to study the paraglottic space and ventricles.

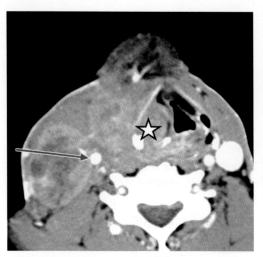

Fig. 18: Axial CT image showing mass in the right pyriform sinus with extralaryngeal extension.

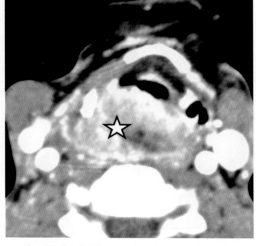

Fig. 19: Axial CT image showing mass from the posterior pharyngeal wall.

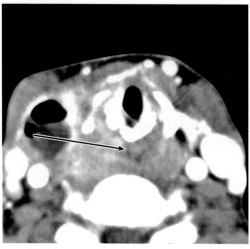

Fig. 20: Axial CT image showing mass in the postcricoid pharynx with cervical adenopathy.

● CONCLUSION

Imaging plays a significant role in staging of the laryngeal or hypopharyngeal cancers, in assessing the true extent of the disease which is crucial in guiding the management. Thorough understanding of the anatomy and imaging protocols are important to interpret the imaging.

● FURTHER READING

1. Becker M, Burkhardt K, Dulguerov P, et al. Imaging of the larynx and hypopharynx. Eur J Radiol. 2008;66(3):460-79.
2. Connor S. Laryngeal cancer: How does the radiologist help? Cancer Imaging. 2007;7:93-103.
3. Gilbert K, Dalley RW, Maronian N, et al. Staging of laryngeal cancer using 64-channel multidetector row CT: Comparison of standard neck CT with dedicated breath-maneuver laryngeal CT. AJNR Am J Neuroradiol. 2010;31(2):251-6.
4. Kuno H, Onaya H, Fujii S, et al. Primary staging of laryngeal and hypopharyngeal cancer: CT, MR imaging and dual-energy CT. Eur J Radiol. 2014;83(1):e23-35.
5. Richards PS, Peacock TE. The role of ultrasound in the detection of cervical lymph node metastases in clinically N0 squamous cell carcinoma of the head and neck. Cancer Imaging. 2007;7:167-78.
6. Schwartz DL, Rajendran J, Yueh B, et al. FDG-PET prediction of head and neck squamous cell cancer outcomes. Arch Otolaryngol Head Neck Surg. 2004;130(12):1361-7.
7. Som PM, Curtine HD. The Larynx. Head and Neck Imaging, 4th edition. London: Mosby Publishers; 2003. pp. 1595-699.

CHAPTER 30

Guidelines in the Management of Laryngeal Cancers

Akshay Kudpaje, Krishnakumar Thankappan

● INTRODUCTION

Laryngeal cancer is one of the most common malignancies in head and neck. It accounts for approximately 1% of all new cancer diagnosis. The total incidence has been reported to be rising in recent years. It accounts to 2.3% of all malignant tumors in males and about 0.4% of all malignant tumors in females. Histologically, squamous cell carcinoma is the most common (85%).

The main risk factors for laryngeal cancer are habits of tobacco smoking and alcohol consumption, and their effects are synergistic. For the causation of glottic cancer, smoking is considered the main risk factor. In contrast, alcohol usually has higher risk for supraglottic cancers.

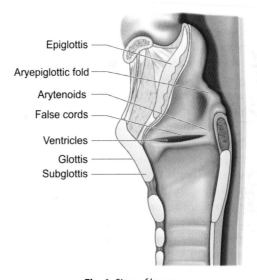

Epiglottis

Aryepiglottic fold

Arytenoids

False cords

Ventricles

Glottis

Subglottis

Fig. 1: Sites of larynx.

● ANATOMY

The larynx is divided into the supraglottic, glottic, and subglottic subsites **(Fig. 1)**. The supraglottic region extends from the hyoid bone superiorly to a horizontal line drawn through the apex of the ventricle inferiorly. It has five subdivisions: epiglottis, false cords, the ventricles, the aryepiglottic folds, and the arytenoids **(Fig. 2)**. The subglottis is located below the vocal cords; it extends from about 5 mm below the free margin of the vocal cord up to the inferior border of cricoid cartilage.

The glottis consists of the true vocal cords and anterior commissure. The most common site for the cancer is glottis (49%) followed by supraglottis (16%).

Larynx is formed by hyoid bone, thyroid cartilage, and the cricoid cartilage which are held together by ligaments and membranes. The more mobile inner side of laryngeal framework consists of the epiglottis, arytenoids, corniculate, and cuneiform cartilages. The conus elasticus (cricovocal ligament) extends from the upper surface of cricoid cartilage to

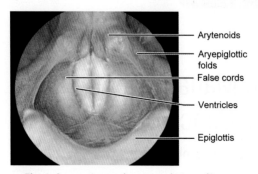

Fig. 2: Scopy picture showing subsites of larynx.

Arytenoids
Aryepiglottic folds
False cords
Ventricles
Epiglottis

Early glottic carcinoma

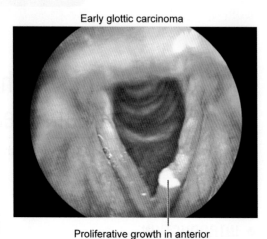

Proliferative growth in anterior third of left cord

Fig. 3: Scopy picture showing an early glottic lesion.

Advanced glottic carcinoma

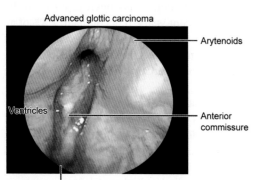

Arytenoids
Ventricles
Anterior commissure

Transglottic growth with subglottic extension

Fig. 4: Scopy picture showing advanced transglottic tumor.

vocal process of arytenoid and lower third of the thyroid cartilage; upper free border of this membrane is thickened to form the vocal ligament. The pre-epiglottic and paraglottic spaces are continuous spaces lying between the external framework of the thyroid cartilage and hyoid bone and the inner framework of the epiglottis and intrinsic muscles.

Lymphatic drainage is fairly predictable, with supraglottic region draining mainly to lateral neck nodes (Level II–IV). In contrast, true vocal cords have very sparse lymphatics, and nodal spread occurs when tumor extends to supraglottic or subglottic regions. The subglottic region drains primarily to level VI region. The submandibular nodes are rarely involved in laryngeal cancers, and there is small risk of involvement of level V node. The incidence of clinically positive nodes is 55% at time of diagnosis. Elective neck dissection shows pathologically positive nodes in 16% of cases and clinically node negative neck if observed, eventually identifies appearance of positive nodes in 33% of cases.

● CLINICAL FEATURES

The cardinal symptom of laryngeal cancer presentation is hoarseness of voice. As the lesion increases in size patients may present with breathing difficulty and stridor. Associated symptoms may include dysphagia, odyno-phagia, otalgia, and weight loss. Examination should begin with systematic examination of all sites of head and neck, with special attention to assessment of larynx in patient presenting with hoarseness. It can be done using Hopkins scope or a fiberoptic nasolaryngoscope to evaluate the most likely subsite, the extent of tumor, and vocal cord mobility **(Figs. 3 and 4)**. The vocal cord mobility has pivotal role in determining the T staging. The performance status of the patient and the comorbidities has to be evaluated. Neck has to be examined to look for palpable nodes and larynx has to be examined for laryngeal crepitus and widening.

Radiological

A contrast enhanced CT scan of head, neck, and chest is the imaging method of choice for evaluating the larynx. It helps to determine the extent of tumor, in particular the inferior extent, invasion of paraglottic and pre-epiglottic spaces and/or extension through the thyroid cartilage to paralaryngeal soft tissues. The presence of nodal metastasis and its relation with great vessels can also be studied. The chest has to be screened for any abnormalities in the lung, the most common site of distant metastasis and second primary tumors in this group of patients. If early extralaryngeal spread is suspected, MRI scan may be useful. Sagittal MRI may be useful in detecting early invasion of the base of tongue **(Figs. 5A and B)**.

Direct Laryngoscopy

Direct laryngoscopy examination done under general anesthesia helps to see the ventricles, subglottis, apex of pyriform fossa, and the postcricoid area. These areas are not consistently seen by indirect examinations. A biopsy is taken from the obvious lesion and from the suspicious areas.

● TREATMENT

Tables 1 and 2 give the TNM staging and prognostic stage groups according to the AJCC 8th edition. The management of laryngeal cancers primarily depends on stage at presentation. Early stage tumors (stage I, II) are treated with single modality treatment either by radiotherapy or transoral laser surgery. Advanced stage tumors (stage III, IV) are treated with multi-modality treatment. The decision making depends on variety of factors like the age of patient, performance status, comorbidities, surgical access issues, the skills, and the preferences of the multidisciplinary board, and, importantly, the wishes of the patient. The primary aim of the treatment is cure with the best functional outcome and least risk of serious complication. Patient may be considered as early group if chance of cure with larynx preservation is high; a moderately advanced group if the likelihood of local control is 60–70%, but the chance of cure is still good; and an advanced group if chance of cure is moderate and likelihood of laryngeal preservation is relatively low **(Flowchart 1)**.

Endolaryngeal growth with paraglottic extension

Transglottic with extralaryngeal extension

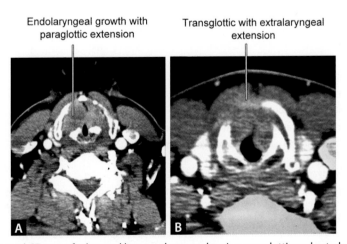

Figs. 5A and B: Axial CT scan of advanced laryngeal cancer showing paraglottic and extralaryngeal spread.

Table 1: TNM staging larynx cancers (AJCC, 8th edition).

T Stage	
Supraglottis	
TX	Primary tumor cannot be assessed
Tis	Carcinoma in situ
T1	Tumor limited to one subsite of supraglottic with normal vocal cord mobility
T2	Tumor invades mucosa of more than one adjacent subsite of supraglottis or glottis or region outside the supraglottis (e.g. mucosa of base of tongue, vallecula, medial wall of pyriform sinus) without fixation of the larynx
T3	Tumor limited to larynx with vocal cord fixation and/or invades any of the following: postcricoid area, pre-epiglottic space, paraglottic space, and/or inner cortex of thyroid cartilage
T4	Moderately advanced or very advanced disease
T4a	*Moderately advanced local disease:* Tumor invades through the outer cortex of the thyroid cartilage and/or invades tissues beyond the larynx (e.g. trachea, soft tissues of neck including deep extrinsic muscle of the tongue, strap muscles, thyroid, or esophagus)
T4b	*Very advanced local disease*: Tumor invades prevertebral space, encases carotid artery, or invades mediastinal structures
Glottis	
TX	Primary tumor cannot be assessed
Tis	Carcinoma in situ
T1	Tumor limited to the vocal cord(s) (may involve anterior or posterior commissure) with normal mobility
T1a	Tumor limited to one vocal cord
T1b	Tumor involves both vocal cords
T2	Tumor extends to supraglottis and/or subglottis, and/or with impaired vocal cord mobility
T3	Tumor limited to the larynx with vocal cord fixation and/or invasion of paraglottic space and/or inner cortex of the thyroid cartilage
T4	Moderately advanced or very advanced disease
T4a	*Moderately advanced local disease:* Tumor invades through the outer cortex of the thyroid cartilage and/or invades tissues beyond the larynx (e.g. trachea, cricoid cartilage, soft tissues of neck including deep extrinsic muscle of the tongue, strap muscles, thyroid, or esophagus)
T4b	*Very advanced local disease*: Tumor invades prevertebral space, encases carotid artery, or invades mediastinal structures
Subglottis	
TX	Primary tumor cannot be assessed
Tis	Carcinoma in situ
T1	Tumor limited to the subglottis
T2	Tumor extends to vocal cord(s) with normal or impaired mobility
T3	Tumor limited to larynx with vocal cord fixation and/or invasion of paraglottic space and/or inner cortex of the thyroid cartilage
T4	Moderately advanced or very advanced disease
T4a	*Moderately advanced local disease:* Tumor invades through the outer cortex of the thyroid cartilage and/or invades tissues beyond the larynx (e.g. trachea, cricoid cartilage, soft tissues of neck including deep extrinsic muscle of the tongue, strap muscles, thyroid, or esophagus)
T4b	*Very advanced local disease:* Tumor invades prevertebral space, encases carotid artery, or invades mediastinal structures

Contd...

Contd...

Clinical N (cN)

NX	Regional lymph nodes cannot be assessed
N0	No regional lymph node metastasis
N1	Metastasis in a single ipsilateral lymph node, 3 cm or smaller in greatest dimension and ENE (–)
N2	Metastasis in a single ipsilateral node larger than 3 cm but not larger than 6 cm in greatest dimension and ENE (-); or metastases in multiple ipsilateral lymph nodes, none larger than 6 cm in greatest dimension and ENE (–); or in bilateral or contralateral lymph nodes, none larger than 6 cm in greatest dimension and ENE (–)
N2a	Metastasis in a single ipsilateral node larger than 3 cm but not larger than 6 cm in greatest dimension and ENE (–)
N2b	Metastasis in multiple ipsilateral nodes, none larger than 6 cm in greatest dimension and ENE (–)
N2c	Metastasis in bilateral or contralateral lymph nodes, none larger than 6 cm in greatest dimension and ENE (–)
N3	Metastasis in a lymph node larger than 6 cm in greatest dimension and ENE (–); or metastasis in any node(s) with clinically overt ENE (+)
N3a	Metastasis in a lymph node larger than 6 cm in greatest dimension and ENE (–)
N3b	Metastasis in any node(s) with clinically overt ENE (+)

Pathological N (pN)

NX	Regional lymph nodes cannot be assessed
N0	No regional lymph node metastasis
N1	Metastasis in a single ipsilateral lymph node, 3 cm or smaller in greatest dimension and ENE (–)
N2	Metastasis in a single ipsilateral node, 3 cm or smaller in greatest dimension and ENE (+); or metastasis in a single ipsilateral node larger than 3 cm but not larger than 6 cm in greatest dimension and ENE (–) or metastases in multiple ipsilateral lymph nodes, none larger than 6 cm in greatest dimension and ENE (–); or in bilateral or contralateral lymph nodes, none larger than 6 cm in greatest dimension and ENE (–)
N2a	Metastasis in a single ipsilateral node, 3 cm or smaller in greatest dimension and ENE (+); or metastasis in a single ipsilateral node larger than 3 cm but not larger than 6 cm in greatest dimension and ENE (–)
N2b	Metastasis in multiple ipsilateral nodes, none larger than 6 cm in greatest dimension and ENE (–)
N2c	Metastasis in bilateral or contralateral lymph nodes, none larger than 6 cm in greatest dimension and ENE (–)
N3	Metastasis in a lymph node larger than 6 cm in greatest dimension and ENE (–); or in a single ipsilateral node larger than 3 cm in greatest dimension and ENE (+); or multiple ipsilateral, contralateral, or bilateral nodes any with ENE (+)
N3a	Metastasis in a lymph node larger than 6 cm in greatest dimension and ENE (–)
N3b	Metastasis in a single ipsilateral node larger than 3 cm in greatest dimension and ENE (+); or multiple ipsilateral, contralateral, or bilateral nodes any with ENE (+)

Note: A designation of "U" or "L" may be used for any N category to indicate metastasis above the lower border of the cricoid (U) or below the lower border of the cricoid (L). Similarly, clinical and pathological ENE should be recorded as EN E (–) or ENE (+)

Distant metastasis M

M0	No distant metastasis
M1	Distant metastasis

(AJCC: American Joint Cancer Committee)

Table 2: AJCC prognostic stage groups.

When T is ...	And N is ...	And M is ...	Then the stage group is ...
Tis	N0	M0	0
T1	N0	M0	I
T2	N0	M0	II
T3	N0	M0	III
T0, T1, T2, T3	N1	M0	III
T4a	N0,N1	M0	IVA
T0, T1, T2, T3,T4a	N2	M0	IVA
Any T	N3	M0	IVB
T4b	Any N	M0	IVB
Any T	Any N	M1	IVC

(AJCC: American Joint Cancer Committee)

Flowchart 1: Management of carcinoma in situ.

Early Stage (T1N0 and T2N0)

These lesions are treated often by radiotherapy or transoral endolaryngeal surgery. Both these treatment modalities have similar cure rates; however, there is no direct comparison of the efficacy of these two modalities. Both treatment modalities have advantages and disadvantages. The main advantage of radiotherapy is that it is thought to have better voice outcomes and can treat patients with poor performance status. For endolaryngeal surgery, advantages include treatment is single setting, cheaper, certainty of removal of specimen and ability to access margins surgically; disadvantage is that it can affect the voice quality and access can sometimes be difficult **(Flowchart 2)**.

Moderately Advanced Tumors (T1T2T3 any N)

These patients have advanced stage tumors and have to be treated with multimodality treatment. The options are concurrent chemoradiation or total laryngectomy. The preferred treatment is concurrent chemoradiation, since cure rate is similar as compared to traditional surgical approach, i.e. laryngectomy with

Flowchart 2: Management of early vocal cord tumors.

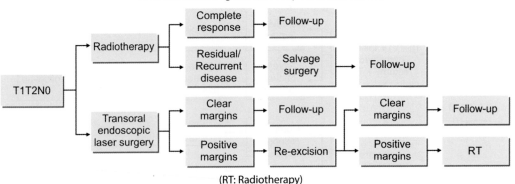

(RT: Radiotherapy)

Flowchart 3: Management of moderately advanced laryngeal cancers.

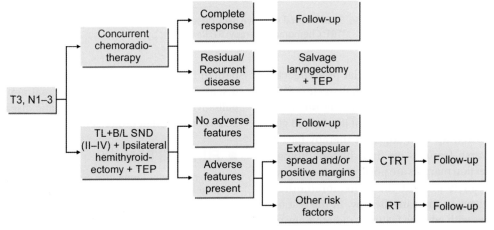

(CTRT: Chemoradiotherapy; TEP: Transesophageal puncture; TL: Total laryngectomy;
B/L SND: Bilateral selective neck dissection; RT: Radiotherapy)

additional benefit of organ preservation in significant number of patients. This additional benefit of organ preservation has significant impact on quality of life (QOL). The concurrent chemoradiation most commonly is conventional fractionation at 2 Gy per fraction to a typical dose of 70 Gy in 7 weeks with single agent cisplatin given every 3 weeks at 100 mg/m^2 **(Flowchart 3)**. Partial laryngectomy surgeries including vertical partial, horizontal partial, and supracricoid laryngectomies are also an option. But such surgeries are being done less,

with the advent of chemoradiotherapy. Total laryngectomy is rarely done in this situation, especially if the larynx is dysfunctional at the onset; the patient having a pretreatment tracheostomy, dysphagia, and aspiration.

Advanced Laryngeal Tumors (T4a any N)

The patients who have a frank extralaryngeal spread treatment with chemoradiation are not optimal. The treatment for this group of patients

Flowchart 4: Management of advanced laryngeal cancers.

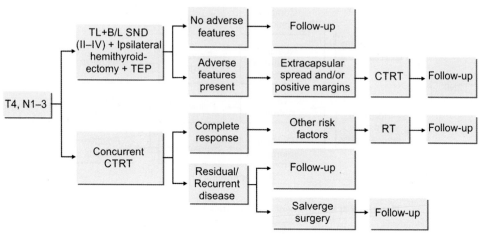

(TL: Total laryngectomy; B/L SND: Bilateral selective neck dissection; TEP: Transesophageal puncture; CTRT: Chemoradiotherapy; RT: Radiotherapy)

is laryngectomy with partial pharyngectomy with bilateral selective neck dissection (II–IV), hemithyroidectomy (depending on the side and extent of involvement of the thyroid gland) followed up with adjuvant therapy based on adverse features on final histopathology. If resection margins are positive and/or perinodal spread is present then chemoradiotherapy is given as adjuvant therapy. In the rest of the cases with adverse features, radiotherapy alone is given as adjuvant **(Flowchart 4)**. Concurrent chemoradiotherapy may be an option only when the patient is not fit for surgery.

Very Advanced Tumors (T4b any N)

This group includes newly diagnosed locally advanced T4b(M0), newly diagnosed unresectable nodal disease, metastatic disease, recurrent or persistent disease or patients unfit for surgery. The aim of treatment is cure for patients with newly diagnosed but unresectable disease. Chemoradiotherapy protocols can be given depending on the performance status of the patient. For patients with recurrent disease, goal is cure, if surgery or radiation is feasible. If patient has received previous radiotherapy or disease is unresectable, mode of treatment is palliative. For patients with metastatic disease, goal is palliation or prolongation of life.

● **FURTHER READING**

1. American Joint Committee on Cancer. Larynx. In: Edge SB, Byrd DR, Compton CC, Fritz AG, Greene FI, Trotti A (Eds). AJCC Cancer Staging Manual, 7th edition. New York, NY: Springer; 2010. pp. 81-92.
2. Forastiere AA, Goepfert H, Maor M, et al. Concurrent chemotherapy and radiotherapy for organ preservation in advanced laryngeal cancer. N Eng J Med. 2003;349(22):2091-8.
3. Mendenhall WM, Morris G, Amdur RJ, et al. Parameters that predict local control after definitive radiotherapy for squamous cell carcinoma of the head and neck. Head Neck. 2003;25(7):535-42.
4. Pignon JP, Bourhis J, Domenge C, et al. Chemotherapy added to locoregional treatment for head and neck squamous-cell carcinoma: Three meta-analyses of updated individual data. MACH-NC Collaborative Group. Meta-Analysis of Chemotherapy on Head and Neck Cancer. Lancet. 2000;355(9208):949-55.
5. Wolf GT, Fisher SG, Hong WK, et al. Department of Veterans Affairs Laryngeal Cancer Study Group. Induction chemotherapy plus radiation compared with surgery plus radiation in patients with advanced laryngeal cancer. N Engl J Med. 1991;324(24):1685-90.

CHAPTER 31

Guidelines in the Management of Hypopharyngeal Cancers

Akshay Kudpaje, Krishnakumar Thankappan

● INTRODUCTION

Carcinoma of the hypopharynx usually presents with advanced stage disease. Patients usually have significant comorbidities: Respiratory, cardiac, and nutritional, which may restrict the therapeutic options leading to suboptimal oncologic outcomes in advanced stage disease.

Tobacco and alcohol use is most commonly associated with carcinoma of hypopharynx. In addition, patients are typically elderly, with dysphagia and weight loss as a result of their tumor burden, and/or a poor baseline diet.

Squamous cell carcinoma (SCC) accounts for 95% of cancers in the hypopharynx; field cancerization is a common phenomenon in these patients. The wide mucosal exposure to carcinogens results in a field of diseased mucosa characterized by high-grade dysplasia, giving rise to the index hypopharyngeal tumor. Therefore, these patients have high rates of synchronous and/or metachronous upper aerodigestive primary tumors. Approximately 10% of patients may be found to have synchronous primary tumors and up to 20% will develop a metachronous second primary tumor.

● ANATOMY

The hypopharynx is interposed between the oropharynx superiorly and the upper esophagus inferiorly, with the larynx located anteriorly. In the adult, the hypopharynx extends from the hyoid bone above to the cricopharyngeus muscle and lower border of the cricoid cartilage below. The cervical esophagus extends from the lower border of the cricoid cartilage into the thorax. The hypopharynx includes the posterior pharyngeal wall, the pyriform fossae or sinuses, and the postcricoid region as subsites (**Figs. 1A and B**).

Lymphatic drainage of the hypopharynx terminates in the lymph nodes along the jugular vein (levels II, III, and IV) and appears to a lesser extent in the nodes along the spinal accessory nerve (level V), and even less frequently in the submandibular area (level Ib). Significant lymphatic drainage occurs from the posterior pharyngeal wall and drains to the retropharyngeal lymph nodes. Lymphatics from the inferior part of the pyriform sinus, the postcricoid area, and the upper esophagus often drain to the nodes along the recurrent laryngeal nerves to the paratracheal lymph nodes (level VI).

About 83% of tumors arise from the pyriform sinus, 9% from posterior pharyngeal wall, and about 4% from the postcricoid region. Hypopharyngeal cancers are prone for submucosal spread. Studies have shown, on serial sectioning 60% of hypopharyngeal cancers demonstrate significant submucosal spread, which can contribute to local recurrence and poor outcomes after definitive treatment.

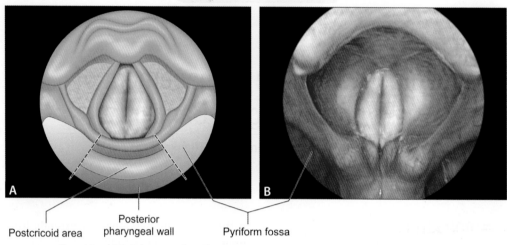

Postcricoid area · Posterior pharyngeal wall · Pyriform fossa

Figs. 1A and B: Schematic diagram showing subsites of hypopharynx with scopy picture.

Lymphatic spread occurs in majority of tumors by the time of diagnosis. More than 50% of patients present with clinically positive cervical nodes at the time of diagnosis. In addition 30–40% of N0 necks are found to have pathological involvement when dissected electively, rendering 65–80% of patients ultimately node positive.

● CLINICAL FEATURES

Patients with hypopharyngeal cancers often initially present with nonspecific symptoms, which are commonly attributed to infection or gastrointestinal causes, leading to frequent delay in diagnosis. Hence, they usually present with advanced disease. Some patients may present palpable nodes as the only symptom. Dysphagia is most common presenting symptom in up to 85% of cases, although palpable neck mass is the most common physical finding. Other findings include odynophagia, weight loss, hoarseness, referred otalgia, and neck pain.

Assessment should start with global evaluation of their general health, nutritional status, and anemia. History regarding smoking and alcohol has to be taken in detail, as this has an effect on respiratory and hepatorenal systems. Evaluation of primary tumor can be done using either a Hopkins scope or flexible nasopharyngoscope to study the extent; mucosa spread to adjacent sites mobility of vocal cord, and narrowing of the airway is noted. Neck examination is done to determine the enlarged nodes to record their number, size, and distribution. Laryngopharyngeal mobility over the cervical vertebra is examined to rule out prevertebral muscle involvement **(Fig. 2)**.

Radiological Findings

Computed tomography scan is currently the most frequently employed imaging study used initially in the work up of hypopharyngeal cancers **(Fig. 3)**. It helps us determine the exact three-dimensional extent of tumor; to detect the presence of locoregional neck metastasis; to detect pulmonary metastasis or synchronous second primary. One of the limitations of CT scan is that it is difficult to differentiate between tumor and soft-tissue edema. MRI helps to resolve this issue in doubtful cases. PET-CT scan has important role in evaluating recurrent and residual tumor from edema and scarring in patients treated with definitive therapy including, surgery and/or chemoradiotherapy. **Tables 1 and 2** show the TNM staging of the hypopharyngeal cancers and prognostic stage groups according to the AJCC 8th edition.

Advanced pyriform fossa tumor with paraglottic extension

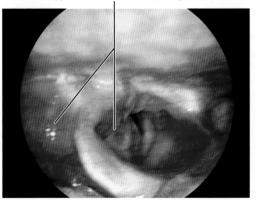

Fig. 2: Scopy picture showing an advanced pyriform tumor with paraglottic extension.

Advanced pyriform fossa tumor with paraglottic extension

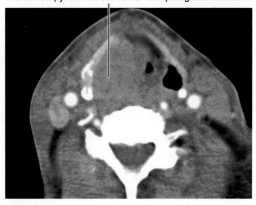

Fig. 3: Axial scan CT scan picture of advanced hypopharyngeal tumor with paraglottic extension and extralaryngeal spread.

Table 1: TNM staging hypopharynx cancers (AJCC, 8th edition).

T Stage	
TX	Primary tumor cannot be assessed
Tis	Carcinoma in situ
T1	Tumor limited to one subsite of hypopharynx and/or 2 cm or smaller in greatest dimension
T2	Tumor invades more than one subsite of hypopharynx or an adjacent site, or measures larger than 2 cm but not larger than 4 cm in greatest dimension without fixation of hemilarynx
T3	Tumor larger than 4 cm in greatest dimension or with fixation of hemilarynx or extension to esophagus
T4	Moderately advanced or very advanced disease
T4a	*Moderately advanced local disease:* Tumor invades thyroid/cricoid cartilage, hyoid bone, thyroid gland, or central compartment soft tissue*
T4b	*Very advanced local disease:* Tumor invades prevertebral fascia, encases carotid artery, or involves mediastinal structures
	*Note: Central compartment soft tissue includes prelaryngeal strap muscles and subcutaneous fat
Clinical N (cN)	
NX	Regional lymph nodes cannot be assessed
N0	No regional lymph node metastasis
N1	Metastasis in a single ipsilateral lymph node, 3 cm or smaller in greatest dimension and ENE (–).
N2	Metastasis in a single ipsilateral node larger than 3 cm but not larger than 6 cm in greatest dimension and ENE (–); or metastases in multiple ipsilateral lymph nodes, none larger than 6 cm in greatest dimension and ENE (–); or in bilateral or contralateral lymph nodes, none larger than 6 cm in greatest dimension and ENE (–).
N2a	Metastasis in a single ipsilateral node larger than 3 cm but not larger than 6 cm in greatest dimension and ENE (–).
N2b	Metastasis in multiple ipsilateral nodes, none larger than 6 cm in greatest dimension and ENE (–).

Contd...

Contd...

Clinical N (cN)	
N2c	Metastasis in bilateral or contralateral lymph nodes, none larger than 6 cm in greatest dimension and ENE (–)
N3	Metastasis in a lymph node larger than 6 cm in greatest dimension and ENE (–); or metastasis in any node(s) with clinically overt ENE (+)
N3a	Metastasis in a lymph node larger than 6 cm in greatest dimension and ENE (–)
N3b	Metastasis in any node(s) with clinically overt ENE (+)
Pathological N (pN)	
NX	Regional lymph nodes cannot be assessed
N0	No regional lymph node metastasis
N1	Metastasis in a single ipsilateral lymph node, 3 cm or smaller in greatest dimension and ENE (–)
N2	Metastasis in a single ipsilateral node, 3 cm or smaller in greatest dimension and ENE (+); or metastasis in a single ipsilateral node larger than 3cm but not larger than 6 cm in greatest dimension and ENE (–) or metastases in multiple ipsilateral lymph nodes, none larger than 6 cm in greatest dimension and ENE (–); or in bilateral or contralateral lymph nodes, none larger than 6 cm in greatest dimension and ENE (–)
N2a	Metastasis in a single ipsilateral node, 3 cm or smaller in greatest dimension and ENE (+); or metastasis in a single ipsilateral node larger than 3 cm but not larger than 6 cm in greatest dimension and ENE (–)
N2b	Metastasis in multiple ipsilateral nodes, none larger than 6 cm in greatest dimension and ENE (–)
N2c	Metastasis in bilateral or contralateral lymph nodes, none larger than 6 cm in greatest dimension and ENE (–).
N3	Metastasis in a lymph node larger than 6 cm in greatest dimension and ENE (–); or in a single ipsilateral node larger than 3 cm in greatest dimension and ENE (+); or multiple ipsilateral, contralateral, or bilateral nodes any with ENE (+)
N3a	Metastasis in a lymph node larger than 6 cm in greatest dimension and ENE (–)
N3b	Metastasis in a single ipsilateral node larger than 3 cm in greatest dimension and ENE (+); or multiple ipsilateral, contralateral, or bilateral nodes any with ENE (+)

Note: A designation of "U" or "L" may be used for any N category to indicate metastasis above the lower border of the cricoid (U) or below the lower border of the cricoid (L). Similarly, clinical and pathological ENE should be recorded as ENE (–) or ENE (+).

Distant metastasis M	
M0	No distant metastasis
M1	Distant metastasis

(AJCC: American Joint Cancer Committee)

• TREATMENT

Early Stage (Stage I–II, T1, T2, N0)

These tumors cannot be treated with a single modality, either surgery or radiotherapy. Both have similar cure rates. In general, curative radiation therapy is preferred as the definitive treatment approach for patients with early-stage tumors, as it provides a good chance for organ preservation. Alternatively, open or endoscopic surgery (partial laryngopharyngectomy) with ipsilateral or bilateral neck dissection may be performed. More recently, transoral laser microsurgeries have been performed with promising results in selected early-stage lesions.

Table 2: AJCC prognostic stage groups.

When T is ...	And N is ...	And M is ...	Then the stage group is ...
Tis	N0	M0	0
T1	N0	M0	I
T2	N0	M0	II
T3	N0	M0	III
T0, T1, T2, T3	N1	M0	III
T4a	N0, N1	M0	IVA
T0, T1, T2, T3,T4a	N2	M0	IVA
Any T	N3	M0	IVB
T4b	Any N	M0	IVB
Any T	Any N	M1	IVC

(AJCC: American Joint Cancer Committee)

Radiation is commonly favored as surgery in this region is morbid; often results in chronic aspiration due to injury/sacrifice of the superior laryngeal nerve. Additionally, given that concerning pathologic features (positive margins, node positivity, pathologic T3 or T4 status, perineural invasion, and lymphovascular invasion) often prompt postoperative (chemo) radiation following surgery. Definitive radiation may allow patients to forgo the toxicities associated with multiple treatment modalities. Radiotherapy consists of a 6–7-week course, with treatment delivered 5 days per week. The dose delivered to the primary tumor is 66–70 Gy and the neck is delivered dose of 54–60 Gy. Lymphatic coverage from the skull base to the clavicle is routine for patients undergoing radiation for hypopharyngeal cancer. The delivery of radiation can be either three-dimensional conformal radiotherapy (3DCRT) or intensity-modulated radiation therapy (IMRT); the latter is commonly used for radiotherapy in hypopharynx. The dose received by high risk primary tumor and involved lymph nodes is 66–70 Gy/fraction. The low and intermediate risk (sites of suspected subclinical spread) receives dose of 44–50 Gy and 54–63 Gy, respectively.

Primary surgical management of patients with early-stage cancer of the hypopharynx is indicated in patients who refuse radiation, have had previous radiotherapy, or those patients in which organ preservation is feasible, and postoperative radiation is unlikely to be used. As submucosal spread of tumor is common (making margin-negative resections difficult) and 30–40% of clinically N0 patients will have pathologically involved lymph nodes that may warrant postoperative radiotherapy, careful patient selection is necessary before attempting organ-preservation surgery.

Transoral methods, including transoral laser microsurgery (TLM) and transoral robotic surgery, have been recently employed in attempt to achieve margin-negative tumor resection while minimizing damage to adjacent normal tissues. With these approaches, neck dissection is often deferred until final margin analysis is performed on the primary tumor specimen, with delayed neck dissection performed if margins are negative, or more radical open surgery (or radiation ± chemotherapy) entertained when primary margins are positive. This approach may facilitate surgery without the need for tracheostomy and feeding tubes, and oncologic outcomes appear similar to open surgical approaches for appropriately selected Tl–2 lesions **(Flowchart 1)**.

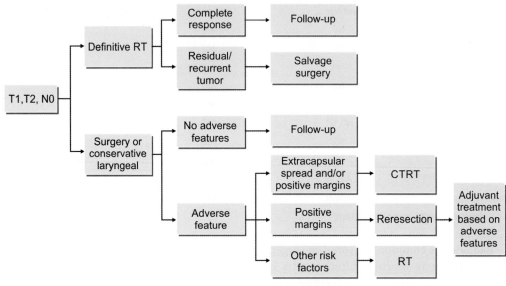

Flowchart 1: Management of early-stage hypopharyngeal tumors.

(CTRT: Chemoradiotherapy; RT: Radiotherapy)

Moderately Advanced Tumors (T1, T2 Node Positive or T3 N⁺)

Patients with T3 hypopharyngeal tumors generally require laryngopharyngectomy for surgical management and adjuvant (chemo) radiotherapy. Therefore, given the need for radiotherapy and goals of organ preservation, definitive chemoradiotherapy is the treatment of choice in stage III and IV hypopharyngeal cancers. Conventional radiotherapy, with or without chemotherapy, is utilized in this scenario and typically aims to deliver 70 Gy in 2 Gy daily fractions to gross disease, with 50–60 Gy delivered to areas at risk for microscopic disease. This can be delivered either by 3DCRT or IMRT. The high risk regions, i.e. primary tumor and involved lymph nodes will receive 70 Gy (2 Gy/fraction) and low/intermediate risk areas will receive 44–50 Gy (2 Gy/fraction) and 54–63 Gy (1.6–1.8 Gy/fraction), respectively along with weekly or three weekly cisplatin based on performance status of patient **(Flowchart 2)**.

Advanced Tumors (T4A)

Total laryngectomy and partial pharyngectomy (laryngopharyngectomy) with bilateral neck dissections with TE prosthesis for voice restoration with adjuvant chemo (radiation) based on final histopathology is the treatment of choice in advance hypopharyngeal cancers with extralaryngeal spread. The indication of adjuvant chemoradiation is either positive margins, perinodal spread in the nodes or both. Indications for postoperative radiation include pathologic T3–T4 tumors, N2–3 nodal disease (>1 involved lymph node), perineural invasion and tumor emboli in adjacent vasculature **(Flowchart 3)**.

Postoperatively ideal time to start radiotherapy is within 6 weeks. The high risk regions such as positive margins will receive dose of 60–66 Gy (2 Gy/fraction). Low to intermediate risk (i.e. sites of suspected subclinical spread) will receive dose of 44–50 Gy to 54–63 Gy, respectively. When concurrent chemotherapy is planned single agent cisplatin is given every 3 weeks at 100 mg/m².

Flowchart 2: Management of moderately advanced stage hypopharyngeal tumor.

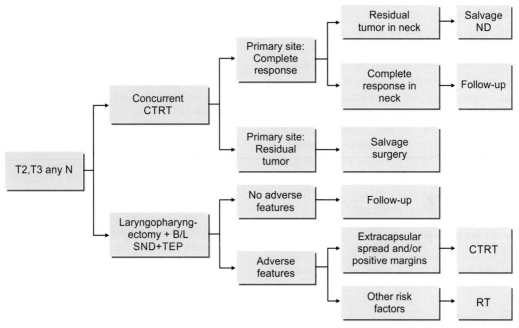

(CTRT: Chemoradiotherapy; B/L SND: Bilateral selective neck dissection; TEP: Transesophageal puncture; ND: Neck dissection; RT: Radiotherapy)

Flowchart 3: Management of advanced stage hypopharyngeal tumor.

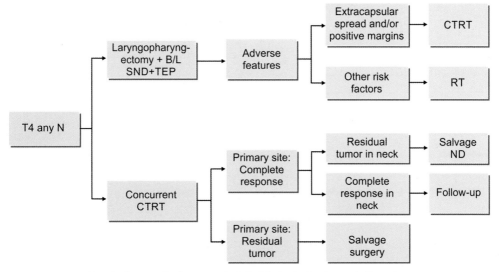

(CTRT: Chemoradiotherapy; B/L SND: Bilateral selective neck dissection; TEP: Transesophageal puncture; ND: Neck dissection; RT: Radiotherapy)

Very Advanced Stage Tumors (Stage IVb)

This group includes newly diagnosed locally advanced T4b (M0), newly diagnosed unresectable nodal disease, metastatic disease, recurrent or persistent disease or patients unfit for surgery. The aim of treatment is cure for patients with newly diagnosed but unresectable disease. For patients with recurrent disease, goal is cure if surgery or radiation is feasible. If patient has received previous radiotherapy or disease is unresectable, mode of treatment is palliative. For patients with metastatic disease, goal is palliation or prolongation of life.

● FURTHER READING

1. Bernier J, Cooper JS, Pajak TF, et al. Defining risk levels in locally advanced head and neck cancers: a comparative analysis of concurrent postoperative radiation plus chemotherapy trials of the EORTC (#22931) and RTOG (# 9501). Head Neck. 2005;27(10):843-50.
2. Bernier J, Domenge C, Ozsahin M, et al.; European Organization for Research and Treatment of Cancer Trial 22931. Postoperative irradiation with or without concomitant chemotherapy for locally advanced head and neck cancer. N Engl J Med. 2004;350(19):1945-52.
3. Cooper JS, Pajak TF, Forastiere AA, et al.; Radiation Therapy Oncology Group 9501/Intergroup. Postoperative concurrent radiotherapy and chemotherapy for high-risk squamous-cell carcinoma of the head and neck. N Engl J Med. 2004; 350(19):1937-44.
4. Lefebvre JL, Chevalier D, Luboinski B, et al. Larynx preservation in pyriform sinus cancer: preliminary results of a European Organization for Research and Treatment of Cancer phase III trial. EORTC Head and Neck Cancer Cooperative Group. J Natl Cancer Inst. 1996;88(13):890-9.

CHAPTER 32

Principles of Surgery in Larynx and Hypopharynx Cancers

Akshay Kudpaje, Krishnakumar Thankappan, Subramania Iyer

● INTRODUCTION

Management of laryngeal and hypopharyngeal cancer has evolved with more emphasis to organ preservation without compromising survival. In early stage (T1, T2, N0), laryngeal and hypopharyngeal cancers, transoral laser surgery has similar oncologic and organ preservation outcomes compared to radiotherapy. In locally advanced (T3, T4) tumors, organ conservation can be achieved in selected group of patients by voice conservation surgeries. However, when advanced disease limits the former, then focus shifts from voice conservation surgery to more radical surgery (total laryngectomy with partial pharyngectomy) with voice restoration.

Surgeries for laryngeal and hypopharyngeal cancers include (**Flowchart 1**):

- Transoral surgery—voice conservative surgery:
  - Laser microsurgery
  - Robotic surgery
- Open surgery:
  - Voice conservative surgery:
    - Vertical hemilaryngectomy
    - Supraglottic laryngectomy
    - Supracricoid partial laryngectomy
  - Laryngectomy with voice restoration:
    - Near total laryngectomy
    - Total laryngectomy, partial pharyngectomy with voice prosthesis.

Flowchart 1: Laryngeal surgical procedures.

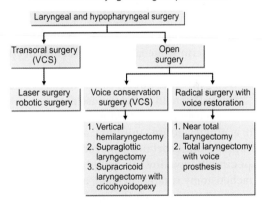

● TRANSORAL LASER MICROSURGERY

Indications for transoral laser surgery are early stage (T1, T2) tumors. This surgery is done using suspension direct microlaryngoscopy coupled with operating microscope the carbon dioxide laser. Transoral laser microsurgery (TLM) may or may not entail a "piecemeal excision" of the laryngeal tumor. Small lesions can be removed en bloc or by dividing the tumor across its main axis. Although this approach violates Halstedian technique, advocates argue that by appreciating the unseen depth of the lesion especially near critical and/or unique anatomy an adequate oncologic resection can be achieved while minimizing the sacrifice of surrounding normal structures. Using the operating room microscope, which provides magnification of 4X to 12X the endoscopic surgeon can have significantly improved visualization and thus more detailed understanding of the interface between tumor and normal tissue.

Hirano in 1977 has described vocal cord, as a five layered unique multilayered structure microscopically with different mechanical properties. The different stiffness characteristics of these layers result in mechanically decoupled groupings of the layers, to form:

- Mucosa (cover)—composed of epithelium and superficial lamina propria (Reinke's space)
- Vocal ligament (transition)—composed of the intermediate lamina propria and deep lamina propria
- Body of the vocal fold—the vocalis (thyroarytenoid muscle) muscle.

The advantages of TLM include treatment in a single sitting, minimal absence from employment, certainty of removal of the specimen, swallowing problems is rare, tracheostomy is rarely needed, and the ability to assess margins surgically. Importantly, it also allows further laryngeal surgery or radiotherapy in case of recurrence.

Although TLM offers many advantages to the surgeon, there are also important limitations. First, not every patient may be a suitable candidate. Inadequate endoscopic exposure due to dental occlusal deformity, retro or micrognathia or macroglossia may limit the number of patients eligible for endoscopic resection. Anterior commissure lesions are associated with glottis webs postoperatively and voice outcome is not so great compared to radiotherapy.

Classification of endoscopic cordectomy by Remacle M et al. is as follows:

- Subepithelial cordectomy
- Subligamental cordectomy
- Transmuscular cordectomy
- Total cordectomy
- Extended cordectomy:
  - Including contralateral vocal fold
  - Including the arytenoids
  - Including the ventricular fold
  - Including the subglottis.
- Anterior commissurectomy with bilateral anterior cordectomy.

Open voice conservative surgery options include vertical partial laryngectomy (VPL), supraglottic partial laryngectomy, and supracricoid partial laryngectomy. This group of surgeries refers to any procedure which maintains physiologic speech and swallow without need for tracheostomy. The goal is to preserve maximum laryngeal function of deglutition, respiration, phonation, and airway protection without compromising cure rate **(Figs. 1 and 2)**.

The four basic principles of conservative laryngeal surgery are:

1. Must know extent of tumor
2. Preserve cricoarytenoid unit the basic functional unit of larynx
3. Resection of normal tissue is necessary
4. Must consent the patient for total laryngectomy

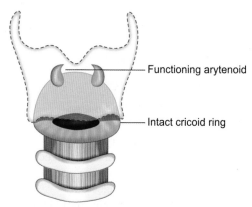

Fig. 1: Schematic diagram showing minimum functioning remnant for a successful voice conservative surgery.

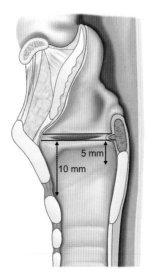

Fig. 2: Schematic diagram showing extent of subglottic spread where partial laryngectomy can be done.

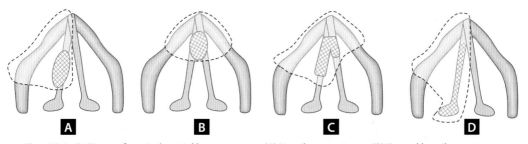

Figs. 3A to D: Types of vertical partial laryngectomy. (A) Hemilaryngectomy; (B) Frontal hemilarygectomy; (C) Frontolateral hemilaryngectomy; (D) Extended hemilarygectomy.

● VERTICAL PARTIAL LARYNGECTOMY

This procedure is rarely done, as the lesions amenable for this procedure can be addressed endoscopically with better functional and similar oncologic results. The extent of resection is dependent on the location of lesion within the glottis, based on the extent of resection. VPL is classified as:

- *Hemilaryngectomy*: For lesion which are limited to vocal cord without anterior commissure or arytenoid involvement **(Fig. 3A)**
- *Frontal hemilaryngectomy*: For lesions with only anterior commissure involvement **(Fig. 3B)**

- *Frontolateral hemilaryngectomy*: For vocal cord lesions with involvement of anterior commissure **(Fig. 3C)**
- *Extended hemilaryngectomy*: For vocal cord lesion involving the arytenoids **(Fig. 3D)**.

Indication

T2 glottic lesions.

Contraindications

- Fixed vocal cord lesions
- Involvement of posterior commissure
- Invasion of arytenoids
- Thyroid cartilage invasion.

● SUPRAGLOTTIC LARYNGECTOMY

Indications

Infrahyoid supraglottic lesions with mobile cords with minimal pre-epiglottic space involvement.

Contraindications

- Extension to petiole of epiglottis to involve anterior commissure, transventricular spread to vocal cord or paraglottis
- Thyroid cartilage involvement
- Anterior commissure involvement
- Vocal cord fixation
- Bilateral arytenoids involvement
- Pyriform apex involvement
- Postcricoid mucosa involvement
- Severe chronic obstructive pulmonary disease (COPD), coronary artery disease (CAD).

Procedure

Under general anesthesia (GA) transverse cervical neck incision is given with tracheostomy site planned separate from the incision. If necessary preliminary tracheostomy is performed, ideally tracheostomy is done just before laryngeal cuts are given. Subplatysmal flaps raised superiorly up to digastric inferiorly up to suprasternal notch. Sternohyoid and sternothyroid muscles are transected in the upper border of the thyroid cartilage to expose the thyroid cartilage. The perichondrium of the thyroid cartilage is incised in the upper border and reflected downward over the upper half of thyroid cartilage. This reflected perichondrium can be used as second layer in the closure. It is critical to preserve the superior laryngeal nerve with its neurovascular bundle. When thyroid cartilage cuts are made, care must be taken to prevent injury to anterior commissure since it results in permanent difficulty in speech and swallowing. The cartilage cuts have to be made at least 1 mm above the estimated level of anterior commissure. The location of anterior commissure varies between males and females. In females, it is located at the junction of upper one-third and lower two-thirds and half way between the thyroid notch and inferior margin in males.

In early tumors, with little or no significant infiltration of pre-epiglottic space the entire hyoid can be preserved by subperiosteal dissection of the pre-epiglottic space which is resected along with the tumor. Preserving hyoid allows more secure closure and hence early rehabilitation. Larynx enters through the valecula after performing a tracheostomy if not previously done. Specimen excised under vision staying above the vocal cords and preserving it. Closure is done from laterally progressing toward center using 1-0 sutures that is passed through thyroid cartilage inferiorly and base of tongue superiorly, if hyoid is preserved sutures are passed around it to secure the closure. The suture line is reinforced using a second layer with the thyroid perichondrium. Drains are placed and wound closed in layers.

Postoperative Care

Nasogastric tube feeds are begun 24–48 hours after surgery. After 4–5 days, decannulation of tracheostomy is tried by changing to metal tube and corking it. After about 7–10 days if wound healing is complete and no signs of pharyngeal leak oral intake is encouraged with swallowing therapy. Return to normal deglutition will take around 2–12 weeks. If aspiration is severe feeding gastrostomy is performed and oral feeding withheld for few days.

● SUPRACRICOID PARTIAL LARYNGECTOMY WITH CRICOHYOIDOEPIGLOTTOPEXY (SCPL-CHEP)

The supracricoid partial laryngectomy (SCPL) includes an en bloc resection of bilateral paraglottic spaces (including the thyroarytenoid musculature), bilateral vocal folds, bilateral vestibular folds, the thyroid cartilage, and at most one arytenoid. Superior part of the resection includes the infrahyoid epiglottis and a portion of the pre-epiglottic space. The suprahyoid third of the epiglottis may be spared and used for reconstruction via CHEP.

Indications

- Early stage T1–T2 glottic, supraglottic, or transglottic cancers that are not suitable to transoral resection (inadequate exposure)
- Select T3 glottic, supraglottic, or transglottic cancers
- Select T4 lesions with thyroid cartilage involvement of the ala, sparing the outer perichondrium.

Contraindications

- Extensive involvement of posterior commissure
- Bilateral arytenoid fixation or extensive mucosal disease
- Extralaryngeal spread
- Invasion of hyoid bone
- Extensive invasion of the pre-epiglottic space to include the epiglottis
- Subglottic extension greater than 10 mm anteriorly, 5 mm laterally, or 2 mm posteriorly
- Massive pre-epiglottic space involvement into the vallecula; lateral pharyngeal wall extension.

Summary of Surgical Steps

- A transverse skin incision
- Subplatysmal flaps are raised exposing the thyroid cartilage
- The trachea is mobilized and released from surrounding tissue to allow the upward mobility
- Tracheotomy
- The thyroid cartilage is released from all lateral attachments

- The cricothyroid joint is disarticulated
- Inferiorly, opening to the endolarynx is got through the cricothyroid membrane
- The thyrohyoid membrane is incised just above the thyroid cartilage (transepiglottic laryngotomy) to complete the resection
- Reconstruction by impaction of cricoid cartilage inferiorly onto hyoid bone and suprahyoid epiglottis remnant superiorly (cricohyoidoepiglottopexy, CHEP) of the pre-epiglottic space to include the epiglottis.

• SUPRACRICOID PARTIAL LARYNGECTOMY WITH CRICOHYOIDOPEXY (SCPL-CHP)

This procedure represents an extension of SCPL-CHEP resection, with added resection of the entire epiglottis and pre-epiglottic space tissue. Reconstruction is performed by cricohyoidopexy (CHP).

Indications

- Early stage T1-T2 glottic, supraglottic, or transglottic cancers not suitable for transoral resection (inadequate exposure)
- Select T3 glottic, supraglottic, or transglottic cancers
- Select T4 lesions with thyroid cartilage ala involvement, sparing outer perichondrium.

Contraindications

- Extensive involvement of posterior commissure
- Bilateral arytenoid fixation or extensive mucosal disease
- Extralaryngeal spread
- Invasion of hyoid bone
- Subglottic extension greater than 10 mm anteriorly, 5 mm laterally, or 2 mm posteriorly
- Massive pre-epiglottic space involvement into the vallecula; lateral pharyngeal wall extension.

Summary of Surgical Steps

- A transverse skin incision
- Subplatysmal flaps are raised exposing upper portion thyroid cartilage
- The trachea is released from surrounding tissue to allow for upward mobilization
- Tracheotomy
- The thyroid cartilage is released from all lateral attachments
- The cricothyroid joint is disarticulated
- Inferiorly, access to the endolarynx is achieved through the cricothyroid membrane
- The thyrohyoid membrane is incised just below the hyoid bone (transvallecular pharyngotomy) to complete the resection
- Reconstruction by impaction of the cricoid cartilage inferiorly onto the hyoid bone and base of tongue superiorly (cricohyoidopexy, CHP).

Postoperative Care

Cuffless tracheostomy tube is used to maintain the airway postoperatively. Intermitted blockage of the tube is encouraged after a week, if tolerating decannulation is tried. Nutrition is maintained by nasogastric tube postoperatively. Swallowing will take days to week with aggressive swallowing therapy.

● NEAR TOTAL LARYNGECTOMY

This surgery is different from voice conservation surgery; in near total laryngectomy (NTL) voice is preserved but not nasal respiration whereas in voice conservation surgery both voice and nasal respiration are preserved. For a conservative laryngeal surgery to be successful laryngeal remnant must have intact cricoid ring and at least one mobile functioning arytenoid. However, when vertical extent of lesion necessitates the resection of the cricoid and one innervated functioning arytenoid is preserved, NTL can be performed.

Indications

- T3/T4 lateralized transglottic lesion of the larynx, with interarytenoid area free. Involvement of contralateral vocal cord, if at all should be such that a voice shunt of adequate size can be created after resection.
- T3/T4 lateralized cancer of the pyriform.
- Sinus with involvement of apex and fixed hemilarynx with interarytenoid, retroarytenoid, and postcricoid area free to enable safe resection preserving the contralateral arytenoid.

Contraindications

- Interarytenoid and postcricoid involvement
- Mucosal involvement of more than one-third of opposite vocal cord.

Procedure

The majority of steps in NTL is similar to that of total laryngectomy, bilateral lateral neck dissection (II–IV) has to be done along with the procedure. Transverse cervical neck incision is planned in such a way to have a separate stoma for side tracheostomy. Skin flap is raised superiorly up to digastric inferiorly up to suprasternal notch. Larynx is skeletonized dividing the straps at the sternal attachment and omohyoid over the internal jugular vein and reflected superiorly to expose the thyroid gland. Next exposure of hyoid and thyroid cartilage is done by dividing the sternohyoid at the hyoid bone; the strap muscles get reflected down on the contralateral side exposing thyroid cartilage after separating the sternothyroid muscles from the oblique line.

Next step is the airway transfer and laryngeal entry; a side tracheostomy is done at a predetermined level with care taken to preserve at least two intact rings above the stoma. Laryngeal entry is now done as in routine laryngectomy, i.e. transvalecullar. Once the lesion is seen the superior thyroid lamina on opposite side is incised preserving the posterior lamina where pharyngeal muscles are inserted ensuring that recurrent laryngeal nerve is not disturbed at the point of entry into larynx. Laryngeal cuts are given with care to preserve one functioning arytenoid and adequate length of vocal cord to create a shunt. The shunt is created by dividing the small wedge of 1st tracheal ring to facilitate closure and continued over a 12 Fr rubber catheter up to the interarytenoid area using interrupted sutures, over which the neopharynx closure is done either with a vertical or T-shaped depending on the amount of mucosa preserved. Tracheostoma is created and wound is closed in layers after placing the drains.

Complications

- Pharyngeal leak
- Shunt stenosis
- Aspiration through the shunt.

● TOTAL LARYNGECTOMY

Indications

- Advanced laryngeal and hypopharyngeal carcinoma with extensive cartilage erosion or significant spread outside the endolarynx into the base of tongue.
- Recurrent or residual laryngeal and hypopharyngeal cancer not amenable for conservation laryngeal surgery after organ preservation radiotherapy or chemoradiotherapy.
- Chondronecrosis of larynx not responding to medical therapy.

Procedure

Under GA transverse cervical neck incision given with stoma planned with the incision or separate from the skin incision. Subplatysmal flaps raised superiorly up to digastrics inferiorly up to suprasternal notch. Open the fascia over the sternocleidomastoid muscle to expose the carotid sheath, the omohyoid muscle dissected and cut using electrocautery. Transect the strap muscles at the sternal attachment to expose the thyroid and divide the thyroid isthmus in midline and reflect laterally with preserved vasculature. Plan the tracheostoma inferiorly at 3rd or 4th ring and change the endotracheal tube to neck if patient was intubated orally.

The constrictor muscles from the thyroid ala is detached using a cautery or scalpel blade. The mucosa of the pyriform sinus on uninvolved side is mobilized for additional mucosa for pharyngeal closure. Suprahyoid muscles are cut and entered into pre-epiglottic space and larynx entered through transvalecullar approach and larynx specimen excised with good margins. Before the closure of the neopharynx cricopharyngeal myotomy is done. Tracheoesophageal prosthesis is placed and neopharynx is closed in layers. Drains are placed and wound is closed in layers.

● ALARYNGEAL SPEECH

The options for speech after a total laryngectomy are:

- *The artificial larynx (electrolarynx):* It is an electronic, battery-powered device that produces vibrations that are transmitted through the external tissues of the neck or cheek or delivered intraorally via a plastic tube into the oral cavity for speech production.
- *Tracheoesophageal voice restoration:* Tracheoesophageal puncture (TEP) is a communication between the trachea and the pharynx. A one way valve that allows the air from the lungs to pass into the pharynx to vibrate it is used. However, the valve does not allow the food or secretions to enter the trachea. The patient closes the stoma to allow the air to enter the pharynx. It may be performed as a primary procedure at the time of total laryngectomy; in other cases,

TEP may be carried out as a secondary procedure at a subsequent time point.

- *Esophageal speech*: The vibratory source is the pharyngoesophageal segment. Oral air that is introduced into the esophagus and expelled past the pharyngoesophageal segment is the driving force for speech production.

● FURTHER READING

1. Laccourreye O. Supracricoid partial laryngectomy with crico hyoidoepiglottopexy for early glottis carcinoma classified as T1-T2 N0 invading the anterior commissure. Am J Otolaryngol. 1997;18(6):385-90.
2. Pradhan S. Voice conservation surgery for laryngeal and hypopharyngeal cancer. New Delhi: Lloyds Publishing House; 2006.

CHAPTER 33

Tracheostomy and Airway Management

Salima Rema Windsor

● INTRODUCTION

Types of surgical airway include:
- Tracheostomy:
  - Open:
    - Cervical
    - Thoracic
  - Percutaneous dilatational tracheostomy
- Cricothyroidotomy.

● TRACHEOSTOMY

Definition

Tracheostomy is the creation of an opening into the trachea. A tracheostomy in its true sense implies that the opening has a connection to an opening in the skin, i.e. creation of a stoma.

Historical Background

Tracheostomy is not a new procedure. It has been depicted in Egyptian tablets dating back to 3600 BC. Asclepiades was recorded as performing the first tracheostomy in 100 BC. Many reputable physicians opposed the procedure due to its high mortality and morbidity. Antonio Musa Brasavola did the first documented case of successful tracheostomy which was published in 1546. In the earlier days trachea was entered through the cricoid cartilage which leads to laryngeal stenosis. It was Chevalier Jackson in 1909 who described the placement of the tracheostomy below the first tracheal ring to avoid this. Due to his contributions in the field he is regarded as the father of modern tracheostomy.

Indications

The conditions that necessitate tracheostomy differ in pediatric and adult population. There are four major indications for tracheostomy.
1. Prolonged ventilation
2. Upper airway obstruction
3. Tracheobronchial toilet
4. Elective.

Prolonged Ventilation

The most common indication for tracheostomy in the current scenario is for prolonged mechanical ventilation in the intensive care setting. The indications for the same include critical illnesses, postoperative complications or head injury. The exact timing of surgery is much debated but should be considered in patients who are unlikely to be extubated within 7 days of intubation. This reduces the irreversible injury to subglottic mucosa from endotracheal tube, allows for pulmonary toilet, and facilitates weaning from mechanical ventilation.

Upper Airway Obstruction

The major causes for upper airway obstruction that demand a tracheostomy in adults are neoplasms of larynx, maxillofacial and neck trauma, infective causes like epiglottitis and abscess, and neurological conditions like bilateral vocal cord paralysis.

Tracheobronchial Toilet

In patients with suppressed cough reflex due to various causes there will be chronic aspiration leading to retained secretions in the tracheobronchial tree. Tracheostomy then allows for suctioning out the secretions and tracheobronchial toilet.

Elective

Tracheostomy may be done as an elective procedure prior to major head and neck surgeries.

Common indications for tracheostomy in children and adults are given in **Table 1**.

Contraindications

Since tracheostomy in most of the cases is a lifesaving procedure there are very few absolute contraindications for conventional tracheostomy. Tracheal stenosis below the site of proposed tracheostomy is an absolute contraindication for the procedure.

Relative contraindication includes severe medically uncorrectable bleeding diathesis where prothrombin time or activated partial thromboplastin time is more than 1.5 times the normal range, platelets below 50,000, and bleeding time more than 10 minutes.

Advantages and Disadvantages

Tracheostomy reduces the anatomical dead space by about 150 mL. This substantially reduces the effort of breathing and airway resistance. This along with better clearance of secretions allows for early weaning off the ventilator. Tracheostomy tube is less irritating to the upper airway than the endotracheal tube and allows the patient to be less sedated. It allows the patient to eat and talk though with a speaking valve.

There are certain disadvantages for the tracheostomy as well. As the airflow bypasses the nose and throat where humidification normally happens unfiltered cold dry air enters the trachea directly. This stimulates the goblet cells in the trachea and disrupts the mucociliary clearance thus producing excess mucus which can block the airway. Also tracheal mucosa undergoes squamous metaplasia over the time.

Table 1: Indications for tracheostomy.

Adult	Pediatric
Neoplasms: • Larynx • Hypopharynx • Oropharynx • Thyroid *Trauma:* • Larynx • Neck • Maxillofacial *Infection:* • Neck abscess • Acute epiglottitis *Others:* • Bilateral abductor paralysis • Foreign body • Angioedema	*Children below 1 year (mostly congenital):* • Subglottic stenosis • Bilateral vocal cord paralysis • Laryngeal cyst • Subglottic hemangioma • Laryngeal web *Children above 1 year:* • Epiglottitis • Acute laryngotracheobronchitis • Diphtheria • Laryngeal edema • Laryngeal trauma • Prolonged intubation • Juvenile laryngeal papillomatosis

The presence of tracheostomy significantly impairs the mechanism of swallowing by splinting the larynx and preventing the upward excursion of larynx. There will be loss of cough reflex following tracheostomy due to inability to generate high intrathoracic pressure. This necessitates the frequent suctioning following tracheostomy. Eventually, the patient develops effective cough and secretions lessen which reduces the need for suctioning.

Procedure

The procedure is performed in emergent, urgent or elective manner. It can be done under local or general anesthesia. The patient is positioned supine with neck extension. The important landmarks like thyroid cartilage, cricoid cartilage, and suprasternal notch are identified and marked. Care should be taken to position the chin, thyroid, and suprasternal notch in the same vertical line.

The Jackson's triangle which is bounded by lower end of thyroid cartilage suprasternal notch and anterior border of sternocleidomastoid on both sides, is infiltrated with 2% lignocaine with adrenaline. The incision can be midline and vertical from the cricoid cartilage to suprasternal notch or horizontal midway between these two landmarks **(Fig. 1)**.

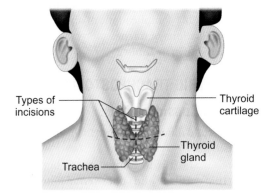

Types of incisions — Thyroid cartilage — Thyroid gland — Trachea

Fig. 1: Skin incisions for tracheostomy.

If the horizontal incisions are made superior and inferior skin flaps are elevated. Further dissection is proceeded in the midline and the strap muscles are retracted. Deep to the strap muscles we can identify the thyroid isthmus in the investing layer of deep cervical fascia. This may be of variable size overlying the second and third tracheal rings. Conventionally, thyroid isthmus is divided. This can be done using diathermy or alternatively it can be clamped, divided and cut edges oversewn and transfixed. Many times this may not be necessary and the isthmus can be dissected and pulled up or down from the trachea. If the trachea is lying low it can be elevated by inserting a cricoid hook under the inferior aspect of cricoid cartilage.

Once trachea is identified and hemostasis is achieved the anesthetist is warned that the surgeon is going to enter the trachea. In an awake patient a further dose of intratracheal infiltration of local anesthetic is given to avoid cough when trachea is incised. Diathermy is avoided further in order to avoid airway fire and patient is ventilated on low flow oxygen. Endotracheal tube is passed downward slightly to avoid inadvertent injury to the cuff.

The trachea is entered between the second and third tracheal ring. The first ring is avoided for fear of late complication of subglottic stenosis. Various options exist for the tracheal opening. They include:

- Vertical cut
- Horizontal incision between the rings
- Removal of a square or circular window of tracheal cartilage centered on second and third tracheal ring
- Bjork flap (inferiorly based U-shaped flap)
- Superiorly based tracheal flap
- H-shaped
- T-shaped
- Cruciate **(Fig. 2)**.

The dead space between the skin and tracheal openings can be avoided by approximating the edges of the tracheal opening to the skin opening with the help of maturation

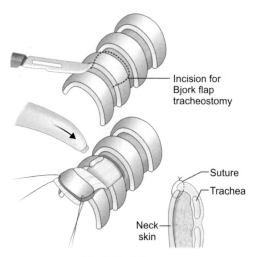

Incision for
Bjork flap
tracheostomy

Suture

Trachea

Neck
skin

Fig. 2: Bjork flap.

sutures. The inferior maturation sutures are most important as they avoid formation of a false track while inserting the tracheostomy tube.

At the end the trachea is cleared of all mucus and blood, and the tracheostomy tube is introduced in a smooth gentle manner. In intubated patient the anesthetist is asked to deflate the cuff and withdraw the endotracheal tube once tracheal lumen is entered. The wound is loosely closed with sutures around the tube. The tube is secured with ties around the neck and sutured to the skin. The suture should be tied snugly in flexed position so as to allow two finger to pass underneath it. The wound is covered with a dressing.

Postoperative Care

Care of a tracheostomized patient requires diligence and patience.

The tracheostomy tube should be kept for 2–3 days before it can be changed as this allows the formation of the tract and as far as possible should be changed by the surgeon who did the tracheostomy.

- A fresh tracheostomy tube and dilator must be kept by the side of the patient.

- As patient cannot speak an alerting device like a bell must be kept by the side.
- Inner tube must be removed and cleaned every 2 hours for the first 48 hours; later, it can be cleaned every 4 hours.
- Cuff pressure should be maintained at 20–25 mm Hg and cuff should be deflated every 2 hours for 10 minutes after proper suctioning of the tube and pharynx.
- Regular suction should be performed with premeasured suction tubes of adequate diameter [2 x (size of tracheostomy tube -2)].
  - Suction pressure—small children 50–100 mm Hg, older children or adults 100–120 mm Hg (or use Y connector)
  - Separate suction tubes for trachea and pharynx
  - Suck only during withdrawal
  - Anesthetize trachea before suction
  - Soften crusts before suction.
- Humidification of inhaled air should be done to avoid tracheitis and crust formation.
- Chest physiotherapy is given to remove accumulated secretions.
- Skin dressing should be changed every day with sterile gauze and antibiotic cream to avoid wound infection.
- Mucolytics and expectorants for management of cough.

Complications of Tracheostomy

Tracheostomy is a safe procedure but still carries a risk for complications of about 5–40%. The complications of tracheostomy fall into the categories shown in **Table 2**.

● PEDIATRIC TRACHEOSTOMY

Anatomic Considerations

Neck of a child differs from adult in the following aspects:

- Neck is short with limited space between thyroid cartilage and suprasternal notch.
- Dome of pleura is easily pulled into the neck with minimal extension.

Table 2: Complications of tracheostomy.

Immediate	Intermediate	Late
• Anesthetic complications • Hemorrhage: 　– Veins: 　　♦ Anterior jugular 　　♦ Jugular venous arch 　　♦ Internal jugular 　– Arteries: 　　♦ Carotids 　　♦ Thyroid arteries 　　♦ Brachiocephalic (children) • Air embolism • Apnea • Cardiac arrest • False passage • Local damage: 　– Thyroid cartilage 　– Cricoid cartilage 　– Recurrent laryngeal nerve 　– Esophagus • Pulmonary edema (POPE)	• Tube obstruction by secretions and crust • Tube displacement • Surgical emphysema • Pneumothorax/ pneumomediastinum • Infection: 　– Tracheitis 　– Tracheobronchitis 　– Stomal 　– Pneumonia 　– Lung abscess 　– Mediastinitis 　– Clavicular/sternal osteomyelitis 　– Necrotizing fasciitis • Tracheoesophageal fistula • Atelectasis • Dysphagia	• Tracheocutaneous fistula • Tracheal stenosis • Laryngeal stenosis • Tracheomalacia • Difficult decannulation • Trachea-innominate artery fistula • Tracheoarterial fistula: 　– Innominate 　– Common carotid 　– Aorta (in aneurysm) • Granuloma formation • Unsightly scar and keloid • Broken tubes (foreign body) • Difficult decannulation: 　– Original pathology 　– Tracheal stenosis 　– Laryngeal stenosis 　– Tracheomalacia 　– Granuloma 　– Psychological dependence 　– Physiological dependence • Depression

- Trachea is soft and pliable and difficult to palpate.
- Cricoid is very soft and difficult to distinguish.

Choice of the Tracheostomy Tube

The correct choice of the tracheostomy tube is extremely important in order to avoid damage to tracheal mucosa. The pediatric tracheostomy tubes are usually cuffless.

Behl and Watt found that the size of the tube can be conveniently calculated by the following formula:

- Inner diameter (mm) = age in years/3 + 3.5
- Outer diameter (mm) = age in years/3 + 5.5

Premature neonates less than 1,000 g	2.5 mm
Premature neonates more than 1,000 g	3.0 mm
Neonates or infants 0–6 months	3.0–3.5 mm

As the child grows tube size need to be adjusted.

Procedure

The following precautions have to be taken in pediatric tracheostomy:

- Head extension facilitated by a chin strap and shoulder bag.
- Horizontal incision preferred.
- Removal of subcutaneous fat with diathermy to improve visibility.
- Lateral stay sutures with nonabsorbable sutures before incising the trachea. This can be used to apply traction and expose trachea during surgery, also can be lifesaving should accidental decannulation occur before stomal maturation.
- Vertical incision of the trachea is preferred and avoids removal of cartilage.
- Stomal maturation sutures from tracheal edge and skin edge using resorbable sutures is important.
- Label the stay sutures right and left and it should be taped to the chest with label a "DO NOT REMOVE".

● TYPES OF TRACHEOSTOMY TUBES

Cuffed and Noncuffed Tubes

A cuffed tracheostomy tube maintains a closed circuit for ventilation. It also protects the airway from the risk of aspiration especially when there is significant bleeding. Cuff pressure should be maintained within a range of 20–25 mm Hg and should be checked at least twice a day. Cuffed tubes bear the disadvantage of causing tracheal necrosis and granulation. Cuff should be deflated when the patient uses speaking valve. Pediatric tubes are usually cuffless to reduce the risk of tracheal stenosis.

Fenestrated and Unfenestrated

Fenestrated have openings in the outer cannula that allow the air to be directed to the oral cavity and nasopharynx. This movement of air allows the patient to speak and produce more effective cough. However, it is associated with the risk of aspiration. So patients with high risk of aspiration and those on positive pressure ventilation cannot use this type of tubes or they should use a nonfenestrated inner cannula along with this.

Single and Double Lumen Tubes

A single lumen tube decreases the airway resistance by maximizing the inner diameter. But this tube gets blocked easily and the whole tube will have to be changed every 5–7 days. Double lumen tubes have an outer cannula that maintains the airway and an inner cannula that can be removed for cleaning. Patients with tracheostomy should ideally be discharged from the hospital with an uncuffed double lumen tube. The presence of inner cannula decreases the diameter by 1–1.5 mm thus increasing the airway resistance.

Special Tubes

Some tubes may have extra length either horizontally or vertically. Tubes with extra horizontal length are used for patients with deep trachea such as obese patients or those with distorted anatomy due to edema or tumors. The tubes with extra vertical length are used in patients with tracheal stenosis, granulation or tracheomalacia. Some tubes have adjustable flanges to allow bedside adjustments of length of the tube. Some have a built in tubing to allow for suctioning out secretions that accumulate above the cuff. This helps in preventing microaspirations and ventilator-associated pneumonia.

● PERCUTANEOUS DILATATIONAL TRACHEOSTOMY

Percutaneous dilatational tracheostomy (PDT) is a bedside procedure usually done in the intensive care unit on intubated patients. PDT over a guidewire was first performed by Ciaglia in 1985. PDT has now become the standard of care in ICU and has replaced surgical tracheostomy in a large subset of patients.

Indications

Percutaneous dilatational tracheostomy in ICU is classically indicated in following situations to facilitate weaning in difficult to wean patients.
- Tracheobronchial toilet
- Reduce sedation
- Anticipated prolonged ventilator stay
- To protect airway from the risk of aspiration.

Percutaneous dilatational tracheostomy is generally avoided as an emergency intervention procedure unless performed by a very experienced surgeon. In case of emergency, cricothyroidotomy is considered as the procedure of choice. Contraindications of PDT are summarized in **Table 3**.

PDT versus Surgical Tracheostomy

The potential benefits of PDT over surgical tracheostomy include:
- Avoid transfer to theatre
- Less operating time

Table 3: Contraindications of percutaneous dilatational tracheostomy.

Absolute	Relative

• Infants
• Infection at tracheostomy site
• Operator inexperience
• Unstable cervical spine injuries
• Uncontrollable coagulopathies
	• Enlarged thyroid
	• Presence of pulsatile vessels at the site
	• High riding innominate artery
	• History of previous tracheostomy
	• *Difficult anatomy:*
	   – Short neck
	   – Morbid obesity
	   – Limited extension of neck
	   – Local malignancy
	• Need for positive end expiratory pressure more than 10 cm of water

■ Fewer intra- and postoperative complications

■ Better cosmesis

■ Reduced incidence of wound infection.

Techniques of PDT

The method is based on Seldinger technique of passing a guidewire to create a passage into trachea and then it is serially dilated or it is gradually dilated using a single tapered horn like dilator.

Ciaglia Serial Dilatational Technique

Ciaglia et al. in 1985 did the first PDT using multiple serial dilators over a guidewire. This procedure has undergone three basic changes since then in terms of levels of tracheal insertion, use of bronchoscopic guidance, and use of a single tapered dilator. Site of insertion moved caudally from cricoid cartilage by one or two tracheal rings.

Ciaglia Single Dilatational Technique

This is popularly known as Ciaglia blue rhino. It was introduced in 1999 more than a decade after initial description of PDT. This involves a much simpler kit. This entails the use of single bevelled hydrophilic dilator. Use of single dilator is associated with less tidal volume loss during the procedure as we need not remove the dilator in between.

Other Techniques

■ Griggs percutaneous technique

■ Balloon dilatational technique (Ciaglia blue dolphin).

Procedural Adjuncts

Bronchoscopy

It has advantage of real time confirmation of needle placement, midline position of needle, tube placement, and avoidance of injury to posterior tracheal wall.

Ultrasound

This is a readily available bedside modality which is especially useful in patients who are morbidly obese and have anatomical abnormalities of neck. This is used to assess the depth of trachea and to identify the tracheal rings. Preoperative identification of aberrant vessels and thyroid isthmus with ultrasound helps to avoid complications.

Cricothyroidotomy

Cricothyroidotomy is an emergent airway procedure done on patients with severe respiratory distress in whom orotracheal or nasotracheal intubation has failed. While cricothyroidotomy may be life-saving in extreme circumstances this technique is intended as temporizing measure until a definite airway is established. There are three main approaches for cricothyroidotomy. In all the approaches the airway is entered through the cricothyroid membrane in the cricothyroid space between cricoid and thyroid cartilage.

Needle Cricothyroidotomy

An angiocatheter is introduced through the cricothyroid space and after withdrawing the needle, catheter can be attached to jet ventilation device.

Percutaneous Cricothyroidotomy (Seldinger Technique)

The airway tube is inserted over a guidewire as we do for PDT.

Surgical Cricothyroidotomy

In this we incise the skin over cricothyroid membrane and airway is entered after incising the cricothyroid membrane.

Rapid Four-step Technique

This requires a scalpel, tracheal hook and a tracheostomy tube. The four steps in this being palpation, stab incision, inferior tracheal traction, and tube insertion. This is faster than standard surgical technique.

Thoracic Tracheostomy

This is done in patients with cervical tracheal stenosis caused by unresectable advanced tumors. This mandates the partial resection of manubrium and clavicle head to approach the uninvolved region of thoracic trachea.

● FURTHER READING

1. Cheung NH, Napolitano LM. Tracheostomy: epidemiology, indication, timing, technique, and outcomes. Respir Care. 2014;59(6):895-915.
2. Cipriano A, Mao ML, Hon HH. An overview of complications associated with open and percutaneous tracheostomy procedures. Int J Crit Illn Inj Sci. 2015;5(3):179-88.
3. Mallick A, Bodenham AR. Tracheostomy in critically ill patients. Eur J Anaesthesiol. 2010;27(8):676-82.

CHAPTER 34

Guidelines in the Management of Carcinoma of the Nasopharynx

Pushpaja KU

● INTRODUCTION

Nasopharyngeal carcinoma arises from the epithelial lining of the nasopharynx, the cuboidal space, behind the nasal cavity. It differs from other head and neck squamous cell carcinomas in epidemiology, etiology, histology, and response to treatment.

● ANATOMY

The nasopharynx is an open space that begins just behind the choana and slopes downward along the airway to the level of the soft palate. The nasal cavity forms the anterior relation via the choana, and inferiorly it continues into the oropharynx. The roof and the posterior wall are formed by the basiocciput, basisphenoid, the clivus, and the first cervical vertebra. The floor is formed by the superior surface of the soft palate. The Eustachian tube opening lies on the lateral wall of the nasopharynx. The posterior portion of the cartilaginous Eustachian tube protrudes into the nasopharynx, making an elevation called the torus tubarius. Posterior to the torus lies a recess called the fossa of Rosenmüller.

Various foramina and fissures located in the base of the skull form important passage for the spread of nasopharyngeal carcinoma (NPC) intracranially and involve cranial nerves. The most important among these are the foramen lacerum and the foramen ovale, which lie in close anatomic relationship with the cavernous sinus and the cranial nerves III–VI in its lateral wall.

● LYMPHATIC DRAINAGE

The nasopharynx is richly supplied by lymphatics, particularly in the roof and in the posterior and lateral walls. These lymphatic channels form have three major pathways:

1. One path is via the lateral pharyngeal wall to the lateral pharyngeal (parapharyngeal) nodes in the lateral pharyngeal or retroparotid space. The uppermost and most prominent of this group of nodes is the lateral retropharyngeal node of Rouvière.

2. From these lateral pharyngeal nodes, efferent channels drain into the jugular chain, especially to the jugulodigastric (subdigastric) nodes. Few lymphatic channels may bypass the lateral pharyngeal wall and drain directly to the jugulodigastric node.

3. Another route is by direct channel to the posterior triangle nodes and the spinal accessory nodes.

● EPIDEMIOLOGY

Nasopharyngeal carcinoma displays a distinct racial and geographical distribution. Nasopharyngeal cancer is endemic disease in Southern China, Southeast Asia, North Africa, and the Arctic, where undifferentiated nonkeratinizing variety is the predominant histology. The major etiological factors for endemic NPC are multifactorial such as genetic susceptibility, early-age exposure to chemical carcinogens, and Epstein–Barr virus (EBV) infection. The male-to-female ratio is 2.5:1. In low-risk populations, a bimodal age distribution has been observed. The first peak incidence is reported at 15–25 and the second peak at 50–59 years of age. In contrast, the incidence in high-risk populations increases after 30 years of age, peaks at 40–60 years, and drops thereafter.

● ETIOLOGY

The cause of NPC is attributed to many factors: EBV infection, genetic predisposition, and environmental factors such as the high intake of preserved food and smoking.

In general causative factors are:
- *Viral:* EBV has long been linked with NPC.
- *Genetic:* Genetic factors may affect the risk of NPC. Nasopharyngeal carcinoma has been associated with certain specific human leukocyte antigen (HLA) haplotypes. Nasopharyngeal carcinoma has also been related with genetic polymorphisms, such as cYP2A6, which is a polymorphism of a nitrosamine metabolizing gene. Copy number losses on chromosomes 1p, 3p, 9p, 9q, 11q, 13q, 14q, and 16q, and recurrent gains on chromosome 1q, 3q, 8q, 12p, and 12q are frequently detected in NPC.
- *Environmental:* Various environmental factors such as improper ventilation, occupational exposures to smoke or dusts, and diet have been implicated.
- *Diet:* Several dietary practices in endemic areas are believed to contribute to the high incidence of NPC. The cooking of salt-cured food, releases volatile nitrosamines that are transmitted by steam and distributed over the nasopharyngeal mucosa. High intake of preserved or fermented foods, including meats, eggs, fruits, and vegetables, which contain high levels of nitrosamines.
- Smoking has also been implicated as a factor in NPC.

● PATHOLOGY

According to the World Health Organization (WHO) classification of NPC, the various pathologic types are given in **Table 1**.

● ROUTES OF SPREAD

Local Extension

Anteriorly, direct spread into the nasal cavity is common. Extension beyond the lateral wall of the nasal cavity may lead to destruction of the pterygoid plates. Invasion of the posterior ethmoid, and maxillary sinuses is less commonly seen. Orbital invasion may occur in advanced disease. Superiorly and posteriorly, the tumor may directly erode the base of the skull, the sphenoid sinus, and the clivus. The foramen lacerum, located directly above Rosenmüller fossa, is a weak area in the base of the skull, through which the tumor can spread into the cavernous sinus and the middle cranial

Table 1: Classification of nasopharyngeal carcinoma.

WHO classification	Former terminology
Keratinizing squamous cell carcinoma	WHO type I (squamous cell carcinoma)
Nonkeratinizing carcinoma*:	
• Differentiated	WHO type II (transitional cell carcinoma)
• Undifferentiated	WHO Type III (lymphoepithelial carcinoma)
Basaloid squamous cell carcinoma	No synonym exists

(WHO: World Health Organization)
*Nonkeratinizing carcinoma is the commonest type of NPC, accounting for 95% in endemic areas

fossa and invade cranial nerves II–VI. Tumor can also extend through the foramen ovale into the middle cranial fossa, the petrous part of the temporal bone, and the cavernous sinus. Inferiorly, direct extension into the oropharynx is not uncommon involving the tonsillar pillars, the tonsillar fossa, and the lateral and posterior oropharyngeal walls. Invasion of the c1 vertebra posteriorly and inferiorly is observed in advanced disease. Direct invasion of the soft palate is rare. Lateral spread into the lateral parapharyngeal space and invasion of the levator and tensor veli palatini muscles can occur early in the disease. Invasion of the pterygoid muscles usually occurs in more advanced disease. Direct tumor extension or lateral retropharyngeal lymph node metastasis in the parapharyngeal space may cause compression or invasion of cranial nerve XII at its exit point through the hypoglossal canal, cranial nerves IX–XI as they emerge from the jugular foramen, and the cervical sympathetic nerves. Compression or direct invasion of the internal carotid artery may also occur in advanced disease. Through the Eustachian tube, tumor can directly gain access to the middle ear.

Lymphatic Spread

Lymphatic spread to the ipsilateral cervical nodes is common and is observed in 85–90% of cases. Bilateral neck nodes are seen in approximately 50% of cases. Spread to the lateral and posterior retropharyngeal lymph nodes occurs early in the disease. Metastasis to the jugulodigastric and superior posterior cervical nodes is also fairly common. From these first echelon nodes, further metastasis to the midjugular and posterior cervical, lower jugular, and posterior cervical and supraclavicular nodes may occur. Occasionally, spread to the submental and occipital nodes occurs because of lymphatic obstruction caused by extensive cervical lymphadenopathy. Metastasis to the mediastinal lymph nodes can occur when supraclavicular lymphadenopathy is present, and occasionally there may be metastasis to the axillary nodes as well.

Hematogenous Spread

Distant metastasis is present in 3% of the cases at presentation and may develop in 18–50% or more of cases during the course of the disease. The incidence of distant metastasis is maximum in patients with advanced neck node metastasis, particularly in the low neck. Bone is the commonly involved distant metastatic site followed by the lungs and liver.

● CLINICAL PRESENTATION

The most frequent presenting complaint in patients with NPC is mass in the neck, due to cervical node metastases. Cervical lymphadenopathy has been observed in 87% of patients. Other common symptoms comprise epistaxis, unilateral hearing loss, nasal obstruction, nasal discharge, headache and facial pain, trismus, and cranial nerve deficits. Most commonly involved nerves are 5th and 6th cranial nerves. Distant metastasis at presentation is detected in approximately 3% of cases. The bones, lungs, and liver are the most common distant metastatic sites.

Tumor–Node–Metastasis Staging [American Joint Cancer Committee (AJCC), 8th Edition]

Major changes are **(Table 2):**

- *Definition of primary tumor (T):*
  - T0 is added for EBV positive unknown primary with cervical lymph node involvement. The stage group is defined in the same way as TI (or TX).
  - Adjacent muscles involvement (including medial pterygoid, lateral pterygoid, and prevertebral muscles) is now designated as T2.

Table 2: TNM staging nasopharynx cancers (AJCC, 8th edition).

T Stage	
TX	Primary tumor cannot be assessed.
T0	No tumor identified, but EBV-positive cervical node(s) involvement.
T1	Tumor confined to nasopharynx, or extension to oropharynx and/or nasal cavity without parapharyngeal involvement.
T2	Tumor with extension to parapharyngeal space, and/or adjacent soft tissue involvement (medial pterygoid, lateral pterygoid, and prevertebral muscles).
T3	Tumor with infiltration of bony structures at skull base, cervical vertebra, pterygoid structures, and/or paranasal sinuses.
T4	Tumor with intracranial extension, involvement of cranial nerves, hypopharynx, orbit, parotid gland, and/or extensive soft tissue infiltration beyond the lateral surface of the lateral pterygoid muscle.
Clinical N (cN)	
NX	Regional lymph nodes cannot be assessed.
N0	No regional lymph node metastasis.
N1	Unilateral metastasis in cervical lymph node(s) and/or unilateral or bilateral metastasis in retropharyngeal lymph node(s), 6 cm or smaller in greatest dimension, above the caudal border of cricoid cartilage.
N2	Bilateral metastasis in cervical lymph node(s), 6 cm or smaller in greatest dimension, above the caudal border of cricoid cartilage.
N3	Unilateral or bilateral metastasis in cervical lymph node(s), larger than 6 cm in greatest dimension, and/or extension below the caudal border of cricoid cartilage.
Distant metastasis M	
M0	No distant metastasis
M1	Distant metastasis

(AJCC: American Joint Cancer Committee; EBV: Epstein–Barr virus)

- The previous T4 criteria "masticator space" and "infratemporal fossa" is now replaced by specific description of soft tissue involvement to avoid ambiguity.
- *Definition of regional lymph nodes (N):*
  - The previous N3b criterion of supraclavicular fossa is now changed to lower neck (as defined by nodal extension below the caudal border of the cricoid cartilage).
  - N3a and N3b are merged into a single N3 category, which is now defined as unilateral or bilateral metastasis in cervical lymph node(s), larger than 6 cm in greatest dimension, and/or extension below the caudal border of cricoid cartilage.

- *AJCC prognostic stage groups* **(Table 3)**:
  - The previous sub-stages IVA (T4N0-2M0) and IVB (any T N3. MO) are now merged to form IVA.
  - The previous IVC (any T any N MI) is now upstaged to IVB.

● DIAGNOSIS

A definitive diagnosis is arrived at by nasopharyngoscopy and biopsy of the primary tumor in the nasopharynx. Thorough physical examination should include careful palpation of the neck, cranial nerve examination, percussion and auscultation of the chest, palpation of the abdomen for possible liver involvement, and percussion of the spine and bones for possible

Table 3: AJCC prognostic stage groups.

When T is ...	And N is ...	And M is ...	Then the stage group is ...
Tis	N0	M0	0
T1	N0	M0	I
T1, T0	N1	M0	II
T2	N0	M0	II
T2	N1	M0	II
T1, T0	N2	M0	III
T2	N2	M0	III
T3	N0	M0	III
T3	N1	M0	III
T3	N2	M0	III
T4	N0	M0	IVA
T4	N1	M0	IVA
T4	N2	M0	IVA
Any T	N3	M0	IVA
Any T	Any N	M1	IVB

(AJCC: American Joint Cancer Committee)

bone metastasis. Routine assessment should include chest radiograph, complete blood counts, and serum biochemistry, including liver function tests and alkaline phosphatase.

Both MRI and CT scans are suitable in diagnostic imaging of the nasopharynx. MRI and CT scans can also detect lymph node metastasis that is not evident on clinical examination. MRI is better than CT for displaying both superficial and deep nasopharyngeal soft tissue detail. MRI is found to be more sensitive for assessment of retropharyngeal and deep cervical nodal metastases. However, it is of limited effectiveness for assessing bone details, and CT scan should be done when the status of the base of the skull cannot be satisfactorily recognized with MRI. In terms of staging, MRI is valuable in detecting marrow infiltration by tumors for patients with clinical or biochemical evidence of distant metastases or otherwise considered at high risk for distant metastases (advanced nodal stage, N3), further imaging with bone scan, CT of chest and upper abdomen or FDG PET-CT imaging may be required.

EBV Biomarkers

The titer levels of immunoglobulin A antibodies to EBV viral capsid antigen (IgA VCA) and early antigen (IgA EA) have been widely used as screening and diagnostic markers for NPC, even though these markers lack specificity. IgA VCA/EA levels usually remain raised even after disease remission is achieved. EBV DNA quantitative testing using a real-time polymerase chain reaction technique is very sensitive and specific for NPC and correlates well with tumor burden. Pretreatment plasma EBV DNA levels have been shown to complement TNM staging, and elevated posttreatment EBV DNA levels at 6 weeks is a powerful prognosticator of recurrence and survival. EBV DNA may be used clinically to monitor disease response and recurrence in the future.

● GENERAL TREATMENT PRINCIPLES

Radiation therapy (RT) is the mainstay of treatment for nasopharyngeal cancer. Surgery of the primary site is not used as first-line treatment because of the deep, complex anatomical location of the nasopharynx and its close proximity to critical neurovascular structures. On the other hand, neck dissection may be indicated after RT for residual nodal disease or for an isolated neck recurrence. Surgery has also been used to salvage certain patients with locally recurrent disease.

T1N0M0 cases are treated with RT alone with good locoregional control. Five-year overall survival rates of 90% for stage I have been reported in the literature.

Concurrent chemoradiotherapy followed by adjuvant chemotherapy has been recommended for T1N1-3, T2–T4, and any N lesions.

The United States Intergroup 0099 trial was the first to demonstrate a beneficial outcome from concurrent and adjuvant chemoradiotherapy for the management of locoregionally advanced nasopharyngeal cancer. In this trial, 193 patients with stage III and IV nasopharyngeal cancer were randomly assigned to two arms—concurrent chemoradiotherapy followed by adjuvant chemotherapy or RT alone. RT schedule consisted of 70 Gy in 35–39 fractions of 1.8–2.0 Gy daily. Chemotherapy included cisplatin (100 mg/m^2 on days 1, 22, and 43) concurrent with RT followed by adjuvant cisplatin (80 mg/m^2 on day 1) and fluorouracil (1000 mg/m^2 daily, days 1–4) repeated every 4 weeks for three cycles. Based upon interim analysis of 147 patients, concurrent chemoradiotherapy and adjuvant chemotherapy was shown to significantly increase 3-year progression-free survival compared with RT alone (69 versus 24%) and overall survival (78 versus 47%). This benefit persevered at 5 years of follow-up.

Chemotherapy (platinum-based) alone or combined with radiation is used for palliation of metastatic disease.

Radiation Therapy

All patients should undergo dental prophylaxis and extraction prior to commencement of RT. They should be advised to stop/abstain from smoking and drinking alcohol. Dietician consultation and relevant instructions regarding nutrition should be given.

CT simulation is used for computerized treatment planning. The patient is made to lie in a supine position with head extended. A customized thermoplastic mask covering the head to shoulder region is used to immobilize the patient. CT images indexed every 3 mm are obtained, extending from the vertex to carina. The target volumes and normal tissue structures are defined using CT images, supplemented with fused diagnostic MRI and/or PET scans.

Tumor Target Volumes

The gross tumor volume (GTV) includes the primary nasopharyngeal tumor and involved lymph nodes as shown by clinical, endoscopic, and radiologic examinations **(Fig. 1)**. The clinical target volume (CTV) covers the GTV, microscopic infiltration and anatomic structures at risk. The CTV targeted at 70 Gy (CTV_70) includes the GTV with a 5–10 mm margin. The CTV targeted at 60 Gy (CTV_60) covers high-risk proximal structures (including the parapharyngeal spaces, posterior third of nasal cavities and maxillary sinuses, pterygoid processes, base of skull, lower half of sphenoid sinus, anterior half of the clivus, and petrous tips), and lymphatic regions (including bilateral retropharyngeal nodes, levels II, III, and VA) **(Fig. 2)**. The CTV targeted at 50 Gy (CTV_50) covers the remaining levels IV–VB. The level I nodes may be spared for patients with N0 disease.

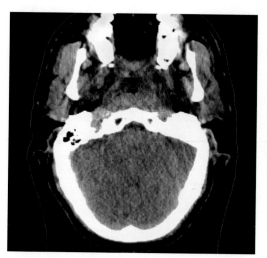

Fig. 1: Computed tomography simulation images showing tumor in the nasopharynx.

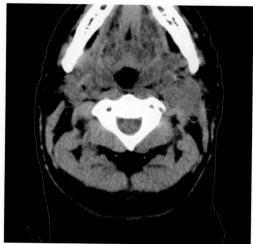

Fig. 2: Computed tomography simulation images showing bilateral level II lymph nodes.

The planning target volume (PTV) comprises of the CTV and the margin needed for systemic and random setup variations.

Dose

Recommended dose is 70 Gy to the gross tumor and nodes, 66 Gy to entire nasopharynx, 60 Gy to high-risk subclinical region and 50 Gy to low-risk subclinical uninvolved nodal region in conventional 2 Gy fractions daily, five fractions in a week schedule.

Intensity-modulated radiation therapy (IMRT) has replaced conventional radiotherapy in the treatment of NPC in many centers throughout the world. With this technique, radiation beams can be modulated in such a manner so that a high dose can be delivered to the tumor with improved target volume coverage while significantly decreasing the dose to the surrounding normal tissues. Two randomized studies have reported that IMRT is superior to conventional 3D-CRT in preserving parotid function and thus resulting in less xerostomia without compromising local control in patients with early stage NPC. Together with

concurrent chemotherapy, all IMRT series have reported excellent results, with local control exceeding 90% at 2–5 years **(Figs. 3 and 4)**.

Treatment-related Complications

Mucositis is the main acute toxicity associated with RT for NPC. Chemotherapy further exacerbates this toxicity and adds the adverse effects of neuropathy, emesis, neutropenia, and other hematologic toxicity. Xerostomia was by far the most common sequel reported with conventional radiotherapy. Dental problems, as a consequence of decreased saliva and altered salivary consistency, occurred in 4–17% of patients treated with conventional radiotherapy. Two randomized trials have revealed the superiority of IMRT over conventional radiotherapy for early-stage NPC in terms of improved salivary function as well as patient quality of life. Other treatment-related complications observed are trismus, Lhermitte's syndrome, temporal lobe necrosis, skull base osteoradionecrosis, pituitary dysfunction, hypothyroidism, carotid stenosis, hearing impairment, and radiation-induced second cancers.

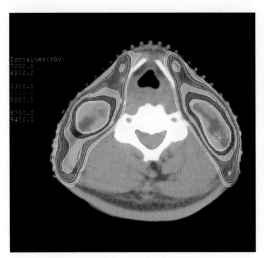

Fig. 3: Intensity-modulated radiation therapy plan showing delineation of target volumes (cTV), the dose distribution, sparing of brainstem, parotids and temporomandibular joints.

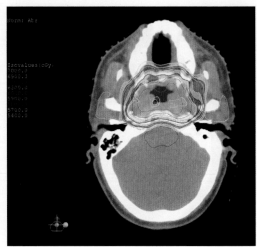

Fig. 4: Intensity-modulated radiation therapy plan showing the dose distribution in the gross lymph node region and bilateral level III, V lymph node region with sparing of larynx and spinal cord.

Follow-up: Periodic clinical and endoscopic examination of nasopharynx and neck is needed to document complete remission of disease. PETCT or MRI for assessment of disease may be scheduled at 3 months post-radiation.

● FURTHER READING

1. Al-Sarraf M, LeBlanc M, Giri PG, et al. Chemoradiotherapy versus radiotherapy in patients with advanced nasopharyngeal cancer: Phase III randomized Intergroup study 0099. J clin Oncol. 1998;16(4):1310-7.

2. Al-Sarraf M, LeBlanc M, Giri PG, et al. Superiority of five year survival with chemoradiotherapy (CT-radiotherapy) vs radiotherapy in patients (Pts) with locally advanced nasopharyngeal cancer (NPC). Intergroup (0099) (SWOG 8892, RTOG 8817, ECOG 2388) phase III study: Final Report. Proc Am Soc Clin Oncol. 2001;20:abstract 905.

4. Chan AT. Nasopharyngeal carcinoma. Ann Oncol. 2010;21(Suppl 7):vii308-12.

6. Kam MK, Leung SF, Zee B, et al. Prospective randomized study of intensity-modulated radiotherapy on salivary gland function in early-stage nasopharyngeal carcinoma patients. J Clin Oncol. 2007;25(31):4873-9.

7. Lee AW, Lin JC, Ng WT. Current management of nasopharyngeal cancer. Semin Radiat Oncol. 2012;22(3):233-44.

8. Lee N, Harris J, Garden AS, et al. Intensity-modulated radiation therapy with or without chemotherapy for nasopharyngeal carcinoma: Radiation therapy oncology group phase II trial 0225. J Clin Oncol. 2009;27(22):3684-90.

9. Pfister DG, Spencer S, Brizel DM, et al.; National Comprehensive Cancer Network. Head and neck cancers, Version 2.2014. Clinical practice guidelines in oncology. J Natl Compr Canc Netw. 2014;12(10):1454-87.

10. Pow EH, Kwong DL, McMillan AS, et al. Xerostomia and quality of life after intensity-modulated radiotherapy vs. conventional radiotherapy for early-stage nasopharyngeal carcinoma: Initial report on a randomized controlled clinical trial. Int J Radiat Oncol Biol Phys. 2006;66(4):981-91.

11. Sun X, Su S, Chen C, et al. Long-term outcomes of intensity-modulated radiotherapy for 868 patients with nasopharyngeal carcinoma: An analysis of survival and treatment toxicities. Radiother Oncol. 2014;110(3):398-403.

General Topics

Chapters

Section 7

General Topics

Chapters

CHAPTER 35

Melanoma and Nonmelanoma Skin Cancers

Divya GM

• INTRODUCTION

Skin cancer is the most common malignancy occurring in humans and it can be divided into two categories—melanoma and nonmelanoma skin cancer (NMSC). The term NMSC practically refers to keratinocyte carcinomas, namely basal cell carcinoma (BCC) and squamous cell carcinoma (SCC), since they account for the 99% of the tumors in this group. The incidence of both has been increasing over the past decades. Currently, between 2 and 3 million nonmelanoma skin cancers and 132,000 melanoma skin cancers occur globally each year. These malignancies can be the source of significant patient morbidity and mortality depending on the histology, stage, and risk features.

• MELANOMA

Melanoma is a malignancy of melanocytes. It accounts for 5% of all skin cancers, but is responsible for >75% of skin cancer-related deaths. Thus, melanoma is the most aggressive form of skin cancer, and it is likely to be an increasingly prevalent problem in the future.

Epidemiology

Melanoma is much more common in whites than in other ethnic groups. The lifetime risk of developing melanoma is about 2.4% in Caucasians, 0.1% in Blacks, and 0.5% in Hispanics. The highest incidence rates have been reported in New Zealand with 50 cases per 100,000 persons and Australia with 48 cases per 100,000 persons. A slight male predominance is consistently reported and the median age of diagnosis is 55 years. Approximately 25% of all cutaneous melanomas arise in the head and neck region, the commonest site being the face. The scalp and ears are the next most common sites of presentation, followed by the skin of the neck.

Risk Factors

Sun and Ultraviolet Light Exposure

Intermittent and intense exposure to sunlight increases the chances of developing melanoma. History of blistering or peeling sunburns, especially during childhood, is at particular risk. Sunbeds and tanning booths are associated with early-onset melanoma, with increasing risk associated with early age of first use as well as with greater use. The first use of a tanning bed before 35 years of age increases the risk for melanoma by up to 75%.

Skin Type

Fair skinned people are at greater risk of developing melanoma. It is rare in non-white people, with 10–20 times less risk.

The phenotype of fair skin, freckling, and red hair has been linked to polymorphisms in the *MC1R* gene, which encodes the melanocortin-1 receptor. These polymorphisms will ultimately result in decreased melanin production.

Family History

Approximately 10% of melanomas are familial and these melanomas are associated with a very early age of onset, frequently in areas without ultraviolet radiation (UVR) exposure. The most common genetic feature in these families is germline deletion or inactivating mutation of the CDKN2A gene on chromosome 9. Inherited photosensitivity disorders such as xeroderma pigmentosum are also associated with a high incidence of melanoma.

Multiple or Dysplastic Nevi

The risk of melanoma is increased in individuals with a large number of moles. Those with more than 100 nevi are seven times more likely to develop melanoma compared to those having less than 15. In people with more than five atypical or dysplastic nevi, there is an increased risk of six fold compared to those with none.

Congenital Nevi

Giant congenital nevi (measures 20 cm or greater) carry a higher risk, with an estimated 4.5–10% of patients going on to develop melanoma. Of these, 70% are diagnosed before the age of 10 years.

History of Prior Melanoma

A prior history of melanoma places a patient at increased risk, with 5–10% of individuals developing a second primary melanoma.

Classification of Melanoma

Based on clinical and pathological features, cutaneous melanoma are divided into four main types. They are:

1. Superficial spreading melanoma (SSM).
2. Nodular melanoma (NM).
3. Lentigo maligna melanoma (LMM).
4. Acral lentiginous melanoma (ALM).

Rarer types include desmoplastic melanoma and metastatic melanoma with no known primary.

Superficial Spreading Melanoma

This is the most common subtype (approximately 70%) of cutaneous melanoma. It generally arises on any skin with intermittent sun exposure and presents initially as a flat lesion that undergoes change in size, shape or color.

Nodular Melanoma

The second most common subtype on the skin and accounts for 15%. This type is characterized by vertical growth without a prior radial growth phase. Nodular melanomas are often highly aggressive and clinically appear as blue-black or blue-red raised nodules **(Fig. 1)**.

Lentigo Maligna Melanoma

These melanomas are associated with chronic sun exposure and are typically located on

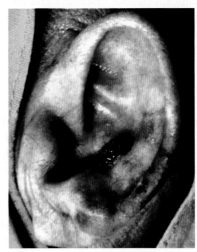

Fig. 1: Nodular melanoma of the pinna.

the head, neck, and arms. They account approximately 10% and appear as flat brown macules, often with hypopigmented areas. It is characterized by asymmetric, subclinical, and often extensive peripheral involvement of atypical junctional melanocytic hyperplasia. Excision with adequate wide margins can be challenging from both a functional and cosmetic point of view.

Acral Lentiginous Melanoma

This is the least common subtype (approximately 5%) among Caucasians. They arise on the palms and soles or in the nail bed and may not be related to ultraviolet light exposure. They appear as a flat lesion, which may be light colored or pink. In the early phase they show horizontal or intraepidermal growth but later nodular growth with invasion is seen.

Desmoplastic Melanoma

Desmoplastic melanoma is rare and accounts for less than 4% of all cutaneous melanomas. Approximately 51% of these lesions occur in the head and neck region. Affected individuals are older and have chronically sun-damaged skin. The appearance of the lesion may be nonspecific and it may look similar to a keloid scar or a benign lesion called dermatofibroma. Up to 73% of desmoplastic melanoma is amelanotic. At the time of diagnosis itself, desmoplastic melanoma demonstrates greater tumor thickness (>5 mm). It is known to be locally aggressive and highly infiltrative and often leads to cranial nerve and skull base involvement.

Metastatic Melanoma with No Known Primary

Most melanomas present as cutaneous lesions, occasionally metastatic deposits (approximately 2–8%) are found without any signs of a primary tumor. The original lesion may be hidden or may have undergone complete regression due to lymphocyte activation by the immune system. Two-thirds of these patients come with regional metastasis and the remaining third involve distant metastasis to sites such as the subcutaneous tissues, lung, and brain. These patients require a search for the primary site with a total body skin and mucosal evaluation.

Diagnosis

Clinical History

Patients should be questioned about the personal and family history of melanoma and information about previous skin biopsies, and details pertaining to the above-mentioned risk factors. A detailed history of the lesion and the changes happened should be taken.

Clinical Examination

The American Cancer Society published the ABCD checklist for the early detection of melanoma. Under these guidelines, concerning signs for melanoma include Asymmetry, Border irregularity, Color variation and Diameter greater than 6 mm. Recently "E" has been added to the ABCD acronym, for Evolving changes.

Biopsy

Any pigmented lesion that demonstrates an ABCD warning sign, has undergone change, or appears different from surrounding nevi on the body necessitates histologic evaluation. This may be performed as either an excisional biopsy or incisional biopsy, depending on the anatomical location and size of the lesion. Ideally, an excisional biopsy with 1–2 mm margins is preferred which will allow adequate pathological analysis of the entire specimen for staging. An incisional or punch biopsy may be performed for large lesions and for those in cosmetically critical areas. Superficial shave biopsy, frozen-section biopsy, and fine-needle aspiration are absolutely contraindicated, because the thickness of the tumor, which dictates treatment, may not be accurately obtained.

Staging

The staging system for cutaneous melanoma was revised by the Melanoma Expert Panel in 2016 and published the eighth edition of the American Joint Cancer Committee (AJCC) melanoma staging system, which was implemented from January 1, 2018 **(Tables 1 to 5)**.

The presence or absence of microsatellite, satellite, or in-transit metastases, regardless of the number of such lesions, represents an N-category criterion. Satellite metastases are defined as grossly visible cutaneous and/or subcutaneous metastases occurring within 2 cm of the primary melanoma. Microsatellites are microscopic cutaneous and/or subcutaneous metastases found adjacent or deep to a primary melanoma on pathological examination. In transit metastases are defined as clinically evident dermal and/or subcutaneous metastases identified at a distance more than 2 cm from the primary melanoma in the region between the primary and the first echelon of regional lymph nodes.

Metastatic Work Up

No special investigations are required for stage I and IIA and B melanoma. Patients with stage IIC or above should have a CT scan of the head, chest, abdomen, and pelvis. Serum lactate dehydrogenase (LDH) should also be measured for those with stage IV disease. Here whole body PET-CT can also be advised.

Prognostic Factors

The most important prognostic factor for patients with melanoma is the clinical stage. The key determinants of outcome for

Table 1: Primary tumor staging.

T category		Thickness	Ulceration status
TX: Primary tumor thickness cannot be assessed.		Not applicable	Not applicable
T0: No evidence of primary tumor (e.g. unknown primary or completely *regressed melanoma*)		Not applicable	Not applicable
Tis (melanoma in situ)		Not applicable	Not applicable
T1		<1.0 mm	Unknown or unspecified
	T1a	<0.8 mm	Without ulceration
	T1b	<0.8 mm	With ulceration
		0.8–1.0 mm	With or without ulceration
T2		>1.0–2.0 mm	Unknown or unspecified
	T2a	>1.0–2.0 mm	Without ulceration
	T2b	>1.0–2.0 mm	With ulceration
T3		>2.0–4.0 mm	Unknown or unspecified
	T3a	>2.0–4.0 mm	Without ulceration
	T3b	>2.0–4.0 mm	With ulceration
T4		>4.0 mm	Unknown or unspecified
	T4a	>4.0 mm	Without ulceration
	T4b	>4.0 mm	With ulceration

Table 2: Nodal staging.

N category		Number of tumor-involved regional lymph node	Presence of in-transit, satellite, and/ or microsatellite metastases
Nx		Regional nodes not assessed	No
N0		No regional metastases detected	No
N1		One tumor-involved node or in-transit, satellite, and/or microsatellite metastases with no tumor-involved nodes	
	N1a	One clinically occult (i.e. detected by SLN biopsy)	No
	N1b	One clinically detected	No
	N1c	No regional lymph node disease	Yes
N2		Two or three tumor-involved nodes or in-transit, satellite, and/or microsatellite metastases with one tumor-involved node	
	N2a	Two or three clinically occult (i.e. detected by SLN biopsy)	No
	N2b	Two or three, at least one of which was clinically detected	No
	N2c	One clinically occult or clinically detected	Yes
N3		Four or more tumor-involved nodes or in-transit, satellite, and/or microsatellite metastases with two or more tumor-involved nodes, or any number of matted nodes without or with in-transit, satellite, and/or microsatellite metastases	
	N3a	Four or more clinically occult (i.e. detected by SLN biopsy)	No
	N3b	Four or more, at least one of which was clinically detected, or presence of any number of matted nodes	No
	N3c	Two or more clinically occult or clinically detected and/or presence of any number of matted nodes	Yes

Table 3: Metastasis staging.

M category		Anatomic site	LDH level
M0		No evidence of distant metastasis	Not applicable
M1		Evidence of distant metastasis	
	M1a	Distant metastasis to skin, soft tissue including muscle, and/or nonregional lymph node	M1a: Not recorded or unspecified
			M1a (0): Not elevated
			M1a(1): Elevated
	M1b	Distant metastasis to lung with or without M1a sites of disease	M1b: Not recorded or unspecified
			M1b (0): Not elevated
			M1b(1): Elevated
	M1c	Distant metastasis to non-CNS visceral sites with or without M1a or M1b sites of disease	M1c: Not recorded or unspecified
			M1c (0): Not elevated
			M1c(1): Elevated
	M1d	Distant metastasis to CNS with or without M1a, M1b, or M1c sites of disease	M1d: Not recorded or unspecified
			M1d (0): Not elevated
			M1d(1): Elevated

Table 4: Clinical TNM staging. It includes microstaging of the primary melanoma and clinical/radiologic/biopsy evaluation for metastases. By convention, clinical staging should be used after biopsy of the primary melanoma, with clinical assessment for regional and distant metastases.

Clinical TNM	T	N	M
0	Tis	N0	M0
IA	T1a	N0	M0
IB	T1b	N0	M0
	T2a	N0	M0
IIA	T2b	N0	M0
	T3a	N0	M0
IIB	T3b	N0	M0
	T4a	N0	M0
IIC	T4b	N0	M0
III	Any T, Tis	≥ N1	M0
IV	Any T	Any N	MI

localized melanoma (stage I and II) are—(1) vertical depth of tumor extension (Breslow tumor thickness), (2) the primary tumor mitotic rate, and (3) presence or absence of surface ulceration. Breslow tumor thickness is measured from the top of the granular layer of the epidermis (or, if the surface overlying the entire dermal component is ulcerated, from the base of the ulcer) to the deepest invasive cell across the broad base of the tumor (in the dermis or subcutis).

In stage III or regional disease, the main predictors of survival are—(1) number of metastatic nodes, (2) tumor burden (microscopic vs. macroscopic disease), and (3) ulceration of the primary melanoma. In stage IV or distant metastatic disease, prognosis varies depending on the site of metastatic disease and elevated serum LDH levels.

Management

Primary

Treatment of primary melanoma is surgical removal. The National Institute for Health and Care Excellence (NICE) recommends at least

Table 5: Pathological TNM Staging: It includes microstaging of the primary melanoma, including any additional staging information from the wide-excision specimen that constitutes primary tumor surgical treatment and pathological information about the regional lymph nodes after SLN biopsy or therapeutic lymph node dissection for clinically evident regional lymph node disease.

Pathological TNM	T	N	M
0	Tis	N0	M0
IA	T1a	N0	M0
IB	T1b	N0	M0
	T2a	N0	M0
IIA	T2b	N0	M0
	T3a	N0	M0
IIB	T3b	N0	M0
	T4a	N0	M0
IIC	T4b	N0	M0
IIIA	T1a/b-T2a	N1a or N2a	M0
IIIB	T0	N1b, N1c	M0
	T1a/b-T 2a	N1b/c or N2b	M0
	T2b/T3a	N1a-N2b	M0
IIIC	T0	N2b, N2c, N3b or N3c	M0
	T1a-T 3a	N2c or N3a/b/c	M0
	T3b/T4a	Any N ≥ N1	M0
	T4b	N1a-N2c	M0
IIID	T4b	N3a/b/c	M0
IV	Any T, Tis	Any N	MI

5 mm margins for stage 0 melanomas, at least 10 mm for stage 1 and at least 20 mm for stage 2. Mohs micrographic surgery can be used to treat lentigo maligna (in situ melanoma), invasive lesions with indistinct margins such as desmoplastic melanoma or for surgery close to important anatomical areas such as eyes or ears.

Lymph Node Disease

Sentinel lymph node biopsy is offered for stage 1B disease or above. The sentinel lymph node is the first node where the skin involved with melanoma drains to and is detected by injecting a blue dye that is visually traced and by detecting the path of a radioactive tracer. When there is clinically enlarged lymph nodes, a fine needle aspiration cytology should be done. If negative or equivocal this may be repeated, or an image-guided core biopsy or open biopsy should be performed. If there is involvement of lymph node, a complete nodal clearance from levels I-V should be done. Depending on the anatomical site of lesion, a superficial parotidectomy may be needed along with the nodal clearance.

Radiotherapy

Although adjuvant radiation has not been shown to have an impact on survival, clinical trials support the efficacy of hypofractionated radiation as an adjuvant treatment to surgery for head and neck cutaneous melanoma patients at high risk for local or regional recurrence. Primary radiation can be used to treat extensive disease in an elderly patient who is not fit for surgery. It can also be administered as palliative treatment in patients who suffer from systemic stage IV disease, especially in the setting of brain or bone metastasis, spinal cord compression, and isolated, symptomatic visceral metastasis.

Chemotherapy

The main role of chemotherapy remains as palliative treatment in the setting of disseminated stage IV disease. Dacarbazine is currently the only chemotherapeutic agent approved for the treatment of advanced stage IV melanoma.

Targeted Therapy

About 40% of the melanomas have BRAF V600E mutations, and on this basis vemurafenib, a selective inhibitor of BRAF with 10-fold greater affinity for BRAF V600E substitution mutation was approved by the FDA for treatment of stage IV melanoma. Both vemurafenib and dabrafenib, another available BRAF inhibitor, are now used along with MEK inhibitors such as trametinib for stage IV melanoma. There are also new immunotherapeutic approaches incorporating anti-CTLA-4 (ipilimumab) and anti-PD1 (pembrolizumab and nivolumab).

● NONMELANOMA SKIN CANCERS

The two most important types of nonmelanoma skin cancers are BCC and SCC. The most common sites of presentation are head and neck regions. It is a multifactorial disease and etiology can be divided into individual, environmental, and genetic factors.

Risk Factors

The individual risk factors include male gender, older age, fair skin with poor tanning ability and immunosuppression. SCC may occur in chronic inflammatory disorders and arise in scars of skin burns or chronic ulcers (Marjolin's ulcer). The main environmental risk factor is solar ultraviolet (UV) radiation; UVB is more carcinogenic than UVA. The other potent environmental risk factors are iatrogenic ionizing radiation and occupational exposure to arsenic and polycyclic hydrocarbons. Infection with HPV has also been definitively linked to the development of both BCC and SCC. Certain genetic syndromes, such as xeroderma pigmentosum, albinism, and epidermolysis bullosa, predispose to all types of NMSCs, and Gorlin's syndrome (nevoid basal cell carcinoma syndrome) is a hereditary disorder characterized by multiple BCCs throughout life.

Staging

In the new AJCC, 8th edition classification, the staging system given for cutaneous squamous cell carcinoma (CSCC) of the head and neck is applicable for all other nonmelanoma skin carcinomas of the head and neck [except Merkel cell carcinoma (MCC)] **(Tables 6 to 10)**.

Table 6: Primary tumor staging.

T category		T criteria
Tx		Primary tumor cannot be identified
Tis		Carcinoma in situ
T1		Tumor smaller than 2 cm in greatest dimension
T2		Tumor 2 cm or larger, but smaller than 4 cm in greatest dimension
T3		Tumor 4 cm or larger in maximum dimension or minor bone erosion or perineural invasion or deep invasion*
T4		Tumor with gross cortical bone/ marrow invasion, skull base invasion and/or skull base foramen invasion
	T4a	Tumor with gross cortical bone/ marrow invasion
	T4b	Tumor with skull base invasion and/ or skull base foramen involvement

*Deep invasion is defined as invasion beyond the subcutaneous fat or >6 mm (as measured from the granular layer of adjacent normal epidermis to the base of the tumor); perineural invasion for T3 classification is defined as tumor cells within the nerve sheath of a nerve lying deeper than the dermis or measuring 0.1 mm or larger in caliber, or presenting with clinical or radiographic involvement of named nerves without skull base invasion or transgression.

Table 7: Clinical staging of regional lymph node.

N category		N criteria
Nx		Regional lymph nodes cannot be assessed
N0		No regional lymph node metastasis
N1		Metastasis in a single ipsilateral lymph node, 3 cm or smaller in greatest dimension and ENE (–)
N2		
	N2a	Metastasis in a single ipsilateral node larger than 3 cm but not larger than 6 cm in greatest dimension and ENE (–)
	N2b	Metastasis in multiple ipsilateral nodes, none larger than 6 cm in greatest dimension and ENE (–)
	N2c	Metastasis in bilateral or contralateral lymph nodes, none larger than 6 cm in greatest dimension and ENE (–)
N3		
	N3a	Metastasis in a lymph node larger than 6 cm in greatest dimension and ENE (–)
	N3b	Metastasis in any node(s) and ENE (+)

Note: A designation of "U" or "L" may be used for any N category to indicate metastasis above the lower border of the cricoid (U) or below the lower border of the cricoid (L).

Table 8: Pathological staging of regional lymph node.

N category		N criteria
Nx		Regional lymph nodes cannot be assessed
N0		No regional lymph node metastasis
N1		Metastasis in a single ipsilateral lymph node, 3 cm or smaller in greatest dimension and ENE (–)
N2		
	N2a	Metastasis in single ipsilateral or contralateral node 3 cm or smaller in greatest dimension and ENE (+); or a single ipsilateral node larger than 3 cm but not larger than 6 cm in greatest dimension and ENE (–)
	N2b	Metastasis in multiple ipsilateral nodes, none larger than 6 cm in greatest dimension and ENE (–)
	N2c	Metastasis in bilateral or contralateral lymph nodes, none larger than 6 cm in greatest dimension and ENE (-)
N3		
	N3a	Metastasis in a lymph node larger than 6 cm in greatest dimension and ENE (–)
	N3b	Metastasis in a single ipsilateral node larger than 3 cm in greatest dimension and ENE (+); or multiple ipsilateral, contralateral, or bilateral nodes, any with ENE (+)

Table 9: Staging of distant metastasis.

M category	M criteria
M0	No distant metastasis
MI	Distant metastasis

Table 10: TNM staging.

TNM stage	T	N	M
0	Tis	N0	M0
I	T1	N0	M0
II	T2	N0	M0
III	T3	N0	M0
	T1	N1	M0
	T2	N1	M0
	T3	N1	M0
IV	T1	N2	M0
	T2	N2	M0
	T3	N2	M0
	Any T	N3	M0
	T4	Any N	M0
	Any T	Any N	MI

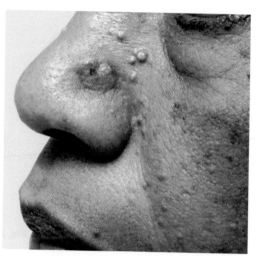

Fig. 2: Early nodular basal cell carcinoma nose.

BASAL CELL CARCINOMA

Basal cell cancer is the commonest type of skin cancer and arises from the basal keratinocytes. They are locally invasive with less propensity for distant metastasis.

Clinical Features

They are slow growing tumors (5 mm or less per year) and typically occur in the head and neck region, most commonly on the nose, but can occur anywhere that is sun exposed. There are five main histological subtypes of BCC—nodular, superficial, basosquamous, pigmented, and morpheic.

The most common form is the nodular BCC; it appears as a raised lesion **(Fig. 2)** with a rolled edge, telangiectasia, and central ulceration—constituting the features of the classical "rodent ulcer".

Superficial BCC is also common and the least aggressive subtype. Features include scaly, dry, and erythematous plaques which are round or oval in shape and typically occur on the limbs and trunk. They may be confused clinically with eczema or psoriasis. Basosquamous BCC is a more aggressive tumor. They are often ulcerated with histologic features of SCC and BCC, and has limited but definite metastatic potential. Pigmented BCC is seen in darker skinned individuals, and this can be easily confused with melanoma. The morpheic BCC, also described as sclerosing type, presents as flat, indurated, whitish, and ill-defined plaques. These are locally aggressive tumors where margin control is particularly difficult and as such have a high propensity for local recurrence.

Basal cell carcinoma (BCC) situated in the H-zone (nose, nasolabial regions, upper lip, columella, periauricular skin, and frontozygomatic area) **(Fig. 3)** is associated with deeper invasion and higher recurrence rates.

Diagnosis

The diagnosis is made based upon the clinical history, physical examination, biopsy, and histological evaluation of lesion. To assess

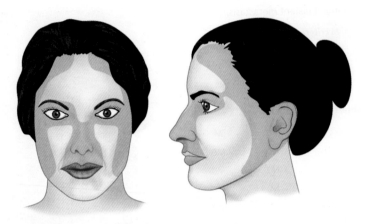

Fig. 3: H zone.

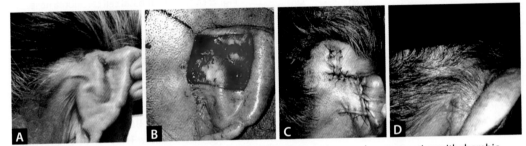

Figs. 4A to D: Surgical excision of nodular basal cell carcinoma pinna and reconstruction with rhombic transposition flap.

invasion of bone, nerves, orbit or parotid gland, either computerized tomography or magnetic resonance imaging may be utilized.

Management

Nonsurgical Treatments

This includes imiquimod cream, topical 5-FU, photodynamic therapy, or cryotherapy. These modalities are mainly employed for superficial BCC.

Surgical Treatment

Surgical excision is the best treatment option for nodular and morpheic BCC. Small, well-defined lesions may be excised with peripheral margins of 4–5 mm and deep margins down to fat **(Figs. 4A to D)**. A histological clearance of at least 1 mm at both the peripheral and deep margins is mandatory.

Lesions which are poorly defined, larger than 2 cm, located on the central face or histologically morpheic or infiltrative are high-risk lesions. These lesions should be considered for Mohs micrographic surgery for the meticulous assessment of the margins.

Radiotherapy

BCCs are highly radiosensitive. It can be used as an alternative to surgery especially for elderly patients or as adjuvant treatment for incompletely excised tumors. It is contraindicated for recurrent tumors in previously irradiated areas. It is usually reserved for elderly patients.

Treatment of Locally Advanced and Metastatic Disease

Targeted molecular therapy for BCC has focused on the Hedgehog signaling pathway. Vismodegib, a Hedgehog inhibitor, can be used for locally advanced or metastatic disease.

Risk Factors for BCC Recurrence

The risk factors for recurrence of basal cell carcinoma includes the following:

- T stage > T1
- *Histology:* Infiltrative/Morpheic/Baso-squamous
- Margin status <4 mm
- *Location:*·H-zone
- Perineural invasion
- Site of prior radiation therapy
- Poorly defined borders
- Recurrent lesion.

● SQUAMOUS CELL CARCINOMA

Squamous cell carcinoma (SCC) is the second most common NMSC. It is a malignant neoplasm of the keratinocytes that may arise de novo or from precursor lesions as actinic keratosis.

Clinical Features

These lesions commonly occur in a typical sun-exposed distribution including the face, scalp, lip, and dorsal hands. Lesions may appear as enlarging plaques, papules or nodules that may be smooth and soft or rough and hardened **(Fig. 5)**. They usually grow quickly over weeks or months. As they progress, they can ulcerate and bleed and may become locally invasive.

Regional metastases are uncommon, occurring in 5% overall and it is usually to the regional lymph nodes. For anterior tumors of

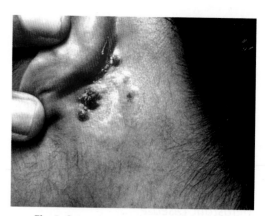

Fig. 5: Cutaneous squamous cell carcinoma post-aural region.

the face, nodal groups at risk include the parotid, external jugular nodes and levels I (including submental and perifacial lymph nodes), II, III, and IV. For posterior tumors of the scalp, nodal groups at risk include the retroauricular, external jugular, occipital nodes, and levels II, III, IV, and V. If distant metastatic disease happens, the most common site is the lungs.

Management

Surgical Treatment

Surgical excision is the treatment of choice. Well-defined T1 lesions should be excised with a peripheral margin of at least 4 mm and down to the subcutaneous fascia. T2 should be excised with a margin of 6 mm or more. SCCs with high-risk features may be excised using Mohs micrographic surgery and this technique is particularly useful for areas where wider margins of excision may be practically difficult or cause significant visual and functional impairment or if there is nerve involvement. Advanced lesions require en-bloc resection of tumor incorporating invaded structures and adequate reconstruction added by adjuvant postoperative radiotherapy. Patients with clinical neck disease should undergo neck dissection.

Radiotherapy

Radiotherapy can be used as a primary treatment for selected patients or adjunct when there is incomplete surgical excision or perineural invasion. Lesions situated at lower eyelid, inner canthus, tip of nose and lip respond well to radiotherapy. Radiotherapy should be avoided in tumors that invade bone or cartilage due to the risk of radionecrosis.

Treatment of Locally Advanced and Metastatic Disease

This includes systemic chemotherapy or treatment with biologic response modifier. The efficacy of these therapies has not been well established. Epidermal growth factor receptor (EGFR) inhibitors are proving effective in the treatment of locally advanced and metastatic cutaneous SCC.

Risk Factors for Cutaneous SCC Recurrence and Metastasis

Rapid growth, size more than 2 cm, location at ear or lip, depth more than 4 mm, perineural invasion, poor differentiation, infiltrative margins, spindle cell and acantholytic histology, local recurrence and immunosuppression are all associated with high risk for recurrence and metastasis in cutaneous SCC.

● FURTHER READING

1. Amin MB, Edge SB, Greene FL, et al. AJCC Cancer Staging Manual, 8th edition. New York: Springer; 2017.
2. Apalla Z, Lallas A, Sotiriou E, Lazaridou E, Ioannides D. Epidemiological trends in skin cancer. Dermatol Pract Concept. 2017;7(2):1.
3. Harrison LB, Mehta PS, Halpern M, Ratner D. Basal and Squamous Cell Skin Cancers. Harrison's Head & Neck Cancer - A Multidisciplinary Approach. Philadelphia: Lippincott Williams & Wilkins; 2014. pp. 635-71.
4. Khan M, Martin-Clavijo A. Benign and malignant conditions of the skin. Scott-Brown's Otolaryngology, Head and Neck Surgery, 8th edition, CRC Press; 2018. pp. 1321-36.
5. Kupferman ME, Davies MA. Melanoma of the Head and Neck. . Harrison's Head & Neck Cancer-A Multidisciplinary Approach. Philadelphia: Lippincott Williams & Wilkins; 2014.pp. 672-96.
6. Schmalbach CE, Durham AB, Johnson TM, Bradford CR. Management of Cutaneous Head and Neck Melanoma. Cummings Otolaryngology–Head and Neck Surgery, 6th Edition. Saunders Elsevier; 2014. pp. 1163-75.

CHAPTER 36

Role of Chemotherapy in Head and Neck Cancer

K Pavithran

● INTRODUCTION

Previously chemotherapy was primarily used for palliation of symptoms in the management of head and neck cancers. With better understanding of the impact of multimodality treatment, chemotherapy is now used as part of both definitive and adjuvant treatment regimens along with radiotherapy. For squamous cell carcinomas of the head and neck (SCCHN), platinum-based compounds (cisplatin or carboplatin) are the most commonly used agents because they have shown the best responses either alone or in combination with other drugs. Platinum compounds are used in combination with antimetabolites such as 5-fluorouracil and taxanes (paclitaxel or docetaxel). Single agent methotrexate is commonly used in the palliative setting **(Table 1)**. Chemotherapy may be used as induction or combined with radiation in one of several sequences, including concurrent, or induction, followed by concurrent chemoradiation therapy or in the metastatic setting. Biological agents that target epidermal growth factor receptors are also used in combination with radiation as well as in the palliative setting.

● INDUCTION CHEMOTHERAPY

The role of induction chemotherapy in the management of locally advanced SCCHN is still debated. Phase III trials have reported

Table 1: Chemotherapeutic agents used in head and neck cancers.

Class of agent	Examples	Main mechanism of action
Platinum	Cisplatin, carboplatin	Forms DNA cross links
Taxane	Paclitaxel, docetaxel	Stabilizes micro-tubules to block M phase
Antifolate (antimetabolite)	Methotrexate	Inhibits DHFR during S phase
Fluoropyrimidine (antimetabolite)	5-fluorouracil	Inhibits during S-phase

(DNA: Deoxyribonucleic acid; DHFR: Dihydrofolate reductase; TS: Thymidylate synthase)

improved local control or survival outcomes in patients with locoregionally advanced SCCHN treated with a taxane (docetaxel is the one most extensively studied) combined with cisplatin and infusional 5-fluorouracil (DPF) compared with patients treated with cisplatin and infusional 5-fluorouracil (PF) alone when followed by the same locoregional treatment. A meta-analysis reported an overall survival benefit when using triplet therapy instead of PF as induction chemotherapy. These studies established that DPF was superior to PF as an induction therapy. However, it did not answer the question whether induction therapy followed by CRT was more effective than proceeding directly to definitive CRT alone.

● INDUCTION CHEMOTHERAPY FOLLOWED BY CRT VERSUS CRT ALONE

The question of whether the use of induction taxane-PF chemotherapy prior to CRT additionally improves outcomes for SCCHN patients has been addressed in two recent randomized trials. The DeCIDE and PARADIGM trials compared induction DPF followed by CRT to CRT alone. Findings from these two studies did not demonstrate improvement in overall survival with DPF induction chemotherapy followed by CRT compared to up-front CRT alone, although the pattern of failure may have been affected. Although there may be a subset of patients (N2c or N3 disease) who may benefit from the integration of induction chemotherapy, its routine application is not supported by the above randomized trials. Studies have also shown that incorporating induction therapy leads to longer treatment duration and the added toxicity of the induction component, compared with chemoradiation alone. Induction chemotherapy is usually given once every 3 weeks for 2–4 cycles before a course of concurrent chemoradiation.

● LOCALLY ADVANCED SCCHN

Concurrent chemoradiotherapy is the standard of care. Many prospective randomized trials have showed that concurrent chemoradiotherapy (CRT) is the most promising approach. There was 6.5% absolute 5-year survival benefit with CRT in the meta-analysis of chemotherapy in head and neck cancer (MACH-NC) and this is due to a reduction in deaths related to HNC. The drugs useful for CRT are cisplatin alone or cisplatin/carboplatin with 5-fluorouracil (5-FU) or other combination chemotherapy. Cisplatin alone is the most commonly used drug in CRT.

Most of the randomized trials of CRT use a dose of cisplatin of 100 mg/m^2 every three weeks during the course of radiotherapy (in USA and Europe). However, the side-effects related to high-dose cisplatin are significant and include peripheral neuropathy, hearing loss, marked nausea and vomiting, and renal dysfunction. However, the most commonly used regimen in India is weekly cisplatin (40 mg/m^2). Weekly carboplatin (at AUC 1.5) is used in CRT in patients who had neoadjuvant chemotherapy or in patients with renal impairment or elderly with other comorbidities. The MACH-NC has also suggested that there is less benefit of CRT in patients older than 70 years age.

Strategies for Organ Preservation in SCCHN

Sequential chemotherapy or CRT, in the form of induction chemotherapy followed by RT or CRT has been a successful strategy for organ preservation in patients with potentially resectable laryngeal and hypopharyngeal SCCHN.

The Veterans Affairs Laryngeal Cancer Study Group (VALCSG) randomized patients with previously untreated advanced (stage III or IV) laryngeal squamous carcinoma to induction chemotherapy followed by definitive radiation therapy vs. those of conventional laryngectomy and postoperative radiation. In the VALCSG trial, the estimated 2-year overall survival was 68% in each arm. More local recurrences and fewer distant metastases were reported in the chemotherapy group than in the surgery group. The larynx was preserved in 64% of the patients overall.

European Organization for Research and Treatment of Cancer (EORTC) 24,891 trial compared induction chemotherapy followed by RT in case of complete response vs. induction chemotherapy followed postoperative RT in patients with hypopharyngeal squamous cell carcinoma. In the 10-year update, treatment failures at local and regional sites occurred at the same frequencies in both groups. The 5- and 10-year estimates of functional larynx in patients who were treated in the induction chemotherapy group were 35% and 26%, respectively.

In the EORTC 24,954 trial, patients with resectable advanced larynx or hypopharynx cancers were included. The control arm was the same as the experimental arm of EORTC protocol 24,891, except that there were four cycles of chemotherapy instead of three cycles and patients in the experimental arm received an alternating schedule of four cycles of chemotherapy and three 2-week courses of radiotherapy, each of 20 Gy. Larynx preservation, progression-free interval, and overall survival were similar in both arms, as were acute and late toxic effects.

The RTOG 91-11 trial had three treatment arms—induction chemotherapy with PF followed by RT, concurrent CRT with high-dose cisplatin, and RT alone. The study accrued patients with stage III or IV laryngeal cancer (T1 and high-volume T4 primary tumors excluded). Follow-up data at 10.8 years showed laryngeal preservation rates and local control was better in the CRT arm. Chemotherapy given concomitantly or as induction showed similar benefit for achieving distant control (7–8% difference compared with RT alone). Overall survival was same among all the three groups.

The Groupe Oncologie Radiotherapie Tete et Cou (GORTEC) 2000–2001 trial investigated TPF induction chemotherapy compared with PF induction chemotherapy followed by RT for larynx preservation in patients with T3 and selected T4 laryngeal or hypopharyngeal cancer. Patients who had induction chemotherapy with TPF had better 3-year larynx preservation rates (70.3%) when compared with those who received the PF induction regimen (57.5%, p = 0.03). Following the results of this study, induction TPF is considered a standard treatment option in Europe for laryngeal and hypopharyngeal cancer.

POSTOPERATIVE CONCURRENT CHEMORADIOTHERAPY

Postoperative concurrent chemoradiotherapy (CRT) in the postoperative setting has been tested in two randomized phase III trials [Radiation Therapy Oncology Group (RTOG) 9,501 study and European Organization for Research and Treatment of Cancer (EORTC) 22,931 study]. Patients with high-risk pathological features were assigned to RT alone vs. RT concurrently with high-dose cisplatin 100 mg/m^2 every 3 weeks. High-risk features were represented by the presence of a positive margin, nodal extracapsular spread, lymphovascular invasion, perineural invasion, and multiple positive lymph nodes. CRT significantly improved progression-free survival in both trials. However, overall survival benefit was seen only in EORTC- 22,931 study. Main side effects in CRT group were mucositis, hematologic toxicity, and muscular fibrosis. In a pooled analysis of data from both trials, two risk factors—extracapsular extension and positive surgical margins were associated with a significant benefit from concurrent CRT.

Targeted Therapy in the Treatment of Locally Advanced HNC

Cetuximab is a chimeric (mouse/human) monoclonal antibody which targets the epidermal growth factor receptor. A phase III trial showed that cetuximab in combination with RT improves locoregional control and overall survival in patients with locally advanced HNC. Cetuximab was initiated 1 week before RT, with a loading dose of 400 mg/m^2, followed by 250 mg/m^2 weekly throughout RT. This study demonstrated that locoregional control, progression-free and overall survival was significantly improved with the combination of RT and cetuximab. Subset analysis showed maximum benefit in oropharyngeal cancer. The side effect profile was similar with the exception of the occurrence of more acneiform rash and infusion reactions in the combination of cetuximab plus RT group than in the group receiving RT alone. Cetuximab with RT is mainly used in situations where cisplatin is contraindicated or in the elderly. The RTOG 0,522 has evaluated RT plus cisplatin with or without cetuximab and has found no improvement in any outcome with the addition of cetuximab for patients with locally advanced HNC treated with definitive CRT. It may be an alternative to cisplatin in HPV + oropharyngeal cancer patients depending on results of RTOG 1,016 study.

NASOPHARYNGEAL CARCINOMA

Patients with T1N0M0 disease is treated with radiotherapy alone. For stage II-IVA, the standard approach is chemoradiation with cisplatin followed by adjuvant chemotherapy with cisplatin or carboplatin with 5FU × 3 cycles. In recurrent metastatic setting, platinum/gemcitabine combination is useful.

RECURRENT OR METASTATIC DISEASE

The prognosis for recurrent or metastatic SCCHN treated with chemotherapy alone is poor. The median survival is usually less than a year even with aggressive combination chemotherapy. Various regimens—both, single-agents or doublets are used in this setting. Although two drugs administered together are more likely to result in a better tumor response than treatment with a single agent, doublets have not been associated with any improvement in overall survival when compared to a single agent. Platinum-based chemotherapy in combination with cetuximab is considered the standard of care in fit patients. Erbitux in First-Line Treatment of Recurrent or Metastatic Head and Neck Cancer (EXTREME) trial showed that the combination of cisplatin or carboplatin with 5-fluorouracil and cetuximab improves OS (median OS is 10.1 months).

METRONOMIC CHEMOTHERAPY

Metronomic chemotherapy is defined as the frequent administration of conventional chemotherapy drugs at low doses with no prolonged drug-free breaks. Its mechanism of action is thought to be due to antiangiogenic and immunomodulatory anti-tumor activities. Metronomic chemotherapy is associated with lower treatment-related toxicity than standard dose chemotherapy. Because of this fact, it is very suitable for elderly and frail patients and who have not yet recovered from the side effects of previous chemotherapy. The drugs commonly used in SCCHN are weekly methotrexate 15 mg/m², or cyclcophosphamide. In one study with methotrexate, the median PFS was about 4 months.

IMMUNOTHERAPY

The immunotherapeutic landscape for HNSCC encompasses a variety of targets that suppress or stimulate the immune system's ability to eliminate neoplastic cells. Activation of checkpoint receptors, such as programmed cell death protein 1 (PD-1) and cytotoxic T lymphocyte-associated protein (CTLA-4), causes T cell suppression. Pembrolizumab is a mAb directed against PD-1 and was first approved for use in metastatic melanoma. In 2016 it was granted accelerated approval as a single agent in patients with recurrent/metastatic HNSCC with disease progression on or after platinum chemotherapy. Nivolumab is another mAb targeting PD-1 and was approved for use as a single agent in patients with recurrent/metastatic HNSCC with disease progression on or after platinum chemotherapy.

SUMMARY

- *Locally advanced SCCHN, unresectable*: Chemoradiation if ECOG performance status (PS) 0-1.
- *PS-2*: Definitive radiotherapy +/- chemotherapy/cetuximab.

- *PS3*: Single agent chemotherapy or best supportive care.
- *Organ preservation strategy for larynx or hypopharynx*: Chemoradiation.
- *Postoperative setting:* SCCHN with high-risk features—positive margins or positive node with extracapsular extension—chemoradiation.
- *Recurrent or metastatic setting*: SCCHN: Cisplatin/carboplatin with 5FU and cetuximab for patients in good performance status. Poor performance status patients—single agent chemotherapy or metronomic chemotherapy.
- *Carcinoma nasopharynx:* For node positive disease or T2–T4 lesions—chemoradiation followed by chemotherapy with cisplatin/carboplatin + 5FU.

● FURTHER READING

1. Al-Sarraf M, LeBlanc M, Giri PG, et al. Chemoradiotherapy versus radiotherapy in patients with advanced nasopharyngeal cancer: Phase III randomized Intergroup Study 0099. J Clin Oncol. 1998;16(4):1310-7.
2. Bernier J, Cooper JS, Pajak TF, et al. Defining risk levels in locally advanced head and neck cancers: A comparative analysis of concurrent postoperative radiation plus chemotherapy trials of the EORTC (#22931) and RTOG (#9501). Head Neck. 2005;27(10):843-50.
3. Blanchard P, Baujat B, Holostenco V, et al.; MACH-CH Collaborative Group. Meta-analysis of chemotherapy in head and neck cancer (MACH-NC): A comprehensive analysis by tumour site. Radiother Oncol. 2011;100(1):33-40.
4. Blanchard P, Bourhis J, Lacas B, et al.; Meta-Analysis of Chemotherapy in Head and Neck Cancer, Induction Project, Collaborative Group. Taxane-cisplatin-fluorouracil as induction chemotherapy in locally advanced head and neck cancers: An individual patient data meta-analysis of the meta-analysis of chemotherapy in head and neck cancer group. J Clin Oncol. 2013;31(23):2854-60.
5. Bonner JA, Harari PM, Giralt J, et al. Radiotherapy plus cetuximab for squamous-cell carcinoma of the head and neck. N Engl J Med. 2006;354(6):567-78.
6. Cohen EE, Karrison TG, Kocherginsky M, et al. Phase III randomized trial of induction chemotherapy in patients with N2 or N3 locally advanced head and neck cancer. J Clin Oncol. 2014;32(25):2735-43.
7. Forastiere AA, Goepfert H, Maor M, et al. Concurrent chemotherapy and radiotherapy for organ preservation in advanced laryngeal cancer. N Engl J Med. 2003;349(22):2091-8.
8. Forastiere AA, Zhang Q, Weber RS, et al. Long term results of RTOG 91-11: A comparison of three nonsurgical treatment strategies to preserve the larynx in patients with locally advanced larynx cancer. J Clin Oncol. 2013;31(7):845-52.
9. Haddad R, O'Neill A, Rabinowits G, et al. Induction chemotherapy followed by concurrent chemoradiotherapy (sequential chemoradiotherapy) versus concurrent chemoradiotherapy alone in locally advanced head and neck cancer (PARADIGM): A randomized phase 3 trial. Lancet Oncol. 2013;14(3):257-64.
10. Kiyota N, Tahara M, Fujii M. Adjuvant treatment for post-operative head and neck squamous cell carcinoma. Jpn J Clin Oncol. 2015;45(1):2-6.
11. Kodaira T, Nishimura Y, Kagami Y, et al. Definitive radiotherapy for head and neck squamous cell carcinoma: Update and perspectives on the basis of EBM. Jpn J Clin Oncol. 2015;45(3):235-43.
12. Lefebvre JL, Andry G, Chevalier D, et al.; EORTC Head and Neck Cancer Group. Laryngeal preservation with induction chemotherapy for hypopharyngeal squamous cell carcinoma: 10-year results of the EORTC trial 24891. Ann Oncol. 2012;23(10):2708-14.
13. Mak MP, Glisson BS. Is there still a role for induction chemotherapy in locally advanced head and neck cancer? Curr Opin Oncol. 2014;26(3):247-51.
14. Petrelli F, Coinu A, Riboldi V, et al. Concomitant platinum-based chemotherapy or cetuximab with radiotherapy for locally advanced head and neck cancer: A systematic review and meta-analysis of published studies. Oral Oncol. 2014;50(11):1041-8.
15. Shang J, Gu J, Han Q, et al. Chemoradiotherapy is superior to radiotherapy alone after surgery in advanced squamous cell carcinoma of the head and neck: A systematic review and meta-analysis. Int J Clin Exp Med. 2014;7(9):2478-87.
16. Vokes EE, Seiwert TY. EGFR-directed treatments in SCCHN. Lancet Oncol. 2013;14(8):672-3.

CHAPTER 37

Principles of Radiotherapy in Head and Neck Malignancies

Anoop R

● INTRODUCTION

Radiation therapy is the clinical specialty dealing with the use of ionizing radiations in the treatment of patients with malignant neoplasm (and certain benign diseases). In early stage of head and neck cancer, it is one of the single modality treatments with a curative intent. In advanced stage disease, it has a definite role in the curative intent multimodality therapy along with concurrent chemotherapy, as definitive organ preserving treatment; or as adjuvant treatment after surgery. It also has an important role in the palliative treatment of incurable cancers.

● GENERAL PRINCIPLES AND RADIOBIOLOGY

Radiation is basically energy traveling through space. This includes high energy electromagnetic radiation such as X-rays, gamma rays, and particulate radiation such as electrons, protons, and neutrons. The photons are produced from the radioactive isotopes or using linear accelerators. If the incident radiation has sufficient energy to dislodge the orbital electrons of the atom, it is called ionizing radiation, as it produces ions in the cells it traverses through. The principal target for radiation damage is the cell DNA. The physical interaction of radiation with the DNA molecule in turn produces biological effects by breakage of chemical bonds by direct and indirect actions, leading to single strand and double strand breaks and thus loss of clonogenic potential. The integrity of the cellular DNA repair mechanism will decide the ultimate biological outcome. If the DNA damage is repaired, the cell will survive; if not, it will perish.

● FOUR R's OF RADIOBIOLOGY

Repair

Most cancer cells have poor DNA repair ability compared to normal cells. Hence, failure to repair the DNA will result in cancer cell death and tumor control, while repair of their DNA will result in tumor progression. Correspondingly, repair of the normal cell DNA will result in survival of the cell, while inability for the same will lead to cell death and normal tissue complications. A minimum gap of 6 hours is required for the normal tissue repair.

Repopulation

It is the compensatory increase in cell proliferation in tissues, in response to an injury that results in a large amount of cell killing. It facilitates the healing of common radiotherapy complications in normal tissues, while in tumor it leads to tumor recurrence and hence is detrimental.

Reoxygenation

Because of the distorted angiogenic attribute of tumors their blood vessels tend to be abnormal functionally and structurally, leading to lack of nutrition and oxygen in certain regions of the tumor. This state of very low tissue oxygenation called hypoxia helps the tumor cell to survive the treatment, as oxygen is essential to fix the DNA damage induced by radiation. Hence, circumventing the hypoxic state by reoxygenation of the tumor is very decisive in the successful outcome of treatment.

Redistribution

Radiation acts on dividing cells. Each cell goes through five phases of cell cycle and radiation is most effective on G2M phase, while the S phase is considered the most radioresistant. Hence when a particular cell dies, there will be redistribution of the remaining cells into G2M phase and this principle is utilized by fractionating radiotherapy.

● FRACTIONATION

The paramount goal in patient care is to optimize treatment efficacy, while minimizing toxicity. In old times, radiation treatment (RT) often used was a single, high-dose sitting. The clinical response was associated with unacceptable normal tissue damage. It was seen later that dividing the total dose into multiple fractions improved the recovery of the normal tissues, without affecting the tumor control. The principles of fractionation are better understood by knowing the 4 Rs of radiobiology. The physicians could improve the therapeutic ratio considerably by effectively utilizing the differential inability of the tumor cells in repairing the DNA damage. Thus the gap between the fractions allows the normal cells to recover, while the tumor cells tend to accumulate the damage and die. Fractionation also allows the redistribution of tumor cells to the sensitive phases of the cell cycle and also improves the reoxygenation of tumor as the number of hypoxic cells decrease with each fraction.

Conventional Fractionation

Conventional fractionation implies dose per fraction of 1.8–2.25 Gy, given once daily, five fractions per week, to total doses determined by the tumor characteristics and the tolerance of critical normal tissues.

Hypofractionation

Hypofractionation implies that dose per fraction is more than 2.25 Gy, given once daily, five fractions per week, while the overall treatment time may be reduced.

Hyperfractionation

Hyperfractionation means a higher total dose is delivered using multiple fractions per day; the dose per fraction is significantly reduced, within the same overall treatment time.

Accelerated Fractionation

Accelerated fractionation implies that the overall treatment time is significantly reduced, the total dose, dose per fraction and the number of fractions, are either unchanged or somewhat reduced, depending on the extent of overall treatment time reduction.

Concomitant Boost

An additional boost dose to the primary tumor region with a smaller field is given as a second fraction after a gap of minimum 6 hours, toward the last part of radiation course.

● METHODS OF RADIATION DELIVERY

Depending on the distance of the radiation source from the target, RT may be divided into:
- External beam radiotherapy, where the radiation is delivered from a distance by a machine outside the body, commonly using linear accelerators

- Brachytherapy, where a sealed radioactive source in the form of wires or seeds is placed near or through the target. These radioactive implants may be temporary or permanent.

  Another form of internal radiation uses unsealed liquid radioactive sources which can be ingested or injected. Radioiodine treatment of thyroid cancers is an example.

● CLINICAL APPLICATIONS

Radical Radiation Treatment

The term is used when RT is used as a single modality with a curative intent in early stage diseases of larynx, nasopharynx, oropharynx, and oral cavity.

Radical Concurrent Chemoradiation

This implies that both radiation and chemotherapy are given concurrently as part of curative intent combined modality treatment, in locally advanced tumors, with the idea of organ preservation.

Radiation dose: 66–70 Gy in conventional fractionation, over a period of 6–7 weeks.

Adjuvant Radiation Treatment

The term is used when RT is given after the definitive treatment, as part of the combined modality treatment in locally advanced head and neck cancers. Postoperatively adjuvant chemoradiation is considered if high-risk features like positive margins or perinodal spread is mentioned in the pathology report.

Radiation dose: 60–66 Gy in conventional fractionation, over a period of 6–7 weeks.

Neoadjuvant Radiation Treatment

The term is used when RT is given preceding the definitive modality.

● RADIATION TREATMENT PLANNING

The RT planning starts with the appropriate patient selection and decision upon the intent of treatment, curative or palliative. A detailed clinical examination along with staging workup is mandatory in all patients with a curative intent treatment **(Flowchart 1)**. Once the treatment decision is made, a proper dental evaluation and appropriate dental prophylaxis and extraction/restoration of the deceased teeth, is a prerequisite for simulation. The nutritional status and swallowing function of the patient should be assessed. Patients are counseled regarding maintaining optimum oral hygiene and bodyweight. Following informed consent, the patient is simulated for the treatment. Two-dimensional planning with fluoroscopy

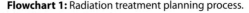

Flowchart 1: Radiation treatment planning process.

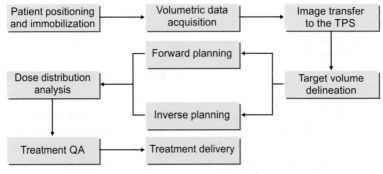

(TPS: Treatment planning system; QA: Quality assurance)

is relatively replaced by a volume based three-dimensional approach using CT scan preferably with contrast **(Fig. 1)**.

The patient is immobilized with a thermoplastic shell, on a flat couch, thereby ensuring reproducible set-up everyday **(Fig. 2)**. Once the treatment position is confirmed, immobilized, and referenced, then the CT scan is taken on a flat couch, which accurately determines the tumor volume as well as three-dimensional relationship of the tumor to normal anatomic structures. Usually scans are obtained with a slice thickness of 3 mm. A slice thickness of 1–2 mm is preferable for delineation of cranial nerves, the skull base, and laryngeal tumors.

The CT scan images are then imported into a RT planning system.

The contours are then drawn on every CT slice by the radiation oncologist, thereby delineating each structure of interest as either the target or the organ-at-risk (OAR).

Any visible tumor is delineated as the gross tumor volume (GTV). A PET or MRI imaging along with endoscope recordings may help the clinician in delineating the tumor extend and anatomy more accurately. The GTV is then encompassed by one or more clinical target volumes (CTV), including the immediate margins beyond the GTV and the lymph node draining regions considered being at high risk of containing tumor cells, the CTV is then expanded to a form a planning target volume (PTV) that accounts for the measured movement of the tumor or organs within the body, in addition to the daily set-up margin. Several beams are then placed and the optimum beam arrangement that covers the target volumes homogeneously to the prescribed dose, while sparing the critical structures to the best is chosen **(Fig. 3)**.

Once the treatment plan is finalized, the patient is then called in and planned verification is done by repositioning the patient with the immobilization device on the treatment machine or conventional simulator. The reference position coordinates of the patient is verified and, using light beams, the geometric parameters are checked. The portal verification images are taken using X-rays and these are compared to the digitally reconstructed radiographs (DRR) to make sure that the isocenter and shape of the fields along with the shielding are consistent with the plan **(Fig. 4)**. The field borders and the patient's bony anatomy are matched with the DRR and any disparity is verified and corrected. The Electronic Portal Imaging Device (EPID) is now available in all linear accelerators **(Fig. 5)**, which facilitate the verification of patient setup before each treatment, matched to the anatomic

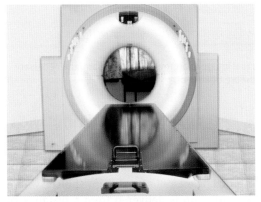

Fig. 1: CT simulator.

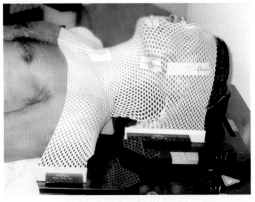

Fig. 2: Patient immobilization.

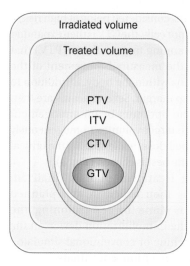

Fig. 3: International Commission on Radiotherapy Units and Measurements (ICRU) definition of GTV, cTV, PTV. Gross tumor volume (GTV) is the volume(s) of known tumor. Clinical target volume (cTV) is the volume(s) of suspected microscopic tumor infiltration. Planning target volume (PTV) is the volume containing the cTV/GTV with enough margins necessary to account for setup variations and organ and patient motion. Internal target volume (ITV) represents the movements of the cTV referenced to the patient coordinate system by internal and external reference points.

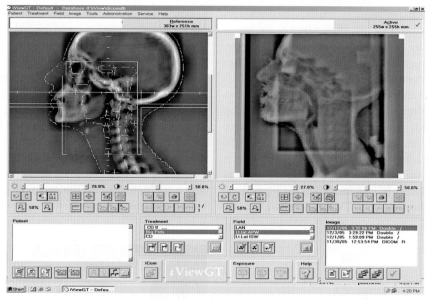

Fig. 4: Portal verification, the reference image, and the actual image anatomy are matched and the necessary correction is applied before treatment.

bony landmarks. More recently, cone-beam CT scanners have been integrated into linear accelerators which generate three-dimensional images of the treatment area, thereby enabling more precise and image-guided patient localization prior to every treatment.

● EXTERNAL BEAM RADIATION THERAPY

Most head and neck cancers are treated with external beam radiation therapy (EBRT), where the radiation is delivered from a distance of

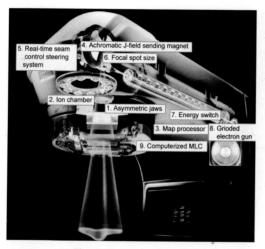

Fig. 5: Linear accelerator.

80–100 cm from the patient. The most frequently used forms of ionizing radiation are high energy photons and electrons. The choice of beams and the beam energy is based upon tumor location and target volume.

Photons

As the photon energy increases, the point of maximum dose absorbed (d-max) occurs at a greater depth. Low energies in the 4–6 MV range typically are used in the head and neck region where tumors are relatively superficial as compared with other areas such as chest or abdomen. As the maximal dose is delivered at a certain tissue depth, megavoltage photon beams have a "skin-sparing" effect. In order to bring up the dose to the surface, especially in superficial lesions, or when the dermis is involved by the tumor, a tissue equivalent material with similar electron density (called "bolus") has to be placed on the skin surface, to ensure adequate dose delivery **(Fig. 6A)**.

Electrons

Skin cancers and other superficial malignancies can be treated with electrons beams. A range of electron energies between 6 and 22 MeV is

available on most linear accelerators. As the electrons travel through tissue they dissipate their energy at much shorter distance. Their dose gradient is often sharp and can only reach a certain depth depending on their initial energy. Hence, tissue beyond their range can be spared while the tumors within their reach get adequate doses. Therefore, they are preferentially used when the treatment targets are superficial to the skin or if there are critical structures deeper to the treatment targets **(Fig. 6B)**.

● THREE-DIMENSIONAL CONFORMAL RADIATION THERAPY (3D-CRT)

Three-dimensional planning is based upon information that is obtained from CT scans, in contrast to older techniques that used two-dimensional planning based upon simulation fluoroscopy and X-ray films. The knowledge of the anatomic relationship of the tumor and normal body tissues, as obtained from the CT simulation, is used to deliver a radiation dose that conforms to the target volume in all the three dimensions and reduces exposure to other critical structures.

● INTENSITY-MODULATED RADIATION THERAPY

Intensity-modulated radiation therapy (IMRT) is an advanced form of 3D-CRT that is advantageous for the treatment of most head and neck cancers. After defining the target volumes and the organs-at-risk, the planning objectives is fed into the planning system, which will generate a treatment plan by multiple iterations, by a process called inverse planning. Nonuniform radiation beam intensities are used to deliver the dose conforming to the geometry of the planning target volume. The dose to the critical structures can be kept much below their tolerance limits. The benefit of IMRT in preventing xerostomia is demonstrated in many clinical trials **(Figs. 7A and B)**.

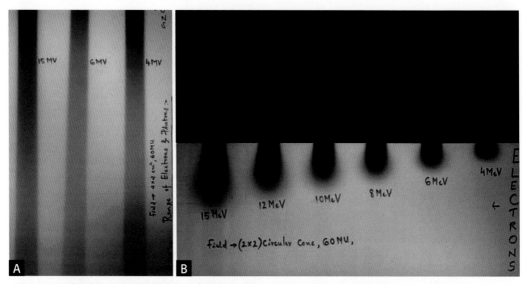

Figs. 6A and B: Beam characteristics—photon and electron, the choice of the beam type and energy is based on the location and geometric parameters of the target volumes.

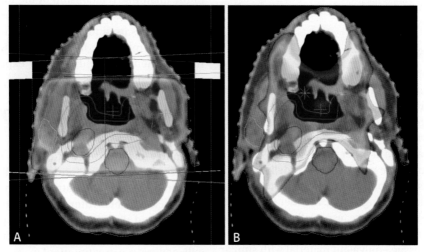

Figs. 7A and B: Intensity-modulated radiation therapy parotid sparing.

IMAGE-GUIDED RADIATION THERAPY

Patient positioning errors during daily RT ranges from 3–5 mm. Hence, a safety margin of 5–10 mm of normal tissue is included in the treatment volume, so that the tumor remains within the target volume. Image-guided radiation therapy (IGRT) utilizes high resolution on-board imaging to guide radiation delivery immediately prior to each RT. These techniques include on-board portal imaging and cone-beam CT scanner.

Treatment replanning and adaptive radiation therapy: Radiation treatments usually use a single treatment plan based on the initial size and shape of the tumor and their anatomic relationship to the normal organs. Since tumor size and the size of the normal organs and body contours can change appreciably during the course of radiation therapy, replanning the treatment, adapting to these changes, may help to reduce the dose to the normal tissue, at the same time ensuring that the tumor gets the prescribed dose.

● BRACHYTHERAPY

In brachytherapy, a radioactive source is placed within or adjacent to the tumor (or tumor bed). It facilitates delivery of a high dose of radiation to the tumor with sudden fall off in the dose toward the periphery. Brachytherapy can be used as a boost technique, to deliver more conformal dose to the target following external beam treatment or as the sole treatment in carefully selected small oral cavity tumors **(Figs. 8A to C)**.

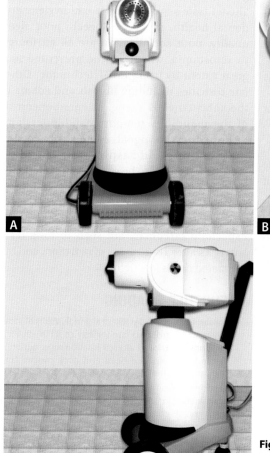

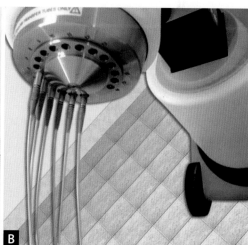

Figs. 8A to C: Brachytherapy machine. High dose rate brachytherapy can be used in interstitial, intraluminal or intracavitary treatment.

Types of Brachytherapy

Brachytherapy is classified according to the dose rate as:

- *High dose rate (HDR)*: Dose rate more than 12 Gy per hour
- *Moderate dose rate (MDR)*: Dose rate less than 12 Gy per hour
- *Low dose rate (LDR)*: Dose rate less than 2 Gy per hour.

Depending upon how the radiation source is placed with respect to the target, it is classified into the following described here.

Interstitial

The radiation source is implanted with needles or catheters through the target to deliver the dose to the target.

- *Permanent implants*: The radiation source is placed permanently in the body.
- *Temporary implants*: The radiation source is removed after a stipulated time.

Intracavitary

The radiation source is placed in the lumen of cavitary structures.

Mould brachytherapy: The radiation source is placed very close to the surface of tumor, such as palate or buccal mucosa to deliver the desired dose to the target.

Radiation Source

- Iridum[192]
- Energy: 0.37 MeV
- Half-life: 74.2 days

● SIDE EFFECTS OF RADIATION TREATMENT

Those complications occurring within the first 6 months of RT are termed as acute complications. Mucositis is the most common acute toxicity during head and neck RT. Pain and odynophagia is usually secondary to mucositis and both usually respond well to conservative medical management. Radiation-induced dermatitis was very common in the earlier time, but with the advent of linear accelerators, the skin toxicity has significantly come down. Other acute complications seen are change in taste sensation and voice.

Xerostomia is the most important late toxicity. The degree of xerostomia is largely dependent on the volume of the gland irradiated and the dose. The loss of function is usually permanent if the mean dose to the parotid gland exceeds 35 Gy. Difficulty in swallowing, altered taste sensation, poor oral hygiene and dental health, impaired speech, poor sleep quality, poor socialization are all attributed to xerostomia, which can be prevented to a great extent by using IMRT technique. Other late toxicities including fibrosis and edema of the subcutaneous tissue, osteoradionecrosis of the mandible, temporomandibular joint dysfunction, laryngeal edema, swallowing dysfunction and aspiration, cochlear dysfunction, can also be conspicuously reduced by the newer techniques and careful RT planning.

Radiation-induced second malignancies, especially sarcomas, are seen in long-term survivors after 10–20 years of radiation, and the estimated risk is less than 1%.

● FURTHER READING

1. Beitler JJ, Zhang Q, Fu KK, et al. Final results of local-regional control and late toxicity of RTOG 9003: A randomized trial of altered fractionation radiation for locally advanced head and neck cancer. Int J Radiat Oncol Biol Phys. 2014;89(1):13-20.
2. Bernier J, Cooper JS, Pajak TF, et al. Defining risk levels in locally advanced head and neck cancers: A comparative analysis of concurrent postoperative radiation plus chemotherapy trials of the EORTC (#22931) and RTOG (#9501). Head Neck. 2005;27(10):843-50.
3. Cooper JS, Zhang Q, Pajak TF, et al. Long-term follow-up of the RTOG 9501/intergroup phase III

trial: Postoperative concurrent radiation therapy and chemotherapy in high-risk squamous cell carcinoma of the head and neck. Int J Radiat Oncol Biol Phys. 2012;84(5):1198-205.

4. Daly ME, Le QT, Jain AK, et al. Intensity-modulated radiotherapy for locally advanced cancers of the larynx and hypopharynx. Head Neck. 2011;33(1): 103-11.

5. Forastiere AA, Zhang Q, Weber RS, et al. Long-term results of RTOG 91-11: A comparison of three nonsurgical treatment strategies to preserve the larynx in patients with locally advanced larynx cancer. J Clin Oncol. 2013;31(7):845-52.

6. Marta GN, Silva V, de Andrade Carvalho H, et al. Intensity-modulated radiation therapy for head and neck cancer: Systematic review and meta-analysis. Radiother Oncol. 2014;110(1):9-15.

CHAPTER 38

Molecular Biology of Head and Neck Cancer

Mayuri Mohan Rajapurkar

● INTRODUCTION

Head neck squamous cell cancers (HNSCCs) are a group of heterogenous tumor involving the mucosa of the upper aerodigestive tract (UADT). Although the etiology is often multifactorial and sometimes unknown, a vast majority of these lesions are attributed to the use of tobacco in its various forms, alcohol which has a synergistic effect when combined with tobacco as a carcinogen and human papillomavirus (HPV). The role of certain types of diets, genetic susceptibility, and viruses other than HPV such as the Epstein–Barr virus (EBV) have also been well described in literature, and are related to certain types of cancer syndromes, and certain subsites within the head-neck region.

Head neck squamous cell cancer is the sixth most common cancer worldwide. In the western world, it is the HPV-related cancers that are increasing in incidence, whereas in India it is the tobacco-related cancers that are the leading cause of oral cancer. The estimated number of new cancers in India per year is about 7 lakhs and over 3.5 lakhs people die of cancer each year. Out of these 7 lakhs new cancers about 2.3 lakhs (33%) cancers are tobacco-related. Oral and pharyngeal cancers are the leading cancers in males in India. Oral cavity is the third most common site of cancer in Indian women, while cervical cancer is the leading cancer site followed by breast, which is the second, most common. India is the oral cancer capital of the world and the majority of the oral cancers in India are caused by the use of smokeless forms of tobacco. 80% of Indian patients present with late or advanced-stage malignancy. In India 71% deaths due to cancer occur in the 30–69 years age group, whereas in the US 50% of deaths due to are above the age of 70 years. 70% of the cancer patients in India die within a year of diagnosis due to late-stage of detection. Thus, the need for early detection and primary prevention cannot be emphasized more.

Even though they originate in the squamous mucosa of the upper aerodigestive tract, there is a lot of heterogeneity in this group of tumors, and thus they can rarely be studied as one entity. This diversity of biology within this group of tumors is due to the fact that the head and neck region consists of several distinct structures (subsites) with distinct anatomic location, microscopic features, lymphatic, and venous drainage. At the molecular level also, these tumors have shown significant heterogeneity, which is independent of their inherent biologic heterogeneity. This was observed in various studies of molecular analyses that showed distinct classes of HNSCCs based on mRNA expression profiles or patterns of DNA copy number alterations that correlate with clinical behavior.

● TOBACCO-RELATED CANCERS

Tobacco use is known to cause mutations in the tumor-suppressor gene TP53, which have been linked to the development of HNSCC. Benzo[α] pyrene diol epoxide (BPDE) is a well-established carcinogen in tobacco. BPDE induces genetic damage by forming covalently bound DNA adducts throughout the genome, including p53.

There are multistep enzymatic complex systems that repair damage caused by carcinogens such as BPDE as well as other insults to the DNA. There may be individual variations in these DNA repair systems that affect the susceptibility to developing tobacco related cancers such as HNSCC. One such example is a particular polymorphism at the ERccl gene, because the ERccl gene product, which is a key enzyme in the nucleotide excision repair system.

● HUMAN PAPILLOMAVIRUS-RELATED CANCERS

Human papillomavirus infection, particularly HPV-16, has been identified to have a causal association with oropharyngeal squamous cell carcinomas. HPV-positive HNSCC is one of the major reasons of increasing cancer incidence among younger men seen lately in the USA and Europe. Patients with HPV-positive HNSCC are diagnosed at a younger age, are less likely to have a history of tobacco use, report a high lifetime number of heterosexual partners, report a young age at first intercourse, and have a history of penetrative orogenital sex. These patients also have a higher frequency of neck node involvement at presentation. HPV-positive HNSCC has been shown to have a better prognosis than HPV-negative HNSCC with a significant reduction in cancer-related mortality.

High-risk HPV strains such as HPV-16 and HPV-18 lead to malignant transformation via inactivation of TP53 tumor suppressor gene by E6 protein encoded in the HPV genome, while E7, which is another HPV protein inactivates the retinoblastoma (Rb) gene product, which is also a tumor suppressor gene. Thus, the cell cycle of the infected cells is disrupted in such a way that it leads to activation of cell growth, and suppression of apoptosis in the affected cell. In addition to inactivation of tumor suppressor genes, there is up-regulation of several genes involved in transcription, and cell-cycle regulation, such as cDKN2A. cDKN2A (cyclin-dependant kinase inhibitor 2A) encodes the tumor suppressor protein p16-INK4A in the Rb tumor suppressor pathway. Overexpression of p16-INK4A correlates strongly with HPV infection in HNSCC and is often used as a surrogate marker for HPV. Detecting p16 overexpression by immunohistochemistry (IHC) is a reliable screening test. Detecting high-risk HPV subtype using in-situ hybridization (ISH) and polymerase chain reaction techniques can be carried out wherever available. HPV vaccine composed of HPV-16 viral capsid proteins has been shown to prevent persistent HPV-16 infection and prevent development of cervical dysplasia. However, there is no data yet on its impact on oral HPV infection. HPV vaccine should be even more effective in HNSCC than cervical cancer, because HPV-16 is responsible only for 50–60% of cervical cancers whereas it is present in 94% of the HPV-positive oropharyngeal cancers. The quadrivalent as well as bivalent vaccines for HPV have been proven to be safe and effective and are now approved for use and easily available.

● GENETIC SUSCEPTIBILITY

The genotype for genes in DNA repair pathways can modify the risk of cancer development even among patients exposed to carcinogens and toxins. Germline mutations have been described that can be sporadic as well as familial. These include the following:

- *Fanconi's anemia*: Germline mutations in caretaker genes *FAA*, *FAD* and *Fcc* leading to lymphoreticular malignancies and second primary cancers in the tongue and pharynx

Bloom syndrome: Helicase gene mutations leading to high risk of tumors at various sites including tongue and larynx

- *Ataxia telangiectasia*: AT-M gene mutation leading to increased risk of T-cell leukemia, solid malignancies of the oral cavity, breast, stomach, pancreas, ovary, and urinary bladder
- *Xeroderma pigmentosum*: This is an autosomal recessive disorder of one or more of the xeroderma pigmentosa genes in the nucleotide excision repair system with a high risk of skin cancer and second primaries in the oral cavity
- *Cowden syndrome*: PTEN gene mutation
- *Multiple endocrine neoplasia Type I*: MEN I gene mutation
- *Multiple endocrine neoplasia Type II*: MEN II gene mutation
- *Neurofibromatosis type II*: NF-2 gene mutation
- *Retinoblastoma*: Rb gene mutation.

These syndromes point towards specific pathways and targets that are essential for development of cancer. Thus, drugs specific to these targets may be developed as in the case of RET.

● CARCINOGENESIS

The following are the six hallmarks of cancer cells, distinguishing them from normal cells:

1. Self-sufficiency in growth signals
2. Insensitivity to growth-inhibitory signals
3. Evasion of programmed cell death
4. Immortality or unlimited replicative potential
5. Sustained angiogenesis
6. Tissue invasion and metastasis.

Carcinogenesis in most HNSCC cases is the result of a stepwise accumulation of genetic alterations which include initiation, promotion, and progression. Initially, there is a critical early genetic change that sets into motion the carcinogenic process, which involves derangements in numerous cellular processes. Carcinogen exposure leads to abnormal expression of tumor suppressor genes or proto-oncogenes or both, and this leads to malignant transformation of cells. This abnormal expression could be a sporadic mutation, deletion, loss of heterozygosity, overexpression or epigenetic modification such as hypermethylation. Some examples include reactivation of telomerase, which is involved in cell-immortalization, deletion of 9p21 found in 70–80% HNSCC, point mutations in TP53 and loss of heterozygosity of 17p in over 50% HNSCCs. This is followed by secondary genetic changes leading to greater genetic instability and a more malignant phenotype. Cellular proliferation continues unregulated, and becomes autonomous due to inactivation of tumor-suppressor genes while proto-oncogenes help maintain the malignant cell phenotype.

● FIELD CANCERIZATION

This concept, first postulated by Slaughter et al. in 1953 refers to large areas of the aerodigestive tract mucosa affected by long-term exposure to carcinogens, resulting in genetically altered fields in which multifocal carcinomas can develop because of independent genetic events. Modern genetic and molecular studies have confirmed the presence of genetic alterations in the mucosa adjacent to primary HNSCCs, thus providing a genetic explanation for this concept. However, these studies strongly suggest that most tumors arising in these abnormal fields are clonally related, and originate from a common preneoplastic progenitor. It has been hypothesized that these multiple tumors are caused by the migration of transformed cells through the upper aerodigestive tract mucosa, either by intraepithelial migration or by saliva (micrometastases). The transformed cells have a survival advantage, eventually displace or replace the surrounding mucosa through a process known as "clonal expansion". In another study, Braakhuis et al. defined field cancerization as mucosa with "the presence of one or more areas consisting of epithelial cells that have genetic alterations. A field lesion (or field) has a monoclonal origin, and does not show invasive growth or metastatic behavior". They have proposed a new classification of secondary HNSCCs arising after treatment of an oral or oropharyngeal carcinoma based on the degree of clonal relation. Tumors with similar genetic profile should be classified as "recurrence" or a metastasis depending on whether the second lesion occurs in the same or a distant anatomical site. If the individual tumors show different genetic alterations, the secondary lesion should be regarded a "true" second primary tumor (SPT). The third group consists of lesions with a common genetic origin but which diverge in later stages; therefore, some show similar allelic imbalances, and mutations but others show different genotypes. This latter group is classified as "second field tumors".

● EPITHELIAL-TO-MESENCHYMAL TRANSITION

Epithelial-to-mesenchymal transition (EMT) is a phenotypic change in cells that provides the epithelial cells an ability to escape from constraints of surrounding tissue architecture. In this way, epithelial tumors invade and metastasize to other tissues. EMT occurs due to protein modifications and transcriptional events in response to extracellular stimuli. Abnormalities in cadherins, tight junctions, and desmosomes lead to a decrease in cell-cell adherence, and loss of polarity in the cells, increasing the mobility of these cells. The epithelial cells disassemble their junctional structures, undergo extracellular matrix remodeling, begin to express proteins of mesenchymal origin, and subsequently become migratory. This process is part of normal embryogenesis as well as inflammatory

response; however in both these cases, it is tightly regulated. During carcinogenesis, EMT causes changes in tumor cell properties that contribute to tumor invasion and metastasis, enabling cancer cell dissemination, and self-renewal capabilities. In HNSCC, EMT has been found to play a role, especially in high-risk tumor subtypes. Genes involved in EMT and nuclear factor-KB (NF-KB) signaling deregulation were the most prominent molecular characteristics of the high-risk tumors in one study.

● EPIGENETIC MODIFICATION

Within a tumor environment, different cancers display varying behaviors, due to multiple epigenetic changes, and genetic mutations. The DNA molecule can be modified, without alteration of the genetic sequence itself, by the addition or subtraction of methyl groups without a change in the base composition. Similarly, histones, the structural proteins found in close association with DNA, can be modified by acetylation, methylation, and ubiquitylation. These non-DNA-encoded modifications can result in heritable changes in gene expression.

● MOLECULAR PATHWAYS INVOLVED IN HNSCC

Molecular and genetic research has led to an increasing understanding of molecular pathways and the discovery of specific gene mutations in HNSCC, and this in turn has resulted in clinical trials of multiple targeted therapies with some promising agents. These are listed below:

- Epidermal growth factor receptor (EGFR)
- Insulin-like growth factor-1 receptor (IGF-1R)
- Phosphatidylinositol-3-kinase/protein kinase B pathway (PI3-K/Akt)
- Mammalian target of rapamycin (mTOR)
- Nuclear factor-kappa B (NF-kB)
- Heat shock protein 90.

Epidermal Growth Factor Receptor

Epidermal growth factor receptor signaling has been strongly implicated in carcinogenesis, tumor progression, and response to therapy in HNSCC. The ErbB family of proteins, a family of four structurally-related receptor tyrosine kinases, is comprised of four receptors (ErbB 1–4, also known as HER 1–4), and 13 polypeptide extracellular ligands. ErbB2 is synonymous with HER2/neu, while ErbB1 is commonly referred to as EGFR. When ligands bind to one of the ErbB receptors, a dimer forms and the receptor's intracellular tyrosine residues then undergo ATP-dependent autophosphorylation. Currently, there are 12 different ligands that are known to activate four known ErbB receptors. Once phosphorylated, the receptor has the potential to trigger a number of different intracellular downstream pathways that can eventually arrest apoptosis, promote cellular proliferation, stimulate tumor-induced neovascularization, and activate carcinoma invasion, and metastasis. The Ras/mitogen-activated protein kinase/extracellular signal-related kinase (Ras-MAPK-ERK) pathway is known to control gene transcription, cell proliferation, and cell-cycle progression, while the phosphatidylinositol-3-kinase/protein kinase B (PI3K/Akt) pathway has been shown to stimulate numerous antiapoptotic signals within the cell. The Janus kinase/signal transducers and activators of transcription (JAK/STAT) and the phospholipase-cγ/protein kinase c (PLcγ/PKc) pathways are also activated in association with EGFR phosphorylation. Thus, EGFR plays a role in carcinoma growth and survival through a multitude of oncogenic downstream signaling pathways.

Currently, there are several EGFR antagonists available for clinical utilization in the treatment of four metastatic epithelial carcinomas, including non-small cell lung cancer, colorectal cancer, pancreatic cancer, and HNSCC. The two classes of therapies that exist to date are monoclonal antibodies (MAbs) to EGFR receptor subunits and small-molecule EGFR tyrosine kinase inhibitors (TKIs). Monoclonal antibodies act by binding the extracellular domain of EGFR and then blocking the ligand-binding region by competitive inhibition. This blocks ligand-induced autophosphorylation through the inability to stimulate tyrosine kinase. The EGFR tyrosine kinase inhibitors act by reversibly competing with ATP in its binding site to the intracellular catalytic domain of tyrosine kinase, therefore inhibiting autophosphorylation of EGFR, and its subsequent downstream signaling.

EGFR overexpression in head and neck cancer cell lines were found to have greater radioresistance compared to cell lines with relatively lower levels of EGFR expression. It was also found that following radiation, EGFR becomes upregulated within the tumor, leading to increased activation of its downstream signaling pathways. Based on this work, Bonner et al. designed and published the landmark randomized controlled trial showing an overall, and progression-free survival advantage with the addition of cetuximab to standard radiation therapy.

Many trials are ongoing and multiple targeted agents are in development currently, however it is difficult to establish the patient population that will specifically benefit from these. Thus, further research into molecular predictors of clinical outcome that would help optimize patient selection and increase therapeutic efficacy is currently an area of intense interest.

● GENETIC EXPRESSION PROFILING AND PROGNOSTIC MARKERS

Large numbers of genetic markers can be tested with greater ease using increasingly sophisticated molecular detection techniques and technologies such as DNA microarrays. As single molecular markers, most of the studies so far have failed to show sufficient predictive potential in terms of the course of disease, prognosis, and survival. However, combinations of different molecular markers and genetic expression patterns may offer more promising diagnostic and prognostic value. Other combinatorial approaches, using biomarkers and traditional clinical markers have been proposed, and will likely gain increasing interest. Selection from among the competing markers and incorporation into clinical practice is another area of intense investigation of our times.

● ROLE OF IMMUNOTHERAPY

Head and neck squamous cell carcinoma evades immune responses via multiple mechanisms. HNSCC has a characteristic immunosuppressive environment with the release of immunosuppressive factors, activation, expansion of immune cells with inhibitory activity, and decreased tumor immunogenicity. Immunotherapeutic approaches designed on the basis of the understanding of these mechanisms led to clinical trials such as the CheckMate-141 and Keynote-012, using the immune-modulating antibodies, Nivolumab and Pembrolizumab, which are now a "fourth" modality in the treatment of HNSCC. These are monoclonal antibodies against programmed cell death protein-1 (PD-1), an "immune checkpoint" receptor found on the surface of T-cells, PD-1 negatively regulates their activation. Nivolumab and Pembrolizumab have been approved by the USFDA in 2016, as new standard-of-care options for the second-line treatment of recurrent and/or metastatic SCC. Checkpoint inhibitor antibodies for the treatment of HNSCC have demonstrated clear benefits in terms of patients' survival and durability of response but can also induce serious immune-related adverse events coupled with an inability to consistently and accurately identify patients

likely to respond to this type of therapy. Many more immunotherapeutic treatment options are currently under investigation. Ongoing trials are investigating immunotherapeutic approaches also in the curative setting and combination therapies using different immunotherapeutic approaches. Understanding the genetic signatures most likely to be associated with a productive response to checkpoint-inhibitor therapy is important along with understanding and developing methods for integrating this modality with the current standard approaches.

● FURTHER READING

1. Perez-Ordoñez B, Beauchemin M, Jordan RC. Molecular biology of squamous cell carcinoma of the head and neck. J Clin Pathol. 2006;59(5):445-53.
2. Stadler ME, Patel MR, Couch ME, et al. Molecular biology of head and neck cancer: risks and pathways. Hematology/Oncology Clinics of North America. 2008;22(6):1099-124.

Tobacco-related Cancers

3. Blot WJ, McLaughlin JK, Winn DM, et al. Smoking and drinking in relation to oral and pharyngeal cancer. Cancer Res. 1988;48(11):3282-7.
4. Hermsen M, Guervós MA, Meijer G, et al. New chromosomal regions with high-level amplifications in squamous cell carcinomas of the larynx and pharynx, identified by comparative genomic hybridization. J Pathol. 2001;194(2):177-82.
5. Leemans CR, Braakhuis BJ, Brakenhoff RH. The molecular biology of head and neck cancer. Nat Rev Cancer. 2011;11(1):9-22.
6. World Health Organization. IARC Monographs on the Evaluation of Carcinogenic Risks in Humans. Lyon, France: World Health Organization; 2014. pp. 1-54.

HPV-related Cancers

7. Fakhry C, Gillison ML. Clinical implications of human papillomavirus in head and neck cancers. J Clin Oncol. 2006;24(17):2606-11.
8. Kreimer AR, Clifford GM, Boyle P, et al. Human papillomavirus types in head and neck squamous cell carcinomas worldwide: a systematic review. Cancer Epidemiol Biomarkers Prev. 2005;14(2):467-75.
9. Slebos RJ, Yi Y, Ely K, et al. Gene expression differences associated with human papillomavirus status in head and neck squamous cell carcinoma. Clin Cancer Res. 2006;12(3 Pt 1):701-9.

9. Tran N, Rose BR, O'Brien CJ. Role of human papillomavirus in the etiology of head and neck cancer. Head Neck. 2007;29(1):64-70.

10. Zhang MQ, El-Mofty SK, Dávila RM. Detection of human papillomavirus-related squamous cell carcinoma cytologically and by in situ hybridization in fine-needle aspiration biopsies of cervical metastasis: a tool for identifying the site of an occult head and neck primary. Cancer. 2008;114(2):118-23.

Genetic Susceptibility

11. Hecht F, Hecht BK. Cancer in ataxia-telangiectasia patients. Cancer Genet Cytogenet. 1990;46(1):9-19.

13. Keukens F, van Voorst Vader PC, Panders AK, et al. Xeroderma pigmentosum: squamous cell carcinoma of the tongue. Acta Derm Venereol. 1989;69(6):530-1.

Carcinogenesis

14. Argiris A, Karamouzis MV, Raben D, et al. Head and neck cancer. Lancet 2008;371(9625):1695-709.

15. Fearon ER, Vogelstein B. A genetic model for colorectal tumorigenesis. Cell. 1990;61(5):759-67.

16. Weinberg RA. Oncogenes, antioncogenes, and the molecular bases of multistep carcinogenesis. Cancer Res. 1989;49(14):3713-21.

Field Cancerization

17. Braakhuis BJ, Tabor MP, Leemans CR, et al. Second primary tumors and field cancerization in oral and oropharyngeal cancer: molecular techniques provide new insights and definitions. Head Neck. 2002;24(2):198-206.

18. van Oijen MG, Slootweg PJ. Oral field cancerization: Carcinogen-induced independent events or micrometastatic deposits? Cancer Epidemiol Biomarkers Prev. 2000;9(3):249-56.

19. Worsham MJ, Wolman SR, Carey TE, et al. Common clonal origin of synchronous primary head and neck squamous cell carcinomas: Analysis by tumor karyotypes and fluorescence in situ hybridization. Hum Pathol. 1995;26(3):251-61.

Epithelial-Mesenchymal Transition

20. Hugo H, Ackland ML, Blick T, et al. Epithelial—mesenchymal and mesenchymal—epithelial transitions in carcinoma progression. J Cell Physiol. 2007;213(2):374-83.

Epigenetic Modification

21. Worsham MJ, Chen KM, Meduri V, et al. Epigenetic events of disease progression in head and neck squamous cell carcinoma. Arch Otolaryngol Head Neck Surg. 2006;132(6):668-77.

Epidermal Growth Factor Receptor (EGFR)

22. Ang KK, Berkey BA, Tu X, et al. Impact of epidermal growth factor receptor expression on survival and pattern of relapse in patients with advanced head and neck carcinoma. Cancer Res. 2002;62(24):7350-6.

23. Bonner JA, Harari PM, Giralt J, et al. Radiotherapy plus cetuximab for squamous-cell carcinoma of the head and neck. N Engl J Med. 2006;354(6):567-78.

24. Ciardiello F, Tortora G. EGFR antagonists in cancer treatment. N Engl J Med. 2008;358(11):1160-74.

25. Thariat J, Milas L, Ang KK. Integrating radiotherapy with epidermal growth factor receptor antagonists and other molecular therapeutics for the treatment of head and neck cancer. Int J Radiat Oncol Biol Phys. 2007;69(4):974-84.

Genetic Expression Profiling and Prognostic Markers

26. Chung CH, Parker JS, Karaca G, et al. Molecular classification of head and neck squamous cell carcinomas using patterns of gene expression. Cancer Cell. 2004;5(5):489-500.

27. Roepman P, Wessels LF, Kettelarij N, et al. An expression profile for diagnosis of lymph node metastases from primary head and neck squamous cell carcinomas. Nat Genet. 2005;37(2):182-6.

28. Thomas GR, Nadiminti H, Regalado J. Molecular predictors of clinical outcome in patients with head and neck squamous cell carcinoma. Int J Exp Pathol. 2005;86(6):347-63.

Immunotherapy

29. Ferris RL, Blumenschein G Jr, Fayette J, et al. Nivolumab for recurrent squamous-cell carcinoma of the head and neck. N Engl J Med. 2016;375(19):1856-67.

30. Seiwert TY, Burtness B, Mehra R, et al. Safety and clinical activity of pembrolizumab for treatment of recurrent or metastatic squamous cell carcinoma of the head and neck (KEYNOTE-012): an open-label, multicentre, phase 1b trial. Lancet Oncol. 2016;17(7):956-65.

CHAPTER 39

Recent Advances in Management of Head and Neck Cancer

Deepak Balasubramanian

● INTRODUCTION

Head and neck oncology has been at the crossroads with regards to their management. With the advent of modern surgical techniques, reconstruction, and organ preservation, there has been a shift in the focus to include the reduction of the treatment morbidity. The move from more radical neck dissection to the more functional neck dissections, the use of transoral and endoscopic procedures, and the adoption of chemoradiotherapy protocols reflect the change in the management of these tumors.

● HUMAN PAPILLOMAVIRUS AND HEAD AND NECK CANCER

The identification of the human papillomavirus (HPV) as an etiological agent in cervical cancer tumorigenesis heralded a new era in the management. This allowed for the development of vaccines, which could potentially decrease the chance of genital infection and thereby reduce the incidence of cervical cancers. Recently, there has been a focus on the role of HPV types 16 and 18 in the etiology of oropharyngeal cancers. This arose from the similarity in the pathological features between oropharyngeal tumors and genital lesions and the identification of p16 expression and HPV RNA in the oropharyngeal lesions. Major studies done in the United States have indicated that HPV-associated oropharyngeal tumors in patients with no other risk factors and habits have a better outcome compared to patients with risk factors and HPV negative tumors. This has allowed for risk stratification in oropharyngeal tumors. Such risk stratification has allowed for potential de-escalation of treatment in the low risk group. Currently, trials are underway using transoral robotic surgery (TORS), single agent chemotherapy, and radiotherapy alone for these HPV negative low risk tumors. Also, the role of HPV in nonoropharyngeal tumors is being investigated.

Transoral Robotic Surgery

With the recent literature revealing the relationship of HPV virus to oropharyngeal cancers and studies proving better outcomes, there has been a move to de-escalate the HPV positive oropharyngeal tumors. Surgical treatment, though possible, had been limited by the transoral exposure, the need for open cervical approaches and instrumentation. Also, the treatment of the neck always necessitated a neck dissection due to the high propensity of nodal metastasis from oropharyngeal primary. However, in the 2000s the surgical robot (DaVinci) had been developed and increasingly used for gynecological and urological procedures. The use of the robot was extended to oropharyngeal primaries with good results and has been approved by the Food and Drug Administration (FDA) for T1 and T2 tumors in 2009.

The currently universally used system is the Da Vinci System. The robot has a console in which the surgeon sits and operates, an instrument cluster which includes the camera and instrumentation. The instruments are positioned transorally after the mouth is opened with a retractor. The surgical arms allow for 360° rotation and the camera is able to see beyond the line of normal sight allowing for unparalleled visualization. The advantages of transoral oropharyngeal surgery include avoiding an open approach (usually a lip split and mandibulotomy), avoidance of tracheostomy, improved visualization and magnification, limited blood loss, and equal results to open approaches. The disadvantages include the cost of the equipment, the need for adjuvant treatment in certain patients (based on the histopathology report which makes it a combined modality treatment), and the learning curve. Though popular in the United States, TORS is yet to become popular in the developing countries.

Sentinel Node Biopsy

The management of the node negative neck has always been controversial in head and neck squamous cell carcinomas (SCC). Due to the high risk of occult node metastasis, an elective neck dissection has been advocated to improve local control. There have been trials and meta-analysis supporting the role of elective neck dissection for N0 oral SCC. Elective neck dissection allows for accurate staging of the neck and allows for planning of adjuvant treatment. However with the improvements in imaging, it is possible to surgically treat a neck after the recurrence with acceptable results.

One of the ways to accurately stage the N0 is to perform a sentinel node biopsy (SLNB). Sentinel node biopsy has been accepted and used in penile, breast, and malignant melanoma. The concept of sentinel node is to identify the first echelon node in the nodal basin. A radio labeled dye namely radio labeled sulfur colloid is injected to the bed of the tumor. The neck is then imaged using a gamma camera and the nodes, which are hot on the scan, are marked on the skin. This region is surgically explored. One of the ways to aid in the identification of the nodes is to inject methylene blue along the margins of the tumor and this will drain to the lymph node blue and stain the node blue. Using a combination of methylene blue and radio labeled colloid is preferred to identify the lymph nodes. Once the nodes are identified, they are dissected in isolation and subjected to histopathological assessment particularly serial step sectioning. This allows for accurate diagnosis regarding the presence of metastasis. Three major trials have been done in the field of oral cavity SCCs and they have indicated a high sensitivity for the technique.

There have been no major trials comparing the SLNB to elective neck dissections. Also the role of SLNB in previously treated oral SCCs is also under investigation. So, currently SLNB is an investigative tool in a trial setting and may become the standard of care in the future.

● MOLECULAR DIAGNOSTICS IN THYROID CANCER

The incidence of thyroid cancer is rapidly increasing worldwide. This is partly due to the increased detection of smaller nodules and improved imaging and pathological diagnosis. A majority of these nodules are differentiated thyroid cancers. The fine needle aspiration cytology (FNAC) is used as the initial diagnostic test for the diagnosis of the thyroid nodules. The American Thyroid Association and the Bethesda classification have categorized the FNAC diagnosis. One such result is the indeterminate FNAC which can be up to 30% of the thyroid nodules reported on FNAC.

These indeterminate nodules pose a problem in their management, as patients inadvertently prefer to undergo surgery to pathologically confirm the diagnosis.

BRAF genetic mutation is the most common mutation causing activation of the MAP kinase pathway in human cancers and is of particular importance in thyroid cancers (T1799A mutation). BRAF mutation has a tumorigenic potential and is associated with aggressive behavior, metastasis, tumor dedifferentiation, and recurrence. Currently, BRAF mutation studies are being done in indeterminate FNACs in an attempt to identify malignant behavior. In the future, it might be a potent tool for the identification of aggressive thyroid tumors.

● NEWER SYSTEMIC AGENTS (EPIDERMAL GROWTH FACTOR RECEPTOR AND TYROSINE KINASE INHIBITOR)

With better understanding of the molecular pathways in head and neck cancer, newer systemic agents have been developed. One of the pathways affected in head and neck cancers includes the epidermal growth factor receptor (EGFR). This receptor is activated in most head neck cancers. Blocking of the EGFR has been tried with monoclonal antibodies against the receptor (e.g. cetuximab) and tyrosine kinase inhibitors (TKIs) (e.g. gefitinib). Currently, cetuximab is indicated for nonsurgical management (unresectable) of recurrent or metastatic SCC along with cisplatin based chemotherapy. The TKIs namely lapatinib and geftinib are used in advanced metastatic salivary gland tumors to arrest disease progression.

Sorafenib and sunitinib have also been tried for advanced radiorefractive and untreatable differentiated thyroid cancer.

● ADVANCES IN RADIATION DELIVERY TECHNIQUES

There has been a shift in the mode of delivery of radiation namely, conformal radiation techniques. The conformal radiation allows for more precise targeting of the tumor and sparing of the adjacent structures. Intensity-modulated radiotherapy is one such technique. A more detailed explanation of the technique is available in the chapter on radiation therapy.

● FURTHER READING

1. Blitzer GC, Smith MA, Harris SL, et al. Review of the clinical and biologic aspects of human papillomavirus-positive squamous cell carcinomas of the head and neck. Int J Radiat Oncol Biol Phys. 2014;88(4):761-70.
2. De Ceulaer J, De Clercq C, Swennen GR. Robotic surgery in oral and maxillofacial, craniofacial and head and neck surgery: a systematic review of the literature. Int J Oral Maxillofac Surg. 2012;41(11):1311-24.
3. Gold KA, Neskey M, William WN Jr. The role of systemic treatment before, during, and after definitive treatment. Otolaryngol Clin North Am. 2013;46(4):645-56.
4. Kuriakose MA, Trivedi NP. Sentinel node biopsy in head and neck squamous cell carcinoma. Curr Opin Otolaryngol Head Neck Surg. 2009;17(2):100-10.
5. Patel KN. Genetic mutations, molecular markers and future directions in research. Oral Oncol. 2013;49(7):711-21.

CHAPTER 40

Head and Neck Reconstruction

Mohit Sharma, Abhijeet N Wakure, Sivakumar Vidhyadharan, Subramania Iyer

● INTRODUCTION

Reconstruction after resection is an integral part of the management of head and neck malignancies. Due to the complicated nature of these defects, head and neck reconstruction should be undertaken only by a team adequately equipped and trained to perform any of the various procedures described below. Furthermore, the team should also include personnel who can provide adequate rehabilitation to the patient during and after reconstruction.

● PRINCIPLES OF RECONSTRUCTION

- Protect and maintain the vital functions at all times viz., airways and enteral nutrition.
- Accurately assess the complete extent of the defect, i.e. the anatomical subunits that are lost and their relationship to one another.
- Use the most appropriate tissue for reconstruction (like for like) within the limits set by the patient's physiology.

● GOALS OF RECONSTRUCTION

- To provide stable coverage of important vital structures.
- To achieve restoration of function viz., speech, mastication, and swallowing.
- To maintain aesthesis.

● RECONSTRUCTIVE STRATEGIES

- *Healing by secondary intention*: This strategy is rarely used; used in cases of small defects of the tongue and very small defects over the scalp.
- *Primary or delayed primary wound closure*: Small defects can be primarily closed taking advantage of the skin laxity of the head and neck region. Care must be taken that closure does not distort other important structures, e.g. the lower lid (which may lead to ectropion). Wide undermining and scoring the galea parallel to the long axis of the defect can help mobilize tissues enough to be able to close scalp defects.
- *Nonvascularized grafts (skin, fat, cartilage, bone, nerve or tendon)*: A graft is a piece of tissue transferred without its blood supply from one part of the body to another where it must derive its nutrition from the native tissue bed. Presence of a healthy and well vascularized bed is essential for the successful "take" of a graft.

  Skin grafts may be split thickness skin graft (STSG) which contains epidermis and a portion of the dermis or full thickness skin graft (FTSG) which contains epidermis and entire dermis. STSG gives poor color and texture match, causes contraction of the wound, and are prone to break down with trivial trauma but are available plentifully, and takes up well. FTSG, on the other hand, gives a good color and texture match, and gives a strong and stable coverage without wound contraction. However, the donor sites are limited (postauricular region and supraclavicular region for the head and neck), and the "take" of the graft may be precarious.

Fat grafts (harvested by liposuction) are used for filling contour defects as soft tissue filler to restore volume. It has been used extensively in aesthetic surgical procedures of the face. Presence of adipose derived stem cells in the lipoaspirate has generated much interest in fat grafting.

Cartilage grafts are used in nasal and auricular reconstruction. Potential donor sites are nasal cartilage, ear cartilage, and costal cartilage. Bone grafts are used in the reconstruction of the facial skeleton. Typical donor areas are the iliac crest, outer table of the calvarium, rib, fibula, etc. Nerve grafts are used typically for bridging nerve gaps (e.g. in facial nerve palsy) either for primary repair, neurotization or functioning muscle transfer. Tendon grafts are rarely used.

- *Vascularized flaps (local flaps, regional flaps, and distant or free flaps):*
  - *Local flaps*: These may be random pattern flaps like the rotation, advancement or transposition flaps. Since the vascularity of the head and neck region is excellent, longer flaps with narrow pedicles can be safely raised. Some of the commonly used local flaps which are based upon named vessels are:
    - *Submental flap*: It is a flap from the submental area which is based upon the submental branch of the facial artery. It is useful for surfacing defects on the lower third of face, floor of mouth, and buccal mucosal defects.
    - *Nasolabial flap*: It is raised from the nasolabial crease and is based upon the angular branch of the facial artery. The flap may be superiorly or inferiorly based. It is commonly used to resurface nasal defects as well as intraoral defects.
    - *Forehead flap*: The median forehead flap is based upon the supraorbital artery and is commonly used to resurface the defects on the dorsum of the nose.
- *Regional flaps*: The commonly used regional flaps in head and neck reconstruction are the pectoralis major myocutaneous flap and the deltopectoral flap. Other flaps that are rarely used include the trapezius flap and the latisimus dorsi flap.
  - *Pectoralis major myocutaneous flap*: The flap is based on the thoracoacromion vessels that run beneath the pectoralis major muscle at the midpoint of the clavicle. The skin paddle receives its blood supply from the underlying muscle. The flap can provide coverage of the middle and lower third of the face, the neck and the oral cavity. It can also provide bone reconstruction if a segment of the 5th or 6th rib or the lateral sternum is harvested along with it. In situations where microvascular free tissue transfer is not possible, this flap is the work horse flap for head and neck reconstructions. Excess bulk, nonpliability, and donor site deformity are the chief drawbacks of this flap.
  - *Deltopectoral flap*: It is based on the internal mammary artery perforators; this flap extends from the parasternal region till the deltoid

region. The second intercostals space perforater is most commonly used. The flap can reach up to the lower third of the face, oral cavity, and neck. To obtain a longer flap, a delay procedure can be performed. A second surgery is needed 3 weeks later to divide the flap pedicle and do the final insetting.

- *Free flaps*: Commonly used free flaps in head and neck reconstruction are the radial forearm flap, anterolateral thigh flap, rectus abdominis flap, fibular flap, Iliac crest flap, and the scapular flap.

  ♦ *Radial forearm flap*: The radial forearm flap is one of the most common flaps used in head and neck reconstruction. It is a fasciocutaneous flap based on the radial artery and it vena comitantes. The cephalic vein provides another source of venous drainage. It provides a large area of thin and pliable skin with a long pedicle. Harvesting the radial bone (approximately 40% of its circumference) between the insertions of pronator teres and brachioradialis can be done to raise an osteocutaneous flap although it is not commonly performed. Lack of tissue bulk, less bone stock, donor site morbidity, and poor aesthesis are the main drawbacks.

  ♦ *Anterolateral thigh flap*: This is a fasciocutaneous flap based on the perforating vessels from the descending branch of the lateral circumflex femoral vessels. The perforator may be musculocutaneous (piercing the vastus lateralis muscle) or less commonly septocutaneous (running through the septum between the rectus femoris and the vastus lateralis muscles. A large flap of up to 25 × 15 cm can be raised. The ALT flap can be raised with the vastus lateralis muscle if a bulky flap is needed or can be thinned if a thin flap is needed. There is minimal functional loss and the aesthesis is good especially if the donor site can be closed primarily.

  ♦ *Fibular flap*: The free fibular flap is the most commonly used flap for reconstruction of the bony defects of the head and neck. The flap is based on the peroneal vessels. The fibula provides good bone stock and its robust periosteal supply ensures that multiple osteotomies can be performed for contouring the bone. The flexor hallucis longus muscle and a skin paddle (based on the peroneal septocutaneous perforater) can be harvested along with the flap to provide soft tissue reconstruction along with bone. Up to 25 cm of the bone length is available and it has a long pedicle with good vessel caliber.

  ♦ *Iliac crest flap*: This flap can be raised on the deep circumflex Iliac vessels which arise from the external Iliac vessels. The bone quality is excellent and good height of the bone can be obtained. Internal oblique muscle can be harvested to reconstruct associated soft tissue defects. Short length of vessels, donor site morbidity (deformity, hernia formation, nerve injury, lateral cutaneous nerve of thigh, etc.), and tenuous blood supply to its skin paddle are the disadvantages of this flap.

  ♦ *Rectus abdominis flap*: The rectus abdominis myocutaneous flap is based upon the deep inferior epigastric vessels. It provides a bulky flap with a long pedicle. Donor site morbidity (hernia formation) and excessive bulk at the pedicle are the disadvantages of the flap.

- *Scapular flap*: The scapular flap is based on the circumflex scapular vessels. Two separate skin paddles with independent mobility can be harvested along with the flap based on the transverse and the descending branches of the parent vessel. This makes it a truly chimeric flap. The short bone length, short pedicle, and need for change in position for harvesting (thus precluding a two team approach and increasing operating time) are the chief disadvantages.

■ *Tissue expansion and distraction osteogenesis*: Tissue expansion makes use of the plastic nature of the human integument to create new autogenous skin. Placement and gradual inflation of prosthesis under the skin and subcutaneous tissue allows the surgeon to expand the skin and subcutaneous tissue which can be used to reconstruct adjacent defects. External hardware is used to gradually distract the bones of the craniofacial skeleton for inducing osteogenesis in cases of bone defects (hemifacial microsomia, fractures, etc.). The surface area as well as the vascularity of a free flap can be increased manifold by placement of a tissue expander underneath it. Color matched FTSGs essential for aesthetic resurfacing of the face are scanty. This problem can be circumvented by expanding the supraclavicular areas and harvesting large amount of FTSG from there.

Tissue expansion takes long time and multiple stages and may produce a temporary but obvious deformity. It cannot be used when an urgent cover is essential

(e.g. when vital structures are exposed) or in presence of infection. It is best performed as a secondary procedure. However, it has the advantage of providing large amounts of local tissue which may be the best match for the defect by providing like for like tissues.

Proper planning is essential to ensure that correct size and shape of expander is chosen, correctly matching donor area is chosen, placement of the expander and its port is in the correct area and the correct tissue plane without damaging the important structures, and the final scars are as inconspicuous as possible. Flaps should be planned for advancement, transposition, or rotation. Access incision for insertion or removal of the expander is usually a pre-existing scar or an edge of the planned flap. Optimal aesthetic reconstruction of the head and neck region is achieved by mobilization of adjacent local tissues which provide good match of color, texture, and hair bearing capability rather than distant tissues. The head and neck region can be subdivided into five tissue specific areas:

- The scalp contains specific hair-bearing qualities that cannot be mimicked by any other tissue of the human body hence defects of the scalp are optimally reconstructed by expanding the remaining area of the scalp and using it to cover the defect. The expander is usually placed in the supra-galeal plane.
- The forehead, although a continuation of the scalp, is distinguished by its thick skin, large number of sebaceous glands, and lack of hair. Defects of the forehead can be reconstructed by expanding the remnant forehead or by utilizing expanded supraclavicular FTSGs. Defects near the hairline may be reconstructed using the expanded scalp although this may bring the hairline bit lower. Care should be taken not to

cause distortion of the brows. The plane of insertion of the tissue expander is above the frontalis muscle.

- The nose being embryologically related to the forehead closely mimics it in color, texture, and sebaceous gland content. Hence, the expanded forehead flap is used for nasal reconstruction.
- The lateral cheek, neck, and upper lip have fewer sebaceous glands, thin skin, and a unique hair-bearing pattern which is significantly different in quality and quantity from that on the remainder of the body. Hence, defects in these areas are adequately reconstructed by expanding local flaps from the adjacent areas. For example, a large Mustarde rotation flap (based inferiorly and medially) can be designed over the neck for cheek reconstruction. The expander is usually placed above the superficial musculo-aponeurotic system (SMAS) layer in the cheek and above the platysma in the neck.
- The skin of the periorbital areas is extremely thin and pliable, containing a minimal number of sebaceous glands. Optimal skin cover of this area is achieved by skin grafts from a color matched area like the postauricular region or the supraclavicular area. Large skin grafts can be harvested by pre-expanding these areas.

Complications of tissue expansion include failure of the device, infection, extrusion, inadequate expansion, improper expansion, and ischemia and necrosis of the expanding tissues. The last one can be prevented by slow expansion and watching for signs of ischemia and urgently deflating the device if present.

- *Facial prosthetics*: Tissue-based reconstruction remains the standard of care for management of defects of the head and neck region. In cases where it may be contraindicated, technically impossible, or may solve the problem only partially, prosthesis based reconstruction offers solutions. Craniofacial prosthesis can be adhesive based or osseointegrated. The advent of osseointegrated prosthetic implants has revolutionized the field of craniofacial prosthetics and has significantly improved aesthetic acceptability, functional performance, biocompatibility and desired retention of the prosthetic implants.

The advantages are:

- Short outpatient procedures with short learning curve
- Minimal morbidity and postoperative pain
- Allows examination of tumor resection sites
- Can be used in compromised tissues
- Can be used for salvage of tissue-based reconstruction
- Excellent and predictable aesthetics

The disadvantages are:

- Does not use living tissue
- Need for multidisciplinary team
- Need for a committed patient
- On-going expenses for remakes and maintenance
- Need for multiple visits for maintenance of the prosthesis
- Need to replace the prosthesis every 2–5 years.

Indications: Craniofacial osseointegration can be of particular benefit for reconstruction of selected defects involving the ear, orbit, nose, and combined midfacial defects.

- Following major cancer resection
- Compromised local tissues due to radiotherapy, burns or trauma
- Failed autogenous reconstruction
- Patient preference
- Poor operative risk
- Nonavailability of donor tissue (e.g. calcified costal cartilage in ear reconstruction).

The implants are usually made up of titanium. Other materials like vanadium, tantalum, and aluminum oxide or ceramics like hydroxyapatite are used less frequently. After the first phase of implant placement, a period of 3–6 months is needed for adequate osseointegration. In the second phase, the soft tissues over the implant are debrided to expose the implant and create a flat nonhair-bearing area of 1 cm around the implant. The prosthesis is created and fixed 4–6 weeks later after adequate healing.

Diligent maintenance is essential to avoid failure of the implants and prosthesis. The usual life of the prosthesis is 2–5 years after which it has to be changed.

- *Composite tissue transplantation:* Partial and complete face transplantation for severely mutilated facial defects has become a clinical reality. As of February 2012, 20 facial transplants have taken place in the world. The obvious advantage is provision of exact tissues that have been lost and that they are dynamic. This result cannot be replicated by any reconstructive method available as of today.

The surgery is immensely complex and has not yet been performed in India. Life-long immunosuppression and strict vigilance to look for rejection is essential as with any organ transplant. The indications for a face transplant are essentially nonlethal. Use of immunosuppression (with its potential toxicity and complications, some of them life-threatening) for a nonlethal condition is questionable. Ethical and psychological issues also need to be addressed since the identity of the donor as well as recipient is at stake. Unless these questions are conclusively answered, facial transplant will not become a commonly performed procedure.

- *Tissue engineering:* The ideal reconstructive technique should be able to exactly replicate the lost tissues with minimal donor site morbidity and no systemic side effects. Although such a technique is not available clinically, tissue engineering promises to provide an effective answer to the reconstructive dilemma.

A scaffold is constructed based on the tissue to be reconstructed, which is then seeded with stem cells or committed progenitor cells. In presence of appropriate environmental signals, the cells differentiate into mature cells of the tissue while also secreting the extracellular matrix. This matrix gradually replaces the original scaffold which slowly gets degraded and disappears totally. Finding compatible scaffolds, appropriate signals, and ensuring cellular proliferation without inducing carcinogenicity are the challenges that are faced by tissue engineering scientists.

Reconstructive Options Based on Each Region

Scalp and Forehead Reconstruction

Small defects of the scalp can be left to heal by secondary intention or closed primarily. Wide undermining of the scalp and scoring the *galea aponeurotica* can help to mobilize the scalp tissue and aid primary closure. Temporary coverage of scalp defects with vascular bed can be achieved by split skin grafting. For small to medium sized defects, local flaps can be useful. These include the rotation, advancement, and transposition flaps. Multiple local flaps may be used for a single defect, e.g. the three flap technique of orticochea. Tissue expansion (see above) enables the surgeon to expand the available scalp tissue in a way that local flaps can be fashioned out of the expanded tissue to cover the defect. Regional flaps have limited role in scalp reconstruction. The trapezius flap may be used to cover the occipital or temporal areas. The pedicled latissimus dorsi flap may be used to cover the temporal area. For large scalp defects, free latissimus dorsi muscle flap covered with a skin graft remains the reconstructive method of choice. Calvarial defects need to be reconstructed either with bone graft (calvarial outer table graft, rib graft) or with titanium mesh. Regardless of which modality is used, this needs to be covered with vascularized tissue **(Figs. 1A to D)**.

Maxillary Reconstruction

Aims of maxillary reconstruction are to close the wound, obliterate the maxillary cavity, restore facial shape, provide support to the orbital contents if preserved or obliterate the cavity if the globe is exenterated, maintain a barrier between nasal sinuses and the brain, and to reconstruct the palate.

Maxillary defects have been traditionally reconstructed by lining the defect with a skin graft and after healing, providing an obturator-prosthesis. Recent literature, however, shows a trend towards reconstruction with autologous tissue. The flap used for reconstruction depends upon the amount of resected skin, soft tissue, and bone. The reconstructive options vary from center to center but certain general principles are followed.

Smaller defects involving only the palate can be reconstructed with local palatal flaps, regional flaps like the temporalis flap or free radial forearm flap. Larger maxillary defects not involving the orbital floor may be reconstructed with a soft tissue free flap to provide bulk and

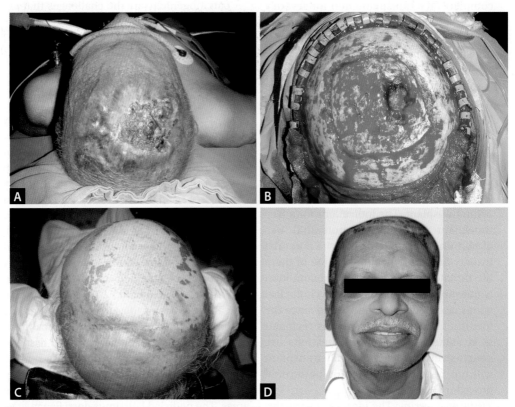

Figs. 1A to D: (A) Squamous cell carcinoma of scalp; (B) Intraoperative photo showing the defect after resection; (C) Postoperative photo of the reconstructed defect using anterolateral thigh flap; (D) Frontal view of the patient with the anterolateral thigh flap reconstruction of the scalp.

oronasal separation (e.g. rectus abdominis myocutaneous flap/anterolateral thigh flap) if dental implants are not to be provided. Vascularized bone flap may be needed if the alveolar arch needs to be reconstructed for dental rehabilitation. The orbital floor has to be reconstructed if the globe is preserved to provide support to the globe. This can be done with bone grafts, fascial slings, titanium mesh (which do not tolerate radiation well), or with vascularized bone flaps (treatment of choice). Large maxillary defects with orbital exenteration are reconstructed with large soft tissue flaps to provide bulk as well as cover **(Figs. 2 and 3)**.

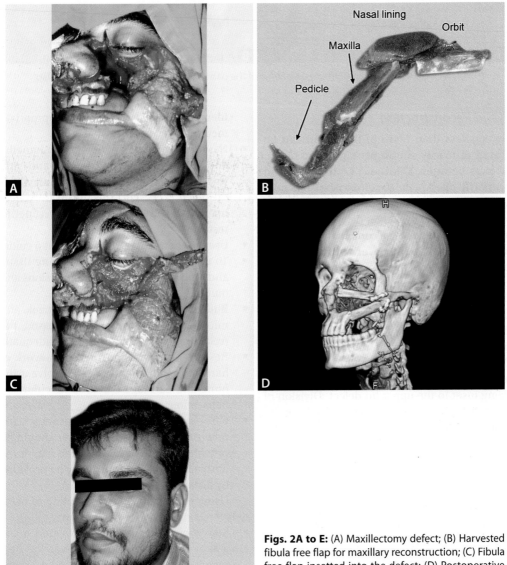

Figs. 2A to E: (A) Maxillectomy defect; (B) Harvested fibula free flap for maxillary reconstruction; (C) Fibula free flap insetted into the defect; (D) Postoperative 3-D reconstructed image; (E) 3 month postsurgery.

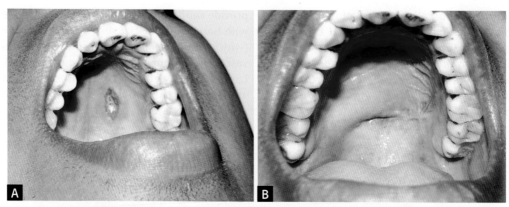

Figs. 3A and B: (A) Mucoepidermoid carcinoma of the palate; (B) Reconstruction with palatal flap.

Eyelid Reconstruction

Defects less than 1/4th of the eyelid can be closed primarily after a pentagonal excision. Defects between 1/3rd and 1/4th are closed primarily after pentagonal excision but only after a lateral cantholysis which allows the lid to advance medially. Larger defects of lower lid are reconstructed using a combination of cheek advancement flap for cover and a chondro-mucosal graft (from the nasal septum) for lining. Large defects of the upper lid are reconstructed using lid sharing techniques using full-thickness tissue from the lower lid. These may be inferiorly based (e.g. the cutler beard flap) or laterally based (e.g. the mustarde flap). The flap is sutured across the globe and remains attached to the lower lid (pedicle) while also being inset in the upper lid defect. Division of the pedicle is done after 3 weeks. The lower lid defect is closed as described above.

Nasal Reconstruction

Goal of nasal reconstruction is to restore normal appearance and patent airways for comfortable breathing.

Principles of Nasal Reconstruction

- The reconstruction of nose can be subdivided into lining, support, and cover.

Identify what is lost and use the appropriate method to reconstruct what is lost.

- Nasal subunits are tip, dorsum, columella, and paired alae, soft triangles and side walls. Reconstruct the entire subunit where the defect is present. This means the defect may have to be enlarged but gives a superior result.
- Use the contralateral normal side as a guide.
- To create a template of the missing tissue and replace tissues in exact dimensions and outline.
- Build on a stable platform of lip, cheek, and mid-face. Unless these are addressed, the nasal reconstruction can never be adequate.
- Restore proper supporting framework of hard and soft tissue. This may involve using bone and cartilage either as vascularized flaps or free grafts.
- Choose appropriate material for reconstruction. The nasal cover should be provided by skin of the forehead flap or the nasolabial flap. The lining may be provided by distant tissues.

Using these principles, an outline of nasal defect reconstruction is given below:

- Superficial defects can be covered using a skin graft. Forehead skin gives the best match in color and texture and is the favored donor site.

- Small defects less than 1.5 cm can be adequately reconstructed using local flaps from the nose like the dorsal nasal flap, single lobe transposition flap, or the bilobed flap.
- Larger defects more than 1.5 cm cannot be closed by local flaps and need regional tissue. The forehead flap or the nasolabial flap is used for reconstructing these defects. Tissue expansion may be needed to increase the size of the forehead flap in case of larger defects.

In case of deep defects that involve the supporting structure of the nose, the skeletal framework has to be restored. A complete framework must extend from the nasal bone above to the base of the columella below and from one alar base and nasal sidewall to the other. The framework supports the nose and its airway, provides shape to its external appearance and protects the repair against gravity, tension and wound contraction. Ideally missing portions of the framework should be provided at the time of flap transfer. Sources of cartilage grafts for recreating the framework are the nasal septum, ear concha, and the costal cartilage.

- For through and through defects, the lining of the nose has to be recreated. This can be done by composite skin graft, FTSGs, advancement of the remaining lining, hinge-over lining flaps, folding the distal part of the forehead or nasolabial flap, prelaminating a forehead flap, or using a second flap (regional flap or distant free flap).
- A subtotal or total nose defect is a challenging problem addressed by a staged repair. In the first stage, a radial forearm flap is transferred and used to cover the defect. In the second stage, this flap is thinned and hinged down to form the lining of the nose. Cartilage grafts are used to create the dorsum, columella, sidewalls, and alae of the nose. The whole structure is covered with a forehead flap. In the third stage, the forehead flap is elevated

and thinned. Further refinements in the cartilage framework may be done at this time. In the fourth stage, the forehead flap pedicle is divided and final insetting is done.

Ear Reconstruction

Ear defects can be either congenital (microtia) or acquired (e.g. postburns or traumatic). Reconstruction may be done using autologus cartilage, implants or prosthesis. Cartilage framework carved out of costal cartilage synchondrosis is placed in a skin pocket and elevated after several months when it gets incorporated well. If native skin is not healthy, the framework may be wrapped in temporoparietal fascia and covered with an FTSG. Medpore or silicon implants can be used but rates of extrusion are high. Alternatively, a prosthetic ear can be fashioned and fitted using osseointegrated implants.

Cheek Reconstruction

Buccal defects are ideally reconstructed with a soft and pliable flap. The defect should be measured with mouth open at maximum to prevent postoperative trismus. If the defect involves gingiva-buccal sulcus, it should be carefully recreated since it acts as a reservoir for food while mastication and helps to direct the food and saliva towards the oropharynx during deglutition. In case of trauma or advanced malignancy, the defect may involve both the skin as well as mucosa (through and through defect). In such a case, the defect may be reconstructed with two flaps (one for the cover and one for lining) or with a single flap folded over an intervening de-epithelialized segment or with a chimeric flap having two skin paddles each perfused by a separate perforator arising from the same parent vessel.

Free flaps that are routinely used for buccal defects are radial forearm flap, anterolateral thigh flap, or rectus abdominis myocutaneous flap (if bulk is needed). The regional flaps that are routinely used are the pectoralis major myocutaneous flap and deltopectoral flap. Local flaps are nasolabial flap, submental flap, buccal fat pad flap, and facial artery myomucosal flap **(Figs. 4A and B)**.

Lip Reconstruction

Since it is a principal aesthetic unit of the lower face, any minor change in the appearance of the lip is readily noticeable. Loss of labial competence may lead to inability to articulate, suck, whistle, and retain food and saliva leading to drooling. The lip consists of three layers, viz. mucosa, muscle, and skin. Accurate closure of the three layers is essential to achieve satisfactory results. The goal of lip reconstruction are prevention of microstomia, recreation of labial sulcus, restoration of the orbicularis oris muscle, accurate alignment of the vermilion, and optimization of cosmesis.

Vermillion defects can be closed by mucosal advancement flaps, buccal mucosa transposition flaps, tongue mucosal flaps or cross lip mucosal flaps. In the upper lip, full thickness defects up to 25% and in the lower lip, full thickness defects up to 30% can be closed primarily with a V or W excision pattern. Intermediate defects can be closed with lip switch flaps (Abbe or Estlander) or by borrowing tissue from the cheeks (Gilles fan flap or Karapandzic flap). Total lip defects are ideally managed by free radial forearm flap with palmaris longus tendon to provide a sling for animation **(Figs. 5A and B)**.

Mandibular Reconstruction

Defects of the mandible can be classified as, central (C)—segment between the canines; lateral (L)—segment lateral to the canine which does not include the condyle, Hemi (H)—the lateral segment including the condyle, or a combination of the above (LC, LCL, etc.). Mandibular reconstruction can be done by a rigidly fixed contoured reconstruction plate which is covered by healthy soft tissue or a soft tissue flap. This method can be used for patients with a lateral defect, who have not and will not receive radiotherapy, and are not suited for long and complex procedures.

Nonvascularized bone grafts can be used for small defects which are less than 6 cm if the surrounding soft tissues are well vascularized and healthy, and the patient has not had, and will not have radiotherapy. Vascularized bone is the optimal method of mandibular reconstruction. This can be achieved with pedicled osseomyocutaneous flaps, viz. pectoralis major with rib or sternum, sternocleidomastoid with clavicle, temporalis

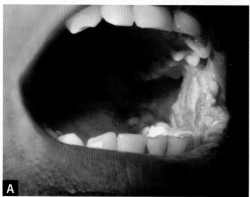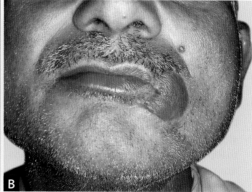

Figs. 4A and B: (A) Squamous cell carcinoma of buccal mucosa involving the commissure of lip (left); (B) Buccal mucosa carcinoma defect (left cheek) reconstructed with radial forearm free flap.

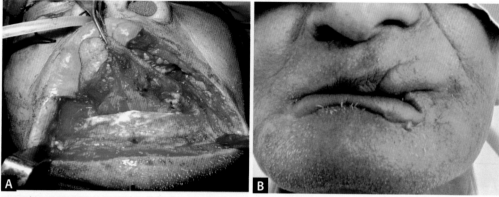

Figs. 5A and B: (A) Postresection defect involving the lower lip extending posteriorly to the ventral tongue, marginal mandibulectomy was included along with the tumor excision; (B) Lower lip reconstructed with radial forearm free flap and palmaris longus tendon sling.

with calvarial bone, or trapezius with spine of scapula. The disadvantages of this method of reconstruction are limited amount and poor vascularity of bone, limited flexibility of bone insetting leading to suboptimal aesthetic and functional outcomes, unwanted soft tissue bulk at the pedicle, and surgical site morbidity.

Free vascularized bone flaps are the method of choice for mandibular reconstruction. The commonly used flaps are fibular flap based on the peroneal vessels, Iliac crest based on the deep circumflex iliac vessels, scapular flap based on the circumflex scapular vessels, and the radial forearm osteocutaneous flap. The fibular flap is the most commonly used free flap for mandibular reconstruction because of its obvious advantages over the other flaps. It has a long vascular pedicle which runs along the bone and gives robust segmental periosteal blood supply. This allows appropriate osteotomies to be performed so as to contour the bone to attain the shape of the mandible. The bone stock is sturdy enough to accept osseointegrated dental implants. The donor site morbidity is minimal. Since it is away from the primary resection site, it allows for a two team approach saving considerable operating time. Finally, it has adequate soft tissue in the form of skin (peroneal

artery perforator based skin paddle) and muscle (flexor hallucis longus or soleus) which can be harvested for complex reconstructions involving the mucosa, and/or the skin of the mandibular region **(Figs. 6 and 7)**.

Tongue and Floor of Mouth Reconstruction

The goals of tongue reconstruction are to enable speech and swallowing while preventing falling back of the neo-tongue and airway compromise. Up to 1/3rd of the tongue defects can be closed primarily without significant functional loss. Hemiglossectomy and higher defects need some form of reconstruction for optimizing function. Various local and regional flaps that are commonly used for tongue reconstruction are infrahyoid flap, pectoralis major myocutaneous flap, and submental flap. The commonly used free flaps are radial forearm flap, anterolateral thigh flap, and rectus abdominis myocutaneous flap.

Tongue defects can be classified as:
- *Hemiglossectomy defects, up to half of the tongue*: These defects need a thin and pliable flap which can maintain mobility of the tongue. Radial forearm free flap is the flap

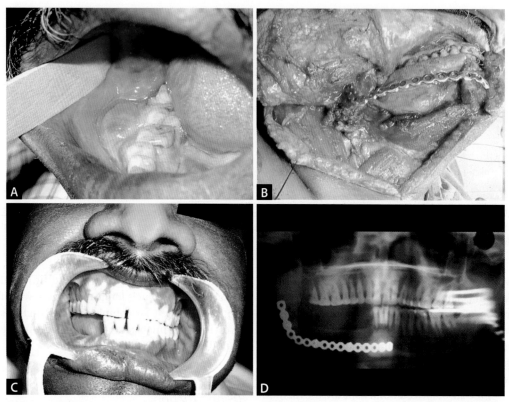

Figs. 6A to D: (A) Squamous cell carcinoma of the right lower gingivobuccal sulcus involving the mandible; (B) Right segmental mandibulectomy defect with intact tongue; (C) Right mandible reconstructed with deep circumflex Iliac artery free flap; (D) OPG showing good union of the deep circumflex iliac artery free flap to the native mandible.

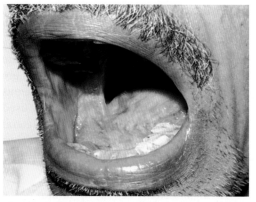

Fig. 7: A segmental mandibulectomy defect reconstructed with osteocutaneous fibula free flap (Intraoral view).

of choice. Alternatively, a thin anterolateral thigh flap may be used.

■ *Defects involving up to 2/3rd of tongue*: The remnant tongue musculature is still able to provide movement to the reconstructed tongue, but we need a slightly bulky flap. Anterolateral thigh flap is the flap of choice.

■ *Defects involving up to 3/4th of tongue*: The remnant tongue is not of any functional use but maintains anatomic continuity with the pharynx and the oral mucosa.

■ *Total glossectomy defects*: Defects more than 2/3rd of the tongue are ideally reconstructed with a bulky flap to provide bulk at the base of the tongue so that it can close off

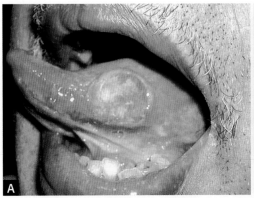
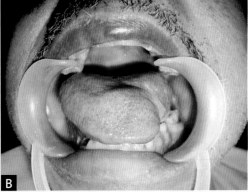

Figs. 8A and B: (A) Squamous cell carcinoma involving the left side of tongue; (B) Tongue defect reconstructed with lateral arm free flap, one-year post-therapy.

the oropharynx while swallowing. These defects can be reconstructed ideally with an anterolateral thigh myocutaneous flap which includes the vastus lateralis muscle to provide the necessary bulk. Alternate flaps are the rectus abdominis myocutaneous flap. Care should be taken to recreate the floor of the mouth and the gingival sulcus, if they are involved. This provides separation of the neck from the oral cavity as well as prevents pooling of saliva and drooling **(Figs. 8 and 9)**.

Pharyngeal Reconstruction

Pharyngoesophageal defects are a result of salvage laryngopharyngectomy following radiotherapy failure for squamous cell carcinoma of the larynx/hypopharynx. Other etiologies include benign strictures, pharyngocutaneous fistulas, and thyroid cancers involving the esophagus. The goals of reconstruction are to provide alimentary continuity, protect the important structures like the carotid artery, and restoration of function like speech and swallowing. Commonly used flaps for reconstruction are the jejunal flap, radial forearm flap, and the anterolateral thigh flap. Speech rehabilitation is typically

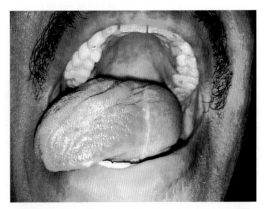

Fig. 9: A case of lateral tongue defect reconstructed with lateral arm flap.

provided with tracheoesophageal puncture and fasciocutaneous flap gives better outcome than visceral flap. Hence, the anterolateral thigh flap is the flap of first choice for pharyngeal reconstruction **(Figs. 10 and 11)**.

● POSTRECONSTRUCTION REHABILITATION

Postreconstructive rehabilitation forms an integral part of overall treatment plan of the patient. This needs a dedicated team of many medical, paramedical, and ancillary personnel.

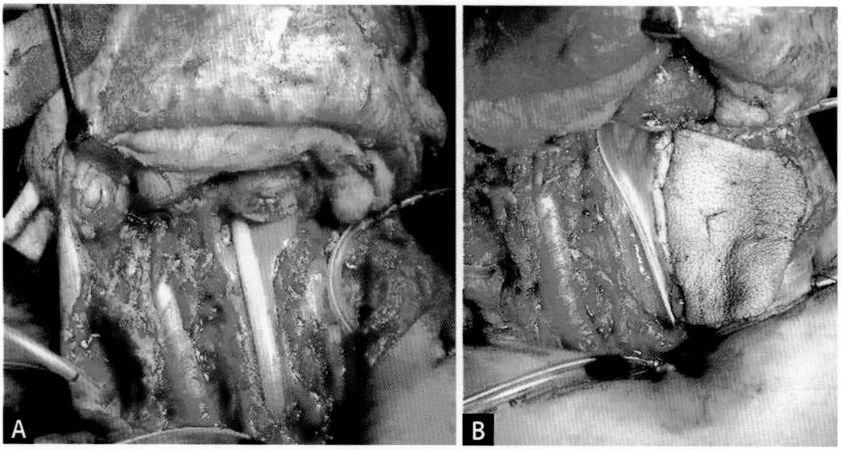

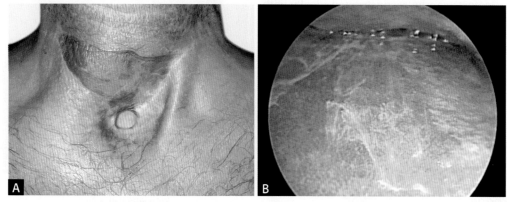

Figs. 10A and B: (A) Pharyngeal defect after laryngectomy with partial pharyngectomy; (B) Laryngectomy with partial pharyngectomy defect reconstructed with radial forearm free flap patch.

Figs. 11A and B: (A) Pharyngeal defect reconstructed with pectoralis major flap patch from inside and skin grafted outside, 6 months after surgery, neck view showing the skin graft above the stoma; (B) Endoscopic view of the throat showing the mucosalized flap.

Functional Rehabilitation

The patient undergoing a major head and neck resection has a major loss of function, viz. speech, swallowing, and mastication. Appropriate reconstruction ensures that the patient sets on a path toward recovery of the lost function. Additional surgical procedures may be needed like thinning of a bulky intraoral flap, vestibule creation, commissuroplasty, etc. Dental rehabilitation with dental prosthesis, speech, and swallowing therapy is essential for functional recovery. This is ensured by a dedicated team of therapists and prosthodontists.

Psychological Support

Undergoing a major head and neck resection and reconstruction gives immense psychological trauma to the patient. Pain, disfigurement, loss of self image, dependence, and loss of livelihood are some of the many emotional problems faced by the patient. Clinical psychologists and social workers have an important role to play in the management of these patients.

Aesthetic Rehabilitation

For the patient to be integrated into the society, aesthesis has to be maintained. Many patients need ancillary surgical procedures like scar revisions, flap thinning, hair transplantation, fat injections, or other forms of tissue rearrangements for achieving a near normal look. Facial prosthetics have an important role in aesthetic rehabilitation of the patient.

Apart from these, adequate social, economic, and occupational rehabilitation of the patient is essential so that the patient may be adequately integrated into the society.

● FURTHER READING

1. Chim H, Salgado CJ, Seselgyte R, et al. Principles of head and neck reconstruction: an algorithm to guide flap selection. Semin Plast Surg. 2010;24(2): 148-54.
2. Iyer S, Thankappan K. Maxillary reconstruction: current concepts and controversies. Indian J Plast Surg. 2014;47(1):8-19.
3. Kuriakose MA, Sharma M, Iyer S. Recent advances and controversies in head and neck reconstructive surgery. Indian J Plast Surg. 2007;40(12):3-12.
4. Nakatsuka T, Harii K, Asato H, et al. Analytic review of 2372 free flap transfers for head and neck reconstruction following cancer resection. J Reconstr Microsurg. 2003;19(6):363-9.
5. Patel KG, Sykes JM. Concepts in local flap design and classification. Operative Techniques in Otolaryngology - Head and Neck Surgery. 2011;22(1):13-23.

INDEX

Page numbers followed by *f* refer to figure, *fc* refer to flowchart, and *t* refer to table.